UNDERSTANDING PRIMING EFFECTS IN SOCIAL PSYCHOLOGY

Understanding Priming Effects in Social Psychology

Edited by
DANIEL C. MOLDEN

THE GUILFORD PRESS
New York   London

© 2014 The Guilford Press
A Division of Guilford Publications, Inc.
72 Spring Street, New York, NY 10012
www.guilford.com

All rights reserved

First published as *Social Cognition*, Vol. 32, Supplement, 2014, in digital format.

No part of this book may be reproduced, translated, stored in a retrieval system, or transmitted, in any form or by any means, electronic, mechanical, photocopying, microfilming, recording, or otherwise, without written permission from the publisher.

Printed in the United States of America

This book is printed on acid-free paper.

Last digit is print number: 9   8   7   6   5   4   3   2   1

Library of Congress Cataloging-in-Publication Data

Understanding priming effects in social psychology / edited by Daniel C. Molden.
    pages cm
  Includes bibliographical references and index.
  ISBN 978-1-4625-1929-3 (paperback)
 1. Social psychology. 2. Priming (Psychology) I. Molden, Daniel C.
HM1033.U653 2014
302—dc23

2014026330

ABOUT THE EDITOR

Daniel C. Molden, PhD, is Associate Professor of Psychology at Northwestern University. His research examines how activating different motivational mindsets influences the ways in which people (1) gather, integrate, and interpret social information, and (2) pursue, represent, and react to social interactions. His work has been featured in publications such as the *Journal of Personality and Social Psychology;* the *Journal of Experimental Psychology: General; Psychological Science;* and *American Psychologist*. Dr. Molden has held fellowships from the National Institute of Child Health and Human Development and the National Institute of Mental Health, and has received funding for his research from the National Science Foundation.

CONTENTS

WHAT IS "SOCIAL PRIMING"?

Understanding Priming Effects in Social Psychology: 3
What Is "Social Priming" and How Does It Occur?
Daniel C. Molden

On the Other Side of the Mirror: 14
Priming in Cognitive and Social Psychology
Stéphane Doyen, Olivier Klein, Daniel J. Simons, and Axel Cleeremans

Effects of Evaluation: An Example of Robust "Social" Priming 35
Melissa J. Ferguson and Thomas C. Mann

Priming Is Not Priming Is Not Priming 49
Dirk Wentura and Klaus Rothermund

Structured versus Unstructured Regulation: 70
On Procedural Mindsets and the Mechanisms of Priming Effects
Kentaro Fujita and Yaacov Trope

WHEN AND HOW SOCIAL PRIMING OCCURS

Prime Numbers: Anchoring and Its Implications 93
for Theories of Behavior Priming
Ben R. Newell and David R. Shanks

Understanding Prime-to-Behavior Effects: 114
Insights from the Active-Self Account
S. Christian Wheeler, Kenneth G. DeMarree, and Richard E. Petty

Replicability and Models of Priming: 129
What a Resource Computation Framework Can Tell Us
about Expectations of Replicability
Joseph Cesario and Kai J. Jonas

Situated Inferences and the What, Who, and Where of Priming 142
Chris Loersch and B. Keith Payne

Priming: Constraint Satisfaction and Interactive Competition 157
Tobias Schröder and Paul Thagard

CONSIDERING NEW SOURCES OF SOCIAL PRIMES

Grounding Social Embodiment 175
Daniël Lakens

Priming from Others' Observed or Simulated Responses 191
Eliot R. Smith and Diane M. Mackie

FROM THE PAST OF SOCIAL PRIMING TO ITS FUTURE

Evaluating Behavior Priming Research: 205
Three Observations and a Recommendation
Ap Dijksterhuis, Ad van Knippenberg, and Rob W. Holland

The Historical Origins of Priming as the Preparation 218
of Behavioral Responses: Unconscious Carryover
and Contextual Influences of Real-World Importance
John A. Bargh

Priming . . . Shmiming: It's about Knowing *When* and *Why* 234
Stimulated Memory Representations Become Active
E. Tory Higgins and Baruch Eitam

Understanding Priming Effects in Social Psychology: 252
An Overview and Integration
Daniel C. Molden

Index 259

WHAT IS "SOCIAL PRIMING"?

UNDERSTANDING PRIMING EFFECTS IN SOCIAL PSYCHOLOGY: WHAT IS "SOCIAL PRIMING" AND HOW DOES IT OCCUR?

Daniel C. Molden
Northwestern University

> How incidentally activated social representations affect subsequent thoughts and behaviors has long interested social psychologists. However, such *priming effects* have recently provoked debate and skepticism. This opening chapter of this volume on understanding priming effects in social psychology identifies two general sources of skepticism: 1) insufficient appreciation for the range of phenomena that involve priming, and 2) insufficient appreciation for the mechanisms through which priming occurs. To improve such appreciation, while previewing the other chapters in this book, this chapter provides a brief history of priming research that details the diverse findings any notion of "social priming" must encompass and reviews developments in understanding what psychological processes explain these findings. Thus, moving beyond debates about the strength of the empirical evidence for priming effects, this volume examines the theoretical challenges researchers must overcome for further advances in priming research and considers how these challenges can be met.

Examining the subtle and unanticipated effects of people's social environments on their thoughts and behaviors has long been an essential goal of research in social psychology. Indeed, one of the most enduring definitions of the field highlights the importance of studying not only the actual presence of others, but their "implied" and "imagined" presence as well (Allport, 1954). Therefore, over time, researchers have progressively pushed the limits of just how fleeting and indirect exposure to social stimuli can be and still affect people's responses, with frequently surprising results (e.g., Bargh, Schwader, Hailey, Dyer, & Boothby, 2012). As a result, it is now virtually axiomatic among social psychologists that the mere exposure to socially relevant stimuli can facilitate, or *prime*, a host of impressions, judgments, goals, and actions, often even outside of people's intention or awareness.

Address correspondence to Daniel C. Molden, Northwestern University, 2029 Sheridan Rd., Evanston, IL 60208. E-mail: molden@northwestern.edu.

However, questions have recently arisen about the evidence for some of these types of priming effects. Growing out of both broad criticisms of research practices in psychology as a whole (see Paschler & Wagenmakers, 2012) and specific failures to replicate particular examples of priming (Doyen, Klein, Pichon, & Cleeremans, 2012; Harris, Coburn, Rohrer, & Pashler, 2013; Shanks et al., 2013), some researchers have expressed doubt about the reliability or even existence of what they have labeled "social priming" (Kahneman, 2012). Further, at times, these criticisms have not only questioned whether the existing evidence supports the proposed processes by which social priming presumably occurs, but even whether these processes are psychologically plausible (Harris et al., 2013).

Whether or not one agrees with these assertions, such challenges to the accepted wisdom on priming effects in social psychology have created healthy debate and provoked a needed reappraisal by social psychologists of their basic assumptions about how and when priming effects occur (e.g., Cesario, 2014). But, at the same time, these challenges have also created confusion about just which of the many phenomena typically described by the now ubiquitous label of "priming" should be subject to the criticisms offered. That is, whereas few doubts seem to exist about whether incidental exposure to certain information can generally prime subsequent responses in ways that are not fully intended (Doyen, Klein, Simons, & Cleeremans, 2014, this volume; Harris et al., 2013; Newell & Shanks, 2014, this volume), no one has clearly specified what distinguishes the priming effects we should trust versus the social priming effects we should doubt. In addition, although some early perspectives on how priming effects occur have not survived closer scrutiny, many new perspectives have recently appeared and contributed to an evolving understanding of such effects. The primary objective of this volume is thus to reduce the confusion surrounding current discussions of priming effects in social psychology in two ways: (1) by more thoroughly considering the many phenomena in social psychology that the term *priming* encompasses, and (b) by more closely examining the psychological processes that explain when and how different types of priming effects occur.

In this opening chapter of this volume, to introduce the first question of what types of effects might be labeled "social priming," I begin with a brief and selective history of priming research in social psychology (for other historical overviews, see Bargh, 2014, this volume; Fujita & Trope, 2014, this volume; Higgins & Eitam, 2014, this volume). Based on the wide range of phenomena that make up this history, I then discuss some common features and basic assumptions social priming effects share, with the caveat that the diversity of these effects prevents any precise definition. Next, to introduce the second question of how social priming effects occur, I provide another brief and selective history of the various explanations that have emerged for such effects and consider some of their limitations. I then conclude by outlining many of the new proposals for priming mechanisms recently developed to address the shortcomings of previous perspectives. Throughout these overviews, in addition to highlighting the questions that are the primary focus of this volume, I also preview all of the other chapters included in this volume—prepared both by those who have produced much of the original work on social priming and by those who have critiqued it[1]—and their specific contributions to the larger discussion.

---

1. Hal Paschler and Daniel Kahneman were also invited to contribute to this volume, but respectfully declined.

A BRIEF HISTORY OF PRIMING RESEARCH IN SOCIAL PSYCHOLOGY

The term *priming* has a long history in the psychological literature and has been used in multiple ways. Although, in all of its forms, priming has generally referred to facilitative effects of some event or action on subsequent associated responses (e.g., Tulving, 1983), within social psychology, this process has specifically come to be defined in terms of how such events or actions influence the activation of stored knowledge (Higgins, 1996; Higgins & Eitam, 2014, this volume). The primary questions pursued by social psychologists studying priming have therefore involved the activation of social representations (e.g., traits, stereotypes, or goals) by exposure to different types of information, and the application of these activated representations in social judgments and behaviors. In addition, due to the separate literatures with even longer traditions in social psychology concerning how people consciously and intentionally use social information when forming attitudes and preferences (Maio & Haddock, 2007) or when judging and responding to others (Hilton, 2007), from the beginning, a primary focus of priming research in social psychology has been on how activated social representations can also have more indirect effects. That is, beyond simply examining the activation of social representations, priming research in social psychology has always considered how these representations influence judgment when people do not versus do consciously associate the activation with the judgment they are making, and do not versus do consciously intend to utilize the activated representation while forming that judgment (see Higgins, 1996).

For example, the earliest work on priming by social psychologists focused on how exposure to trait adjectives in ostensibly unrelated verbal tasks or through subliminal presentation led participants to apply these trait concepts when judging others' behaviors (e.g., Bargh & Pietromonaco, 1982; Higgins, Rholes, & Jones, 1977; Srull & Wyer, 1979). This research soon expanded to examine how other types of primes (e.g., attitude-relevant objects, Fazio, Powell, & Herr, 1983; specific descriptions of behavior, Smith & Branscomb, 1987; and broader social stereotypes, Devine, 1989) altered social impressions, as well as how priming social information influenced other types of judgments (e.g., one's own emotional experiences; Sinclair, Hoffman, Mark, Martin, & Pickering, 1994). The results of these initial studies repeatedly showed that people do appear to utilize activated social knowledge in their judgments, even when the activation arises from unrelated and irrelevant sources and, at times, even after a substantial delay following the initial activation. Given the novelty of these effects at the time and their distinctions from priming effects in other literatures (e.g., Neely, 1977), much of the focus of the early priming research in social psychology was concentrated somewhat narrowly on examining the specific processes by which priming effects on social impressions occurred.

However, beginning in the late 1990s, there was a notable shift in the focus of priming research in social psychology following a series of seminal findings suggesting that the same incidental activation of particular traits or social stereotypes could not only alter the perception of social targets but also the enactment of associated social behaviors (see Dijksterhuis & Bargh, 2001). That is, these new findings indicated that exposure to, for example, African-American faces seemed to increase the likelihood that people would not only form more stereotype-relevant impressions of others' behaviors as hostile, but also behave in ways consistent with hostile stereotypes themselves if the opportunity presented itself. In light of the implications that priming could directly influence actions as well as impressions, social psychologists began concentrating less on investigating the mechanisms of priming effects and more on exploring the boundaries of these effects by documenting (a) what types of behaviors and outcomes could be primed (e.g., Bargh, Gollwitzer, Lee-Chai, Barndollar, & Trötschel, 2001; Hassin, Ferguson, Shidlovski, & Gross, 2007) and (b) from what aspects of the environment these primes could arise (e.g., Williams & Bargh, 2008; Zhong & Liljenquist, 2006). Indeed, in multiple areas of research, rather than the primary focus of the studies itself, priming evolved into more of a tool to study the behavioral effects of activating representations of specific social contexts, such as feeling included versus excluded (e.g., Molden, Lucas, Gardner, Dean, & Knowles, 2009) or high versus low in power (e.g., Galinsky, Gruenfeld, & Magee, 2003), or the effects of inducing specific mindsets, such as a focus on abstract versus concrete representations (e.g., Fujita, Henderson, Eng, Trope, & Liberman, 2006) or on pursuing growth versus maintaining security (e.g., Molden & Finkel, 2010).

Thus, as even this cursory historical review illustrates, the notion of what constitutes a priming effect in social psychology has expanded considerably over time. Research on priming different types of socially relevant stimuli now subsumes an extensive and diverse collection of phenomena, from how the incidental activation of specific social traits alters current impressions, to how the similar activation of general social stereotypes alters current behaviors, to how cues that activate or spur the recall of specific social contexts and events alter current preferences and choices. Overall, priming effects in social psychology therefore encompass a highly diverse set of phenomena and processes whose boundaries are still being explored.

WHAT IS "SOCIAL PRIMING"?

Given this diversity in the priming effects studied by social psychologists, any classification of such effects with the common label *social priming* can only broadly characterize this area of research rather than enumerate necessary and sufficient criteria that precisely define any related phenomenon. Nevertheless, to allow for some generalization across these different types of priming and to identify shared assumptions about how they occur, it is worth at least outlining common features among the various phenomena described thus far.

First, priming effects in social psychology all involve some stimulation of people's mental representations of social targets, events, or situations that then influences subsequent evaluations, judgments, or actions (Eitam & Higgins, 2010; Higgins & Eitam, 2014, this volume). Further, as alluded to earlier, the influence of this priming is assumed to occur outside of *either* (a) awareness of this potential influence *or* (b) intention to utilize the activated representations during judgment or action (Loersch & Payne, 2011; 2014, this volume). That is, the effects of the prime are presumed to arise because people either do not recognize its potential effects on their subsequent responses or, even if they do, still do not intend to utilize the primed representations when making these responses. Thus, in general, priming research in social psychology is largely concerned with how cues that call to mind particular social situations or relationships can subtly influence people's responses even when they do not deliberately connect these cues to their current thoughts and actions.

However, it is important to note that although priming effects in social psychology involve a lack of awareness for the specific influence of the prime on one's responses, they do not also require a lack of awareness for the prime itself (cf. Cleeremans, Destrebecqz, & Boyer, 1998). Many (if not most) examples of these effects involve conscious exposure to or rehearsal of some information prior to the primary measures of interest (see Bargh et al., 2012; Higgins, 1996). Instead, it is people's failure to recognize the possible implications of this exposure that is critical. Moreover, although priming effects in social psychology involve a lack of intention to utilize the primed representations, they do not also require a lack of control over the prime's effects (cf. Posner & Synder, 1975). Indeed, when people do consciously recognize the potential influence of primed social representations on their judgments, the effects of the prime often disappear (if not reverse, creating contrast effects; see Higgins, 1996; Loersch & Payne, 2014, this volume). Thus, although some priming effects studied by social psychologists certainly can operate completely outside of awareness or control (e.g., Payne, Chen, Govorun, and Stewart, 2005), overall, these effects are typically conceptualized as nonconscious, but not as fully automatic (see Bargh, 1989).

The importance of attempting to outline at least some broad characteristics shared by the many different priming effects studied by social psychologists is reinforced by the Doyen, Klein, Simons, and Cleermans (2014) contribution to the opening section of this volume on conceptualizing social priming. As they discuss, part of the current controversy surrounding particular types of priming effects in social psychology is that miscommunications between researchers who study priming within separate research traditions can often arise from a failure to clearly articulate basic assumptions. They thus describe how explicit identification of the qualities of people's exposure to and processing of a prime that are assumed to be critical for the effect of interest, as well as better articulation of the mechanisms required to explain this effect, are necessary to make connections between the various literatures on priming.

However, as noted above and as Ferguson and Mann (2014) also explain in their contribution to opening section, it would be a mistake to use a term like *social priming* to represent a particular set of assumptions or proposed mechanisms that apply to all of the priming effects social psychologists study and can be supported or refuted by any particular set of studies, as some have seemed to suggest (Harris et al., 2013; Kahneman, 2012). Indeed, after elaborating on the lack of precision in the term *social priming*, Ferguson and Mann go on to discuss how a large subset of the priming effects studied by social psychologists that involve evaluative priming closely resembles priming effects studied in other areas of psychology and to argue that the mechanisms for this whole class of effects could even be used to explain some of the priming phenomena that have come under scrutiny.

In their contribution to the opening section of this volume, Wentura and Rothermund (2014) further illustrate the importance of avoiding reliance on the broad label *social priming*. They first detail an under-appreciated distinction within the priming literature in social psychology that involves relatively short-term effects (lasting seconds) from the specific content of the knowledge activated by the prime versus relatively long-term effects (lasting minutes or even days) from how the primed content alters stored representations in memory. They then discuss how and when both of these types of effects may occur and the separate, but equally important, roles they both may play in social judgment and behavior.

Finally, in their contribution to the opening section of this volume, Fujita and Trope (2014) detail yet another important distinction within the priming literature in social psychology that undermines any monolithic application of the term *social priming*. After describing forms of priming that involve more general procedural mindsets rather than the contents of specific representations, they then distinguish between *structured* mindsets that lead people to seek out and construct particular representations of their social environment in a more top-down manner versus *unstructured* mindsets that lead people to attend to whatever salient cues an environment affords in a more bottom-up manner. They also go on to detail the implications of each of these mindsets for how people should respond to different circumstances in which priming might be expected to occur.

Thus, in summary, the many different types of priming effects studied by social psychologists have some prototypical features that separate them from forms of priming studied in other areas of the literature. However, as discussed throughout the opening section of this volume, any use of the term *social priming* to suggest a precise set of common mechanisms across these diverse effects would likely create as much confusion as clarity.

EXPLAINING PRIMING EFFECTS IN SOCIAL PSYCHOLOGY

Although the diverse range of priming effects investigated by social psychologists may not share a common mechanism, identifying the equally diverse range of processes that might explain these effects is a critical goal in understanding how and when priming occurs (Higgins & Eitam, 2014, this volume). Returning to the earliest studies on how priming particular trait categories affects social impressions (e.g., Higgins et al., 1977; Srull & Wyer, 1979), the initial mechanisms proposed all involved two components: (1) the "excitation" of representations in memory by some process of spreading activation through a semantic network of associations, and (2) the use of these excited, or *accessible*, representations to encode information about a social target that was subsequently received. Thus, at the outset, explanations of priming effects in social psychology did not solely rely on the sustained semantic activation of primed categorical knowledge (cf., Neely, 1977). Instead, after the initial influence of this activation on which representations were more ready for use, such efforts were assumed to involve additional interpretive processes to account for the more enduring effects of the prime (see also Wentura & Rothermund, 2014, this volume). The necessity of additional processes beyond semantic activation to explain the influence of trait primes on impression formation was soon reinforced in studies by Smith and colleagues (e.g., Smith & Branscomb, 1987), which suggested that the prolonged effects of priming trait categories relied at least as much on the initiation of inferential procedures involving those trait categories as the activated content of any particular representations (cf. Anderson, 1993).

Yet, once again, studies suggesting that priming could affect social behaviors as well as social impressions (Dijksterhuis & Bargh, 2001) led to a major shift. Beyond generally increasing interest in the outcomes rather than the mechanisms of priming, as discussed earlier, such findings also elevated the importance of spreading activation rather than encoding processes. That is, extrapolating from emerging evidence that imagining actions activates the same areas of the brain as performing them (e.g., Prinz, 1997), researchers proposed that priming particular stereotypes could increase the accessibility of representations of behavior associated with those stereotypes and thus produce the enactment of that behavior if it were applicable to one's present circumstances (Dijksterhuis & Bargh, 2001; see also Bargh, 2014, this volume; Dijksterhuis, van Knippenberg, & Holland, 2014, this volume; Ferguson & Mann, 2014, this volume).

In such *direct expression* explanations for priming effects on behavior, without additional encoding or inference processes to sustain the effects of primed representations, the continued accessibility of the representation itself would appear to determine whether the associated behavior is enacted. Such mechanisms would also seem to imply that, when accessible, primed behaviors should occur whenever the situation allowed. These implications concerning the limited duration and inflexibility of priming effects that are associated with direct expression accounts of priming are a major source of the recent criticism and skepticism of social psychological research on priming. But, an underappreciated body of research by social psychologists themselves has also recently challenged direct expression accounts of priming and reintroduced the important role of encoding and inference in this process (e.g., Cesario, Higgins, & Plaks, 2006; Loersch & Payne, 2011; Wheeler, DeMarree, & Petty, 2007).

The second section of this volume, focused on understanding when and how priming effects in social psychology occur, includes chapters presenting extended discussion of both the criticisms of direct expression accounts and the recent attempts to update these accounts. First, Newell and Shanks (2014) elaborate on the empirical and theoretical limitations of assuming direct, automatic effects of primes on behavior. Arguing that the large literature on anchoring effects in magnitude judgments provides a representative test case for direct expression accounts of priming, they review evidence that questions whether anchoring (a) occurs outside of awareness, (b) is beyond one's control, and (c) produces broad effects on behavior. From this evidence, they further argue that the automatic expression of trait or stereotype primes in behavior across unrelated contexts is theoretically and empirically implausible as well. Next, Wheeler, DeMarree, and Petty (2014) and Cesario and Jonas (2014) also discuss limitations in direct expression accounts of priming effects on behavior and propose additional types of encoding mechanisms that could explain these effects. Wheeler and colleagues describe evidence that priming affects behavior because the representations that become accessible temporarily alter people's *active self-concept*, which then further influences the behaviors they choose. Cesario and Jonas describe evidence that priming social traits or categories triggers an assessment of one's preparation to interact and that the behavior that follows this prime is determined by how people encode the resources they have available in terms of what might be required in this interaction. Following this, Loersch and Payne (2014) describe a broader set of encoding mechanisms that could explain the effects of priming not only on behavior, but also on goals and impressions. They propose that people attribute the increased accessibility that results from priming to a specific source, and that whether this source is, for example, someone else's actions versus one's own choices determines whether the prime affects social impressions versus social behavior, respectively. This broad inferential process thus potentially captures the more specific encoding effects involved in various priming effects studied by social psychologists within a single process model.

In the final chapter of this second section of this volume, Schröder and Thagard (2014) take a somewhat different approach to explaining priming effects by outlining a computational model in which these types of encoding processes could be implemented without awareness or intention. This models relies on processes of parallel constraint satisfaction in a neural connectionist network that includes activated representations of the prime, the self, an applicable behavior, and the potential target of this behavior; it can therefore incorporate the influences of encoding processes such as the active self-concept, perceived behavioral resources, or the inferred source of the prime on how this prime affects judgment or behavior (see also Schröder & Thagard, 2013). Such a perspective answers criticisms that direct expression mechanisms relying on spreading activation from primed representations are too narrow and inflexible by showing that a more sophisticated account of how this activation spreads and what other representations are involved does not possess these limitations.

Considering the chapters in this second section of this volume as a whole, no complete consensus on the mechanisms responsible for various priming effects in social psychology yet exists. However, these chapters do agree that current perspectives on the direct expression of primed representations must be expanded and they each provide insight into emerging evidence that suggests important future directions for building such a consensus.

FUTURE DIRECTIONS FOR PRIMING EFFECTS IN SOCIAL PSYCHOLOGY

Extending this consideration of the future of priming research in social psychology, the final two sections of this volume focus on how this research can best continue to expand. The chapters in the first of these sections, focused on examining new sources from which priming effects might arise, identify several new areas of research that could further extend the range of priming phenomena in social psychology. Lakens (2014) describes emerging perspectives on how, beyond arising from the activation of semantic or symbolic representations, priming effects can also arise from sensorimotor representations (see also Bargh, 2014; Jonas & Cesario, 2013), and critically reviews existing theoretical perspectives on how such *embodiment* effects occur. Going further, Smith and Mackie (2014) discuss how, beyond arising from semantic or sensorimotor information in their present environment, priming effects may stem from people's spontaneous and unintentional simulation of how others might respond.

The chapters in the second of these sections, focused on both the past and future of priming research, all discuss the history of such research in social psychology to clarify the critical issues that new studies on priming should address. After beginning by reviewing the recent history of research on priming behavior and suggesting these effects might be more robust and less counterintuitive than recently portrayed, Dijksterhuis, van Knippenberg, and Holland (2014) discuss several improvements in theory and methodology that promise to strengthen research on priming and the field as a whole. Bargh (2014) next provides a more extensive history of research on priming behavior, arguing that controversial results involving symbolic primes of social traits and stereotypes are but a small piece of this history and only one of the many ways in which primes may influence ongoing behavior. He then reviews what he sees as more important examples of behavior priming that occur in naturalistic social environments and experiences. Finally, Higgins and Eitam (2014), return to the original research on priming social impressions, focusing on how the history of this research informs current discussions of the replicability of priming effects. They then argue that true progress in priming research requires more than just calling for greater attention to moderating variables that might alter such effects, and must involve greater attention to mediating variables that explain these effects (see also Cesario & Jonas, 2014).

On the whole, this volume on understanding priming effects in social psychology provides a comprehensive overview of what has been one of the most central areas of research in social psychology over the past 30 years. Furthermore, although the contributions to this volume identify important challenges that exist in determining the size and range of such priming effects, as well as in clearly explaining how these effects arise, they also illustrate that rather than facing crisis, social priming research is poised to expand and provide new insights on the subtle and pervasive ways in which people's social environments influence their thoughts and actions.

REFERENCES

Allport, G. W. (1954). The historical background of modern social psychology. *Handbook of Social Psychology, 1*, 3-56.

Anderson, J. R. (1993). *Rules of the mind*. Hillsdale, NJ: Erlbaum.

Bargh, J. A. (1989). Conditional automaticity: Varieties of automatic influence in social perception and cognition. In J. S. Uleman & J. A. Bargh (Eds.), *Unintended thought* (pp. 3-51). New York: Guilford.

Bargh, J. A. (2014). The historical origins of priming as the preparation of behavioral responses: Unconscious carry-over and contextual influences of real-world importance. This volume.

Bargh, J. A., Gollwitzer, P. M., Lee-Chai, A., Barndollar, K., & Trötschel, R. (2001). The automated will: Nonconscious activation and pursuit of behavioral goals. *Journal of Personality and Social Psychology, 81*, 1014-1027.

Bargh, J. A., & Pietromonaco, P. (1982). Automatic information processing and social perception: The influence of trait information presented outside of conscious awareness on impression formation. *Journal of Personality and Social Psychology, 43*, 437.

Bargh, J. A., Schwader, K. L., Hailey, S. E., Dyer, R. L., & Boothby, E. J. (2012). Automaticity in social-cognitive processes. *Trends in cognitive sciences, 16*, 593-605.

Cesario, J. (2014). Priming, replication, and the hardest science. *Perspectives on Psychological Science, 9*, 40-48.

Cesario, J., Higgins, E.T., & Plaks, J.E. (2006). Automatic social behavior as motivation to interact. *Journal of Personality and Social Psychology, 90*, 893-910.

Cesario, J., & Jonas, K. J. (2014). Replicability and models of priming: What a resource computation framework can tell us about expectations of replicability. This volume.

Cleeremans, A., Destrebecqz, A., & Boyer, M. (1998). Implicit learning: News from the front. *Trends in Cognitive Sciences, 2*(10), 406-416.

Devine, P. G. (1989). Stereotypes and prejudice: Their automatic and controlled components. *Journal of Personality and Social Psychology, 56*, 5-18.

Dijksterhuis, A., & Bargh, J. A. (2001). The perception-behavior expressway: Automatic effects of social perception on social behavior. In M. P. Zanna (Ed.), *Advances in experimental social psychology* (Vol. 33; pp. 1-40). New York: Academic.

Dijksterhuis, A., van Knippenberg, A., & Holland, R. W. (2014). Evaluating behavior priming research: Three observations and a recommendation. This volume.

Doyen, S., Klein, O., Pichon, C. L., & Cleeremans, A. (2012). Behavioral priming: It's all in the mind, but whose mind? *PLOS ONE, 7*, e29081.

Doyen, S., Klein, O., Simons, D., & Cleeremans, A. (2014). On the other side of the mirror: Priming in cognitive and social psychology. This volume.

Eitam, B., & Higgins, E. T. (2010). Motivation in mental accessibility: Relevance of a representation (ROAR) as a new framework. *Social and Personality Psychology Compass, 4*, 951-967.

Fazio, R. H., Powell, M. C., & Herr, P. M. (1983). Toward a process model of the attitude–behavior relation: Accessing one's attitude upon mere observation of the attitude object. *Journal of Personality and Social Psychology, 44*, 723-735.

Ferguson, M. J., & Mann, T. C. (2014). Effects of evaluation: An example of robust "social" priming. This volume.

Fujita, K., Henderson, M. D., Eng, J., Trope, Y., & Liberman, N. (2006). Spatial distance and mental construal of social events. *Psychological Science, 17*(4), 278-282.

Fujita, K., & Trope, Y. (2014). Structured vs. unstructured regulation: On procedural mindsets and the mechanisms of priming effects. This volume.

Galinsky, A. D., Gruenfeld, D. H., & Magee, J. C. (2003). From power to action. *Journal of Personality and Social Psychology, 85*, 453-466.

Harris, C. R., Coburn, N., Rohrer, D., & Pashler, H. (2013). Two failures to replicate high-performance-goal priming effects. *PLOS ONE, 8*(8), e72467.

Hassin, R. R., Ferguson, M. J., Shidlovski, D., & Gross, T. (2007). Subliminal exposure to national flags affects political thought and behavior. *Proceedings of the National Academy of Sciences, 104*(50), 19757-19761.

Higgins, E. T. (1996). Knowledge activation: Accessibility, applicability, and salience. In E. T. Higgins and A. W. Kruglanski (Eds.), *Social Psychology: Handbook of basic principles* (pp. 133-168). New York: Guilford.

Higgins, E. T., & Eitam, B. (2014). Priming . . . Shmiming: It's about knowing *when* and *why* stimulated memory representations become active. This volume.

Higgins, E. T., Rholes, W. S., & Jones, C. R. (1977). Category accessibility and impression formation. *Journal of Experimental Social Psychology, 13*, 141-154.

Hilton, D. (2007). Causal explanation: From social perception to knowledge-based causal attribution. In A. W. Kruglanski & E. T. Higgins (Eds.), *Social psychology: Handbook of basic principles, second edition* (pp. 232-253). New York: Guilford.

Jonas, K. J., & Cesario, J. (2013). Introduction to the special issue: Situated social cognition. *Social Cognition, 31*(2), 119-124.

Kahneman, D. (2012, September 26). A proposal to deal with questions about priming effects. *Nature.com*. Retrieved January 31, 2014 from http://www.nature.com/polopoly_fs/7.6716.1349271308!/suppinfoFile/Kahneman%20Letter.pdf

Lakens, D. (2014). Grounding social embodiment. This volume.

Loersch, C., & Payne, B. K. (2014). Situated inference and the what, who, and where of priming. This volume.

Loersch, C., & Payne, B. K. (2011). The situated inference model an integrative account of the effects of primes on perception, behavior, and motivation. *Perspectives on Psychological Science, 6*(3), 234-252.

Maio, G. R., & Haddock, G. (2007). Attitude change. In A. W. Kruglanski & E. T. Higgins (Eds.), *Social psychology: Handbook of basic principles, second edition* (pp. 565-586). New York: Guilford.

Molden, D. C., & Finkel, E. J. (2010). Motivations for promotion and prevention and the role of trust and commitment in interpersonal forgiveness. *Journal of Experimental Social Psychology, 46*, 255-268.

Molden, D. C., Lucas, G. M., Gardner, W. L., Dean, K., & Knowles, M. L. (2009). Motivations for prevention or promotion following social exclusion: Being rejected versus being ignored. *Journal of Personality and Social Psychology, 96*, 415-431.

Neely, J. H. (1977). Semantic priming and retrieval from lexical memory: Roles of inhibitionless spreading activation and limited-capacity attention. *Journal of Experimental Psychology: General, 106,* 226-254.

Newell, B. R., & Shanks, D. R. (2014). Prime numbers: Anchoring and its implications for theories of behavior priming. This volume.

Pashler, H., & Wagenmakers, E. J. (2012). Editors' introduction to the special section on replicability in psychological science a crisis of confidence? *Perspectives on Psychological Science, 7,* 528-530.

Payne, B. K., Cheng, C. M., Govorun, O., & Stewart, B. D. (2005). An inkblot for attitudes: Affect misattribution as implicit measurement. *Journal of Personality and Social Psychology, 89,* 277-293.

Posner, M. I., & Snyder, C. R. R. (1975). Attention and cognitive control. In R. L. Solso (Ed.), *Information processing and cognition: The Loyola symposium.* Hillsdale, NJ: Erlbaum.

Prinz, W. (1997). Perception and action planning. *European Journal of Cognitive Psychology, 9,* 129-154.

Schröder, T., & Thagard, P. (2014). Priming: Constraint satisfaction and interactive competition. *Social Cognition.*

Schröder, T., & Thagard, P. (2013). The affective meanings of automatic social behaviors: Three mechanisms that explain priming. *Psychological Review, 120,* 255-280.

Shanks, D. R., Newell, B. R., Lee, E. H., Balakrishnan, D., Ekelund, L., Cenac, Z., ... & Moore, C. (2013). Priming intelligent behavior: An elusive phenomenon. *PLOS ONE, 8,* e56515.

Sinclair, R. C., Hoffman, C., Mark, M. M., Martin, L. L., & Pickering, T. L. (1994). Construct accessibility and the misattribution of arousal: Schachter and Singer revisited. *Psychological Science, 5*(1), 15-19.

Smith, E. R., & Branscombe, N. R. (1987). Procedurally mediated social inferences: The case of category accessibility effects. *Journal of Experimental Social Psychology, 23,* 361-382.

Smith, E. R., & Mackie, D. M. (2014). Priming from others' observed or simulated responses. This volume.

Srull, T. K., & Wyer, R. S. (1979). The role of category accessibility in the interpretation of information about persons: Some determinants and implications. *Journal of Personality and Social Psychology, 37,* 1660-1672.

Tulving, E. (1983). *Elements of episodic memory.* New York: Oxford University Press.

Wentura, D., & Rothermund, K. (2014). Priming is not priming is not priming. This volume.

Wheeler, S. C., DeMarree, & Petty, R. E. (2014). Understanding prime-to-behavior effects: Insights from the active-self account. This volume.

Wheeler, S. C., DeMarree, K. G., & Petty, R. E. (2007). Understanding the role of the self in prime-to-behavior effects: The active-self account. *Personality and Social Psychology Review, 11,* 234-261.

Williams, L. E., & Bargh, J. A. (2008). Experiencing physical warmth promotes interpersonal warmth. *Science, 322,* 606-607.

Zhong, C. B., & Liljenquist, K. (2006). Washing away your sins: Threatened morality and physical cleansing. *Science, 313,* 1451-1452.

ON THE OTHER SIDE OF THE MIRROR: PRIMING IN COGNITIVE AND SOCIAL PSYCHOLOGY

Stéphane Doyen
Consciousness, Cognition & Computation Group (CO3), Center for Research in Cognition & Neurosciences (CRCN), ULB Institute for Neuroscience (UNI), and Center for Research in Social and Cultural Psychology, Université Libre de Bruxelles

Olivier Klein
Center for Research in Social and Cultural Psychology, Université Libre de Bruxelles

Daniel J. Simons
University of Illinois at Urbana-Champaign

Axel Cleeremans
Consciousness, Cognition & Computation Group (CO3), Center for Research in Cognition & Neurosciences (CRCN), and ULB Institute for Neuroscience (UNI), Université Libre de Bruxelles

> Over the past several years, two largely separate traditions have collided, leading to controversy over claims about priming. We describe and contrast the main accounts of priming effects in cognitive and social psychology, focusing especially on the role of awareness. In so doing, we consider one of the core points of contention: claims about the effects of subliminal priming. Whereas cognitive psychologists often are interested in exploring how priming operates with and without awareness, social psychologists more commonly assume subliminality in order to bolster claims about the automaticity of priming. We discuss the criteria necessary to claim that a stimulus was processed entirely without awareness, noting the challenges in meeting those criteria. Finally, we identify three sources of conflict between the fields: awareness, replicability, and the nature of the underlying processes. We close by proposing resolutions for each of them.

All authors contributed equally to composing this chapter. Axel Cleeremans is a Research Director with the Fund for Scientific Research (F.R.S.-FNRS, Belgium). This work was supported by the Belgian Fund for Scientific Research (F.R.S-FNRS) and by IAP Program P7/33 funded by the Belgian Science Policy Office (BELSPO). We are grateful to Daniel Holender and to the referees for their comments on an early version of this manuscript.

Address correspondence to Axel Cleeremans, 50 ave. FD Roosevelt CP191, 1050 Bruxelles, Belgium; E-mail: axcleer@ulb.ac.be.

Priming in Cognitive and Social Psychology

Priming is fundamental in both cognitive and social psychology because it reveals the powerful ways in which our past experiences can influence our present and future behavior. Priming takes many forms, from more efficient processing the second time we encounter a stimulus (repetition priming) to activation of other related concepts (semantic priming) to triggering an associated goal (goal priming). Priming contributes to most human behavior, including perception, memory, decision making, and action.

Priming has been studied extensively by both cognitive and social psychologists. Both fields use similar tasks to prime behavior, both assess whether those influences are automatic, and both posit mechanisms to explain their influence. But they use priming for different purposes. Social psychologists typically use priming as a tool to study the influence of mental representations (e.g., stereotypes, personality traits, or values) on real-world judgments, beliefs, and actions. Cognitive psychologists typically use priming as a tool to study the structure of knowledge representations.

One question looms large over most extant research: Can primes influence behavior in the absence of awareness? This is both the most important question and the most controversial one. Whether our behavior is influenced by events occurring outside of awareness has considerable implications for our concept of free will. It raises issues of personal responsibility (Gazzaniga, 2011; Wegner, 2002) and strikes at the heart of the mind-body problem. Claims about non-conscious priming remain controversial because establishing the absence of awareness is fraught with epistemological and methodological complications.

Social and cognitive psychologists have approached priming without awareness from different perspectives and with different agendas. In social psychology, demonstrating that a prime is processed without awareness is a means to an end (Bargh, 1992). Non-conscious primes presumably influence behavior unintentionally and automatically. For cognitive psychologists, measuring awareness in priming situations often is an end in and of itself. One branch of cognitive psychology has focused extensively on the sorts of priming that operate with and without awareness, debating the criteria needed to claim that a stimulus was processed subliminally (Kouider & Dehaene, 2007; Van den Bussche, Van den Noortgate, & Reynvoet, 2009).

Despite the use of similar methods to induce priming, for the better part of their respective histories, these traditions have proceeded apace, without extensive cross-fertilization. Recently, though, some cognitive psychologists have begun applying the conclusions drawn from cognitive psychology priming research to social psychology priming research, leading to a clash of claims and traditions.

In this paper, we consider differences in how priming is used in cognitive and social psychology in an attempt to deflate the animosity and miscommunication that often spring from a collision of traditions. Specifically, we focus on differences in how cognitive and social psychologists measure and evaluate the role of awareness in priming. We first review the methodological challenges associated with measuring awareness. We then review the sorts of claims about priming and awareness that have been put forward within each field. We conclude by describing three sources of conflict arising from the consideration of priming in social and cognitive psychology, and suggest potential ways to overcome them.

Although priming takes many forms, we focus on a type of study common to both cognitive and social psychology:

1. Experimenters present a prime stimulus, either on a computer display or as part of a task that a participant completes;
2. The prime activates an internal representation;
3. The activated representation influences other representations; and
4. Those other activated representations lead to behavioral changes.

This scope excludes cases of repetition priming, those in which a briefly presented stimulus affects the ability to process *the same stimulus* later. Instead, we focus on what is known as semantic or associative priming in cognitive psychology (and sometimes in social psychology) as well on what social psychologists have sometimes called "goal priming" or "behavioral priming." We include cases in which multiple primes affect a single response as well as studies in which a single experience affects a single behavior.

THE CHALLENGE OF MEASURING AWARENESS

Studies adopting the contrastive approach to assessing awareness (Baars, 1998) typically include two measures, one of the consequences of a prime and one of awareness of that prime. For instance, a subliminal priming paradigm might include a response time task to measure the effects of a prime on processing of a target (i.e., either facilitation or interference) as well as one or more measures of awareness of the prime itself. The awareness measure can take many forms: a forced-choice response in an identification task administered after the main experiment; a qualitative visibility judgment; a confidence judgment; a funnel interview probing participants about their awareness of the link between the prime and their behavior, and so on.

The plurality of forms of awareness (and their associated measures) highlights a core source of disagreement in studies of priming: which measure of awareness is needed to support a particular claim? Subliminal perception (Kouider & Dehaene, 2007) studies explore whether stimuli that have not been consciously encoded can influence subsequent responses. Studies of implicit memory (Schacter, Dobbins, & Schnyer, 2004) examine whether the retrieval process can occur automatically and unconsciously even when the original stimulus was consciously perceived. Implicit learning studies (Cleeremans, Destrebecqz, & Boyer, 1998) are most concerned with whether learning occurs in the absence of awareness of the relationships among ensembles of consciously processed stimuli. Participants might be aware of the presence or absence of a stimulus, they might have conscious memory of a previous experience, they could have an intention to use some information, or they might realize that their judgments are influenced by what they remember.

Thus, consciousness is not a unitary construct. It encompasses many dimensions of experience, each influenced by different processes (Cleeremans, 2003; 2011). Given that its scope ranges from subjective claims of perceptual awareness to metacognition and cognitive control, there is no universally accepted operational definition of what it means for someone to be aware of something. Given the variety of meanings of "awareness," identifying which form of awareness (or lack thereof) is important for a claim is essential (Nisbett & Wilson, 1977). Do claims about awareness refer to encoding or retrieval? Do they involve individual stimuli or relationships among stimuli? Do they require the absence of intentions? Social and cognitive psychology priming studies historically have been interested in different aspects of awareness.

Even with a complete description of the form of awareness that matters for a theoretical claim, measuring awareness presents a greater challenge. Most studies of awareness in priming rely on a form of dissociation logic: The outcome measure is sensitive to the prime even when another measure reveals no awareness. Not all measures provide equally appropriate tests for awareness, though, and this issue remains a point of contention in the literature.

The debate over dissociation logic has long focused on a distinction between subjective and objective measures of awareness. Subjective measures rely on the participant to report what they have consciously perceived on each trial and take that report as an accurate indication of awareness. If the participant claims not to have seen a stimulus, then they did not see it. In contrast, objective measures separate sensitivity to the presence of a stimulus from the confidence of that judgment. The motivation behind the objective approach is that any given self-report of awareness could be influenced by confidence as well as awareness. People might claim not to have seen a stimulus because they are conservative about saying "yes" when they are uncertain, even if they actually did process it consciously. Objective measures typically use a signal detection approach across many trials to show that people were not sensitive to the presence of the subliminal stimuli. They do not take the response on any one trial as indicative of whether or not that stimulus was consciously perceived, because on a single trial, it is not possible to separate sensitivity from their criterion, their default bias to say "yes" or "no."

Subjective measures have been criticized for failing to disentangle conscious processing from differences in confidence. Objective measures have been criticized because behavioral sensitivity does not necessarily imply conscious experience. Nevertheless, any measure of awareness should meet four criteria (Newell & Shanks, 2012; Shanks & St John, 1994) to unambiguously establish that processing was unconscious:

1. The awareness measure should be taken at the same time as the outcome measure, ideally on a trial-to-trial basis (*immediacy*);
2. The awareness measure should tap the knowledge that is relevant to the behavior (*relevance*);
3. The awareness measure should be at least as sensitive to the relevant knowledge as is the outcome measure (*sensitivity*); and
4. The awareness measure should be unaffected by experimental demands or social desirability (*reliability*).

A failure of the immediacy criterion leaves open the possibility that people were aware of the relevant material at the time they performed the outcome measure, but forgot by the time they were tested. Asking participants after a study to report their awareness of primes during the task violates the immediacy criterion. The immediacy criterion is essential in studies of subliminal perception, where the stimulus itself is, by design, weak and fleeting. It is not easy to meet, though, due to the observer paradox: Asking people to report their awareness of a prime on each trial draws attention to the prime, potentially increasing awareness of it.

A failure of the relevance criterion leaves open the possibility that the task measures the wrong form of awareness and that unmeasured aspects of awareness drove any effects of the prime on the outcome measure. For example, studies of implicit learning (for a review, see Cleeremans et al., 1998) examine whether people unconsciously abstract the regularities among sets of stimuli in the same way that natural grammar abstractly describes how words can be combined to form sentences. When asked about the rules they learned, most participants cannot explicitly identify the regularities. But they might perform well on the outcome task based on awareness of the similarities between training and test items. A measure of awareness must check for awareness of any aspect of the primes that might affect performance on the outcome measure.

A failure of the sensitivity criterion means that people were aware, but the measure was not sensitive enough to detect their awareness. If a more sensitive measure could reveal awareness of the relevant information, then claims of nonconscious processing are unmerited. It might seem that asking people to report whether or not they noticed a stimulus would be a highly sensitive measure; presumably, people should be able to report the contents of their own consciousness. But such reports reflect more than just sensitivity to the presence of a stimulus—they also incorporate biases. For instance, people might refrain from reporting on knowledge held with low confidence. Moreover, verbal reports might not be accurate reports of actual experiences, and typical methods cannot distinguish genuine reports from reconstructed ones (Hall, Johansson, Tärning, Sikström, & Deutgen, 2010; Nisbett & Wilson, 1977).

A failure of reliability leaves open the possibility that measures of awareness were influenced by demand characteristics or other biases. A reliable measure should be sensitive only to awareness of the stimulus and not to other factors that could influence reports of awareness. Few studies use measures of awareness that are immune to such biases, and those that do rarely consider the possible contributions of demand characteristics (Klein et al., 2012; Rosenthal, 2009).

Although meeting all four requirements is necessary to unequivocally document the absence of awareness, it is still hotly debated whether any method actually does so (Cheesman & Merikle, 1986; Hannula, Simons, & Cohen, 2005; Holender, 1986; Kouider & Dehaene, 2007; Vermeiren & Cleeremans, 2012). Over the past 30 years, cognitive psychologists have used increasingly refined methods to assess awareness in studies of priming, although all are still subject to criticism based on a failure to meet one or more of these criteria. We explore those developments and this continued debate in the context of the broader study of priming within cognitive psychology. We then turn to the study of priming in social psychology.

PRIMING IN COGNITIVE PSYCHOLOGY

Most modern priming research builds on models of spreading activation (Collins & Loftus, 1975; McNamara, 1992). The core principle underlying such models is that semantic representations are interlinked, with more closely related words and more similar concepts connected more strongly. For example, the representation for the word "nurse" is closely linked to the representation of "doctor," but less tightly linked to "uniform." Activating the word "nurse" activates the word "doctor" strongly, but the more remote the association, the less activation it produces: Activation spreads, but diminishes in potency as it does.

Cognitive psychologists often use priming to infer the structure of semantic representations. For example, they might present the prime word "nurse" and then measure the speed with which people can determine that another word (e.g., "doctor," "uniform," or "house") is a word or non-word (Neely, 1977). The closer the semantic association (determined separately), the faster the response on such a lexical decision task (Collins & Loftus, 1975; McNamara, 1992; Patterson, Nestor, & Rogers, 2007).

In this spreading activation account, priming occurs passively and automatically—as long as the prime word is perceived, it triggers a cascade of semantic associations, leading to faster processing of related words. That automaticity assumption triggered a related question: Could semantic priming occur if people processed the prime but were not aware of having done so?

This question placed the study of semantic associations squarely into a larger, older, and contentious debate about the existence and potency of subliminal perception. That debate has raged for more than 100 years, with a repeating cycle of provocative claims of subliminal perception followed by methodological debunking (Greenwald, Spangenberg, Pratkanis, & Eskenazi, 1991; Holender, 1986). At times, the debate about subliminal perception has veered into domains more commonly studied in social psychology, including persuasion and influence (Strahan, Spencer, & Zanna, 2002). But, within cognitive psychology, the core issues have been the measurement of awareness and the question of what can and cannot occur in its absence.

Although many studies have attempted to document subliminal perception over the past century and a half (e.g., Sidis, 1898), only in the past 30 years has there been a concerted effort to test whether subliminal primes can activate semantic networks, leading to faster judgments for related stimuli. The most prominent early attempts to document semantic processing with methods designed to eliminate awareness were carried out in the 1980s by Marcel (1983). Marcel presented prime stimuli briefly, followed by a visual mask that limited further perceptual information for the prime. For example, participants might view the word "salt" as a prime, followed by a mask, and even though they could neither recall nor identify the prime word, they still were better able to process the subsequently target word, "pepper" (as opposed to the unrelated "lotus"); they showed semantic priming without the ability to identify the prime. This finding reinvigorated the study of semantic priming by subliminal stimuli.

In what might be the most comprehensive critical appraisal of the evidence for subliminal semantic priming, Holender (1986) reviewed all of the primary methods used to measure subliminal semantic processing, identified the criteria necessary to claim that a stimulus actually was processed without awareness, and showed that all prior results failed to meet those criteria. Holender argued for the use of objective measures of awareness: Document that a prime had an effect while also providing direct and objective evidence that the subject could not have consciously perceived the prime at the time it appeared.

At first blush, Marcel's priming studies appear to meet Holender's rigorous criteria, a set similar to the four we described above: Participants processed target words faster following a related prime despite an inability to remember the prime. However, the ability to report a prime's visibility after a study, even a prime that was flashed briefly and masked, fails to meet the immediacy criterion. It might also fail to meet the sensitivity criterion. As a result, it is difficult to distinguish effects that stem from genuinely unconscious processing from effects stemming from weakly conscious and forgotten primes.

Given the challenge of measuring performance at the time of presentation in a way that meets all of the necessary criteria for awareness, many researchers have adopted what is now known as an "objective" assessment of awareness: Show that people are insensitive to the presence of a prime as a way to rule out awareness. If people cannot reliably discriminate the presence of a prime from its absence, then they cannot have conscious access to the meaning of that prime. Objective measures bypass the immediacy requirement by showing that subjects *could* not have consciously detected the prime rather than by arguing that they *did* not detect it. It provides a way to measure awareness reliably, using signal detection methods. Nevertheless, whether this meets the sensitivity criterion can still be debated (e.g., see Dulany, 2001): Is detection necessarily the most sensitive measure of awareness? And, objective measures of awareness potentially fail the relevance criterion: Does a detection task measure the same aspects of awareness as a given outcome measure?

Even studies designed to meet the most rigorous criteria for testing awareness can still fall short, leaving open the possibility that semantic priming effects were consciously mediated. Many recent studies (Dehaene, 2008; Draine & Greenwald, 1998; Naccache & Dehaene, 2001; Snodgrass, Bernat, & Shevrin, 2004) have been subsequently debated, which highlights the continuing challenges involved in ruling out awareness altogether.

In fact, some researchers propose abandoning the attempt to exhaustively eliminate awareness, arguing that doing so may be impossible in principle. If consciousness is not a unitary construct, then there may be no single measure that is adequately sensitive. Moreover, any measure might not be process-pure, tapping exclusively conscious or unconscious processing. If so, then using an adequately sensitive measure of awareness to show that participants could not have seen a prime might have the side effect of also eliminating any unconscious processing of that prime (Reingold & Merikle, 1988).

To address this problem, (Reingold & Merikle, 1988) adopted a different approach, comparing direct measures of performance to indirect ones. Direct measures make explicit reference to the relevant discrimination and include deliberate or explicit judgments (e.g., recognition or recall). Indirect measures make no reference to the relevant discrimination, instead measuring performance (e.g., stem completion in memory tasks). If all measures include both conscious and unconscious components, then by assumption, the direct measures should exhibit a greater conscious component. Presumably, subjects should be more successful in using conscious information when instructed to do so. By this logic, whenever an indirect measure shows greater sensitivity to the prime than a comparable direct one, the difference should be interpreted as evidence of unconscious influences on performance.

The "Process Dissociation Procedure" (Jacoby, 1991) takes this logic a step further. Cognitive control is typically assumed to require consciousness: One cannot control what one is not aware of. Although this claim also is debated (Van Opstal, Gevers, Osman, & Verguts, 2010), Jacoby proposed a method to assess the respective contributions of automatic (unconscious) and controlled (conscious) influences by pitting the direct measure against the indirect one. For instance, participants first memorize a list of words. Then they perform a direct task in which they are asked to complete word stems with words that were *not* on the memorized list. If they still complete the stems with the memorized words, then that provides evidence for the automatic influence of the studied words: The words produced priming when conscious access should have prevented priming.[1]

Procedures like these capitalize on qualitative differences: The pattern of performance differs when people perform the direct task and the indirect task. Such differences add strength to the argument that the tasks tap different underlying mechanisms. Most evidence from the subliminal perception literature finds the same pattern of results with and without awareness, with the purportedly subliminal measures just showing weaker effects (Desender & Van den Bussche, 2012). By demonstrating larger or qualitatively different effects in the task that presumably requires less awareness, researchers can argue that performance on the subliminal task is not just due to reduced (but still present) awareness.

These procedures can produce theoretically important dissociations between tasks, and they provide some suggestive evidence for unconscious processing. However, they too can be criticized for not meeting all four criteria. For example, the direct and indirect measures might just be testing different aspects of awareness, failing the relevance criterion. And, the approach depends on the assumption that the direct measure is more sensitive than the indirect one, but it might just be more subject to explicit reporting biases.

This discussion highlights the prolonged debate within cognitive psychology about subliminal perception and semantic processing in the absence of awareness. Hard-core skeptics can still hold to the claim that there is no indisputable evidence for subliminal semantic priming. And, even proponents of subliminal perception argue that demonstrating the absence of awareness requires exceptional rigor or a set of contentious assumptions.

Nobody doubts the existence of semantic priming. The debate is about the need for consciousness and the claims that follow if subliminal semantic priming occurs. For the vast majority of studies of semantic priming in cognitive psychology, the issue of awareness is of minimal relevance. It is important only for particular types of claims: those arguing that such access is necessarily automatic, those positing routes to behavior that do not require conscious decisions, or those suggesting that much reasoning or deliberation occurs outside of awareness. Most semantic priming effects studied in cognitive psychology, whether they are conscious or unconscious, are small and fleeting.

PRIMING IN SOCIAL PSYCHOLOGY

Although early studies had already suggested that subtle primes could affect social judgment unbeknownst to the subject (e.g., Bargh & Pietromonaco, 1982; Devine, 1989; Higgins, Rholes, & Jones, 1977; Srull & Wyer, 1979), the seminal studies of Bargh, Chen, and Burrows (1996) in the 1990s were the first to show that the automatic effects of primes extended to overt actions. The wealth of studies conducted since then appears to confirm the power of automatic behavioral prim-

---

1. See Payne (2001), Payne, Lambert, and Jacoby (2002), Payne, Jacoby, and Lambert (2004) as well as Stewart and Payne (2008) for the application of the process dissociation procedure in social psychology.

ing. For example, people primed with the concept of professor perform better on knowledge tasks (Dijksterhuis & van Knippenberg, 1998); people primed with the concept of cleanliness or warmth may behave more prosocially (Vohs, Redden, & Rahinel, 2013; Williams & Bargh, 2008); participants primed with a picture of a dog (vs. a cat) behave more loyally (Chartrand, Fitzsimons, & Fitzsimons, 2008), and so on. A recent review of behavioral priming in social cognition concluded, "What were once considered shocking and controversial effects are now widely accepted among social psychologists" (Wheeler & DeMarree, 2009, p. 577).

The discovery of automatic priming effects on behavior triggered the exploration of a variety of prime-to-target relationships with little exploration of the processes underlying each effect. The diversity of these reports gives the impression that priming is ubiquitous and unavoidable. Such "effect" studies continue to appear at a steady rate (e.g., Gibson & Zielaskowski, 2013; Lammers, Dubois, Rucker, & Galinsky, 2013; Shimizu, Sperry, & Pelham, 2013), but theorists have begun to devote more attention to the boundary conditions of priming effects and the processes that may underlie the phenomena (for examples, see Bargh, 2006; Jonas, 2013; Wheeler & DeMarree, 2009).

This sustained interest in priming within social psychology developed from a broader interest in the role of automatic processes. Until the 1970s, many of the phenomena that now fall under the umbrella of social cognition (e.g., causal attribution, person perception, or attitude change) were studied using self-report methods: People were asked to explain why they evaluated, judged, or behaved as they did. In the 1970s, that approach came under fire from Nisbett and Wilson (1977) who showed how wrong we can be about the reasons for our behaviors and beliefs. The critique paralleled earlier criticisms (Mandler & Mandler, 1964) of Titchnerian introspective methods (Titchener, 1902), noting how we often lack introspective access to the mechanisms underlying our cognition.

Nisbett and Wilson's lasting contribution came from their discussion of the different ways in which we can be aware of the causes of our behavior. Their analysis played a central role in the development of social cognition as a field by encouraging the use of methods inspired by cognitive psychology. They put forward that people may be "(a) unaware of the existence of the stimulus that influenced their response; (b) unaware of the existence of the response; (c) unaware that the stimulus has affected the response" (p. 810), a statement that echoes the need to specify the form of awareness being measured.

Nisbett and Wilson (1977) did not focus on subliminal perception, considering the phenomenon to be plausible but not central to their claims. Rather, they addressed how stimuli exert their influence on behavior without this influence being consciously registered or accurately understood by subjects (i.e., point "c" above). From this perspective, priming is theoretically important because it suggests that people's behavior may be influenced by factors they fail to recognize as potential causes of their actions. Thus, what matters chiefly is whether people are aware of the *effect of the prime on the outcome* (e.g., behavior, impression, judgment) rather than whether they are aware of the prime itself. This approach, which accords a peripheral role to issues of awareness of the prime, also characterizes the way social psychologists have approached priming more recently. In the majority of priming studies conducted after Nisbett and Wilson's work, participants actually were aware of the prime (cf. Higgins, 1996).

Still, social psychologists frequently rely on purportedly subliminal stimuli as a way to study how primes influence behavior automatically. In one of the seminal papers on priming in social psychology, Bargh (1992) lists two reasons why social psychologists do so: (1) any influence of a subliminal prime must occur automatically rather than via conscious intervention or deliberation, and (2) the effects of subliminal primes reveal the "way in which social stimuli are interpreted, categorized or evaluated prior to the output of these analyses being furnished to conscious awareness" (p. 238).

The issue of automaticity is central to many areas of social cognition, including dispositional attribution, stereotype activation, impression formation, the effects of attitudes on judgments, and so forth. Automatic processes are those that are unintentional, effortless, outside awareness, and ballistic once initiated (Bargh, 1994). Few processes meet all of these criteria, with most processes in social cognition satisfying a subset of these requirements (Bargh, 1994).

Subliminal priming, though, meets all of these criteria: "Lack of awareness of the stimulus ensures that its subsequent effects were unintended by the subjects" (Bargh, 1994, p. 10). Subliminal effects rule out possible demand effects, strategy shifts, or explicit biases that might otherwise account for a link between the prime and the target behavior. And, if those processes are automatic, then they can reveal the sorts of social processes that are fundamental to how we see the world, those that operate independently of our explicit desires, beliefs, and goals. Thus, even if the use of subliminal priming has not been the norm in social cognition, demonstrating an effect of subliminal primes has been the gold standard for establishing that the underlying process is automatic.

Besides the two reasons mentioned by Bargh, a third appeal of subliminal priming comes from the excitement of showing how subtle factors can have large, counterintuitive effects on behavior (cf. Giner-Sorolla, 2012; Gray & Wegner, 2013, on the role of aesthetic standards in scientific publication). And, no stimulus can be more subtle than a subliminal one. Social cognition is replete with surprisingly powerful and counterintuitive effects of purportedly subliminal stimuli: Subliminally flashed Israeli flags induce changes in political positions and voting behavior weeks later (Hassin, Ferguson, Shidlovski, & Gross, 2007), subliminal fast food logos affect the choice of an interest rate (Zhong & DeVoe, 2010), priming the concept of God makes believers less likely to endorse responsibility for their actions (Dijksterhuis, Preston, Wegner, & Aarts, 2008), and so forth. Such studies, which reveal the powerful real-world effects of seemingly trivial events, are darlings of the media because they provide a compelling narrative that counters the intuitive belief that we know the reasons for our decisions and actions. They regularly appear in top journals and are highly cited, providing an incentive for other researchers to use similar methods.

This broad visibility also contributes to skepticism from cognitive psychologists who study subliminal perception because almost none of these studies meet the criteria necessary to show that the prime fell entirely outside of awareness; most claim that the stimulus is subliminal without directly addressing those criteria.

HOW DO SOCIAL PSYCHOLOGISTS ASSESS AWARENESS?

In many priming studies in social cognition, a single prime influences a single outcome measure, a method that does not permit systematic tests of the detectability of the prime. And, even those studies that use multiple priming trials (e.g., Hassin et al., 2007) typically do not use sensitive measures of awareness of the prime (for exceptions, see Devine, 1989; Hepler & Albarracin, 2013). The most common approach involves using a funneled debriefing, after measuring the outcome behavior, to determine whether participants can guess the purpose of the study, whether they remembered the prime, or if they inferred the link between the prime and the outcome behavior (Bargh & Chartrand, 2000). If a sizable proportion of participants correctly report the link between the prime and behavior, then researchers worry that any effects on the outcome measure were potentially affected by conscious demands. For example, Bargh and Chartrand (2000) question the value of any experiment in which an "alarmingly high proportion" (i.e., > 5%) of participants must be excluded because they report the correct prime-behavior link during debriefing. Note that this method of assessing awareness does not meet any of the criteria for claiming that a stimulus was processed without awareness. The test of awareness was delayed rather than immediate, it relied on verbal reports that might be inadequately sensitive, it might not be reliable because it could be influenced by demands, and it might not be relevant if verbal reports do not tap the same processes thought to be unconscious. The use of verbal reports to assess awareness is ironic in light of the role that Nisbett and Wilson's (1977) criticism of such methods played in the development of priming research in social psychology.

Some studies do go beyond funnel debriefing and use additional methods to assess awareness of the prime. In an influential guide to conducting priming research, Bargh and Chartrand (2000) recommend a follow-up test in which they show primes and ask participants to guess what they are. They conclude that the primes were subliminal "if the participant is not able to guess any of the words or identify the gist of the pictorial content" (p. 10). Again, the test of awareness uses a potentially insensitive measure (verbal report) that might be subject to biases (e.g., subjects might be conservative in their guesses) and that is conducted after the priming episode. Indeed, people may have been aware of the primes but have trouble retrieving them (see Bargh, Bond, Lombardi, & Tota, 1986), or they may simply resort to the most economical option, which is to report that they saw nothing.

Other approaches recommended by Bargh and Chartrand (2000) include conducting an additional experiment to assess awareness of the prime directly (e.g., Bargh et al., 1986; Bargh & Pietromonaco, 1982; Devine, 1989, study 2), an approach common in cognitive psychology as well (Dehaene et al., 2001). For example, in a study of the effect of parafoveally presented stereotype primes on a subsequent impression-formation task (Devine, 1989, study 2), a control condition measured awareness directly. Participants viewed the same words under the same conditions and were asked to guess each word. They successfully guessed fewer than 2% of the stereotype-related words, which was taken as evidence that participants were not aware of the meaning of the primes. Although this method is more rigorous than funnel debriefing, the inability to name words does not exclude all conscious semantic processing.[2] Devine also conducted a recognition test with new participants. At the end of the priming task, participants viewed a list of words (some of which had been presented previously and some not), and they reported which ones they had seen. Their recognition performance did not vary as a function of the priming condition and was no better than chance. Note, though, that this method does not meet the immediacy criterion, and it too might not be optimally sensitive.

In an example of an unusually rigorous test of awareness in a social psychology priming study (Hepler & Albarracin, 2013, study 2), subjects were subliminally primed with words related to action or inaction, which subsequently affected performance on a go/no-go task. In addition to funnel debriefing, participants completed a prime recognition task twice (i.e., identifying primes among distractors) as well as a prime discrimination task in which they viewed primes under the same timing conditions as the primary task and had to make a forced choice identification (which of two words was shown). Participants showed poor recognition and discrimination performance. Moreover, the results were unchanged after eliminating data from those participants who showed better discrimination and recognition accuracy, and performance on the discrimination task was uncorrelated with the effects of priming. It still is possible that the discrimination and recognition tasks were inadequately sensitive to pick up awareness of the presence and conscious influence of a prime, but the approach in this study is laudable for its rigor.

Unfortunately, the use of such a thorough awareness check is rarely reported in social psychology. Many priming studies do not even provide enough detail about the method to determine exactly how awareness was tested. For example, Zhong and Devoe (2010) presented fast food logos or control logos for 12ms in the context of a lexical decision task and showed that the fast food logos made people more impatient (operationalized as the time taken to read a text passage). When reporting how they determined that the primes were subliminal, they state, "When asked after the experiment what they had seen in the flashes, all the participants reported that they had seen color blocks without any meaningful pattern" (p. 620). No information is provided about the nature of the questions, and no systematic tests are conducted to demonstrate that the primes must have fallen outside awareness. Other studies provide no test of awareness at all, simply assuming that the stimulus must have been subliminal because the presentation was brief (e.g., Bargh et al., 1996; Hirschberger, Ein-Dor, Caspi, Arzouan, & Zivotofsky, 2010; Veltkamp, Custers, & Aarts, 2011).

SUMMARY

In cognitive psychology, the question of awareness is paramount; demonstrations of subliminal priming could reveal an alternative mechanism for semantic pro-

---

2. For example, the relevance criterion might not have been met: Social desirability concerns might have discouraged participants from uttering stereotype-related words, thereby explaining lower naming rates for those words than for neutral ones. In some respects, this approach is comparable to a naming task used by Sidis (1898), one considered inadequate by most subliminal perception proponents.

cessing, and if such effects can be explained via explicit processes, the findings themselves may be uninteresting. In social psychology, what counts is whether the prime's influence on behavior happens outside of awareness, and using subliminal presentation is one way to ensure that those effects occur automatically.

Unfortunately, lack of awareness is often assumed rather than tested, and when tests are conducted, they are insufficiently stringent to meet the standards set by subliminal perception researchers (the same holds true for some experiments in cognitive psychology). Claims that a stimulus or its influence fell outside of awareness typically rely on post-experiment funnel debriefing, a procedure that falls short of most established criteria for documenting the absence of awareness.

When a claim rests on the absence of awareness of the primes themselves, researchers must take steps to document the absence of awareness. Those steps could include using signal detection methods to document that participants cannot discriminate the presence of the prime from its absence (i.e., showing that d' for the detection of a stimulus is actually 0 for every subject). Note that this standard is far more challenging to meet than demonstrating an inability to identify or remember a flashed prime, but it provides clear evidence that the observer did not consciously process the prime; if they cannot discriminate the presence of a prime from its absence, then they presumably cannot process the meaning of the prime. Using signal detection analysis across a set of trials also distinguishes discriminability from response bias (i.e., participants might not report a stimulus that they did process with some awareness).

Typically, a signal detection analysis of awareness would be conducted separately from the main priming trials to avoid contaminating the priming measures themselves. Consequently, they do not meet the immediacy criterion. Moreover, people might improve in their ability to detect the primes over the course of a study, so in an ideal design, discriminability would be tested before and after the priming period to verify that d' has not changed.

This objective standard for awareness is perhaps the most stringent, and few studies meet it. But, when a study does not meet this standard, any claims that the prime was processed entirely without awareness must be qualified appropriately. At a minimum, researchers must recognize that a failure to report the presence of a prime or to remember it later is not the same as the ability to consciously process it at the time of presentation. Verbal reports and recognition judgments are influenced both by sensitivity to the presence of the stimulus and by the decision criterion, and claims about awareness require an assessment of whether the prime was consciously perceived, not of whether people neglected to report a low-confidence percept.

In some cases, documenting the complete absence of awareness is not important; the need for such controls depends on the claim the researchers want to make. For example, imagine a simple test in which a subject views a video and then fails to report the presence of a person in a gorilla suit (Simons & Chabris, 1999). If the researcher wants to test whether the gorilla fell entirely outside of awareness but still influenced subsequent performance, then stringent measures of awareness are needed and the verbal report of noticing is inadequate. If, however, the researcher does not wish to explore whether the gorilla was processed unconsciously in the absence of a verbal report, then more stringent tests are unnecessary. For example, they could safely conclude that the gorilla influenced later performance even when it went *unreported*, a claim that might well be informative and interesting (Simons, 2000; Wolfe, 1999; note, though, that there is little evidence for such an effect).

To determine whether awareness matters for a claim, consider whether the finding would be interesting or informative if the crucial aspect of the prime occurred with awareness. For example, take the case in which priming with words related to aging leads participants to walk more slowly (Bargh et al., 1996). In that case, the primes were consciously perceived—subjects descrambled sentences that were fully visible and they had to perceive the relevant words to do so. Unawareness of the stimulus is irrelevant. How about the link between the prime and behavior? If participants were fully aware of the link between the age-related words and their walking speed, the finding would not be as interesting—it could be attributed to task demands, expectancy effects, or other biases. The finding is important only to the extent that it cannot be explained by such explicit biases, so documenting the absence of awareness of the link between the prime and outcome measure is essential.

In most social psychology priming studies, experimenters try to eliminate demand characteristics and other explicit biases in order to show that the prime had its effect automatically. They frequently do so by claiming subjects were unaware of the primes themselves or of the influence of the primes on their behavior. Yet, such claims of awareness require more careful testing and reporting than typically occurs. When evaluating such claims, we should consider whether and in what ways the finding would still be interesting even if subjects were aware.

THREE SOURCES OF CONFLICT AND HOW TO RESOLVE THEM

AWARENESS

Cognitive and social psychologists have focused on different aspects of awareness in the study of priming. Cognitive psychologists have spent decades debating the appropriate way to document subliminal priming because they are fundamentally interested in what unconscious processing would tell us about the mechanisms of semantic processing and representation. In contrast, social psychologists have largely used the absence of awareness as a way to verify that priming effects occur automatically and are not subject to explicit demands and situational biases.

In studies of subliminal perception, researchers decrease stimulus intensity or presentation time until the prime is weakened enough to elude consciousness. In studies of automaticity, the stimuli often are strong, but they exert their influence automatically, in the absence of awareness of the link between the prime and behavior. This difference in emphasis has resulted in a difference in how cognitive and social psychologists verify the absence of awareness in their research. Whereas cognitive psychologists studying subliminal perception typically attempt to meet all four of the criteria for documenting awareness, many priming studies in social psychology rely instead on post-hoc debriefing and verbal reports of awareness.

These differences in approach inspire conflict, largely due to different uses of the term "awareness," but they also could be resolved easily. Priming studies only need to specify the aspect of awareness that is crucial to the claimed effects. Is a lack of awareness of the prime itself essential? Is a lack of awareness of the prime-outcome link essential? Would the finding still be of interest if subjects were aware of the prime or the prime-behavior link?

If the finding would be uninteresting if subjects were aware, the paper should explicitly discuss the ramifications of awareness and note that limitation. If the finding would be interesting regardless of whether or not participants were unaware, the paper can make stronger claims and note how it would be interesting in each case.

Simply increasing the precision of claims about awareness and automaticity would help, but papers also must fully describe how awareness was measured and identify the limitations of those assessments. If an assessment fails to meet one or more of the four criteria necessary to rule out awareness, the paper must acknowledge that failure and discuss its implications for any claims about awareness and automaticity.

PROCESSES

Within cognitive psychology, the presumed mechanism underlying priming is the spread of activation within semantic networks (Collins & Loftus, 1975). In this model, activation diminishes with semantic distance (McNamara, 1992) and fades quickly, often disappearing after a few hundred milliseconds (Muscarella, Brintazzoli, Gordts, Soetens, & Van den Bussche, 2013). From this theoretical perspective, some effects of primes on judgment and behavior seem ungrounded. For example, claims that a subliminal flag can produce long-lasting effects on political attitudes and voting behavior (Hassin et al., 2007) run counter to the limited spread of semantic activation and the duration and potency of such primes in subliminal perception. As social psychologists (e.g., Jonas, 2013) have themselves noted, other findings of strong behavioral consequences of subliminal stimuli or subliminal stimulus-behavior links (e.g., Aarts & Dijksterhuis, 2002) are similarly hard to explain in terms of traditional accounts of spreading activation within semantic networks.

Although several theoretical models have been proposed to account for the substantially more powerful priming in social psychology experiments (e.g., Bargh et al., 1996; Bargh, Schwader, Hailey, Dyer, & Boothby, 2012; Dijksterhuis & Bargh, 2001; Loersch & Payne, 2011), these accounts remain relatively underspecified. For example, the perception-behavior link account claims that primes activate representations that then directly activate relevant behaviors and goals (Bargh et al., 1996; Bargh et al., 2012; Dijksterhuis & Bargh, 2001), but the model does not make explicit predictions about *which* motor behavior will be activated by a given mental representation (e.g., the trait "aggressive" may be manifested in many different motor behaviors) or which of the many environmental primes we experience will exert an effect on behavior (the "reduction problem" highlighted by Bargh, 2006). Although situationally activated goals and motivations seem to play an important role (cf. Bargh, 2006; Wheeler & DeMarree, 2009), current accounts make few a priori predictions, in large part because of their inherent complexity.

For instance, in a review of moderators of priming effects, Wheeler and DeMarree (2009) propose a model[3] that assumes that a prime first activates a construct in memory. The activated construct then directly influences a behavioral representation, which itself directly drives behavior. But its influence can be mediated by many other processes, including how people represent their goals and how they perceive the situation, themselves, or other people. The authors list as many as 16 such moderators, each of which is assumed to modulate some aspect of the complex pathways that link perception to action.

With so many degrees of freedom, it would be unsurprising if priming effects were hard to replicate. Yes, moderators are a possibility, but what is the evidence that they do play a role? Most priming studies are underpowered to detect even medium-sized effects of the prime, and they are massively underpowered to detect an interaction of that effect with one or more moderators (see Simonsohn, 2014). Demonstrating that a moderator matters would require a large-scale, confirmatory study showing how varying the moderator varies the outcome. Without such studies, there would be no way for researchers to know that moderators matter.

REPLICABILITY

At least two factors contribute to the skepticism expressed by some cognitive psychologists about social priming research. First, large priming effects from subtle manipulations are not the norm in cognitive psychology, where weaker manipulations produce weaker, not stronger, effects. The surprisingly large effects (at least to cognitive psychologists) (Pashler, Coburn, & Harris, 2012), coupled with the lack of published direct replications of these findings within the social psychology literature, increase the concern that these effects might not be as robust as a perusal of the literature would suggest (Carlin & Standing, 2013; Doyen, Klein, Pichon, & Cleeremans, 2012; Harris, Coburn, Rohrer, & Pashler, 2013; Pashler et al., 2012; Shanks et al., 2013).

A deeper cause of conflict over replicability follows from differences in the sorts of replications valued by cognitive and social psychologists. Cognitive psychologists historically have tended to devalue individual differences, looking for mechanisms common to most or all people. Consequently, they expect any published effect to be replicable with any reasonably similar population of subjects, provided that the reported methods are followed precisely. Multiple-experiment papers in cognitive psychology often include a direct replication of another finding, followed by extensions of that finding.

In contrast, social psychologists assume that the primes activate culturally and situationally contextualized representations (e.g., stereotypes, social norms), meaning that they can vary over time and culture and across individuals. Hence, social psychologists have advocated the use of "conceptual replications" that reproduce an experiment by relying on different operationalizations of the concepts under investigation (Stroebe & Strack, 2014). For example, in a society in which old age is associated not with slowness but with, say, talkativeness, the outcome variable could be the number of words uttered by the subject at the end of the experiment rather than walking speed.

---

3. Note that Wheeler and DeMarree (2009) prefer the term "descriptive summary" to "model."

The problem with conceptual replication in the absence of direct replication is that there is no such thing as a "conceptual failure to replicate." A failure to find the same "effect" using a different operationalization can be attributed to the differences in method rather than to the fragility of the original effect. Only the successful conceptual replications will be published, and the unsuccessful ones can be dismissed without challenging the underlying foundations of the claim. Consequently, conceptual replication without direct replication is unlikely to change beliefs about the underlying effect (Pashler & Harris, 2012).

Given the existence of publication bias and the prevalence of questionable research practices (John, Loewenstein, & Prelec, 2012), we know that the published literature likely contains some false positive results. Direct replication is the only way to correct such errors (Simons, 2014). The failure to find an effect with a well-powered direct replication must be taken as evidence against the original effect. Of course, one failed direct replication does not mean the effect is non-existent—science depends on the accumulation of evidence. But, treating direct replication as irrelevant makes it impossible to correct Type 1 errors in the published literature.

CONCLUSIONS

Our review of priming research in cognitive and social psychology highlighted important differences in the underlying assumptions, methods, and goals of these fields. Whereas cognitive psychologists historically have used priming to study the structure of mental representations and the extent to which information processing takes place without awareness, social psychologists have used priming to study the automatic effects of a stimulus on behavior. For most studies in social psychology, using subliminal primes is a powerful way to ensure automaticity as well as to eliminate possible demand effects on behavior.

Given evidence from subliminal perception research showing that (1) the effects of primes tend to be small and short-lived, and (2) even the most stringent tests to rule out awareness are controversial, perhaps it is unsurprising that claims of large and lasting effects of primes on behavior have come under scrutiny.

We identified three changes that would help the field move beyond this clash of traditions. First, be more precise in defining what aspect of awareness matters and how it is measured. Second, focus on direct replications and confirmatory tests of proposed moderators. Third, continue to probe the different types of mechanisms that might underlie priming effects.

REFERENCES

Aarts, H., & Dijksterhuis, A. (2002). Category activation effects in judgment and behaviour: The moderating role of perceived comparability. *British Journal of Social Psychology, 41*(1), 123-138.

Baars, B. J. (1998). *A cognitive theory of consciousness*. New York: Cambridge University Press.

Bargh, J. A. (1992). Does subliminality matter to social psychology? Awareness of the stimulus versus awareness of its influence. In R. Bornstein & T. Pittman (Eds.), *Perception without awareness* (pp. 236–255). New York: Guilford.

Bargh, J. A. (1994). The four horsemen of automaticity: Intention, awareness, efficiency, and control as separate issues. *Handbook of Social Cognition, 1*, 1-40.

Bargh, J. A. (2006). What have we been priming all these years? On the development, mechanisms, and ecology of nonconscious social behavior. *European Journal of Social Psychology, 36*(2), 147-168. doi:10.1002/ejsp.336

Bargh, J. A., Bond, R. N., Lombardi, W. J., & Tota, M. E. (1986). The additive nature of chronic and temporary sources of construct accessibility. *Journal of Personality and Social Psychology, 50*(5), 869-878.

Bargh, J. A., & Chartrand, T. L. (2000). Studying the mind in the middle: A practical guide to priming and automaticity research. *Handbook of Research Methods in Social Psychology*, 1-40.

Bargh, J. A., Chen, M., & Burrows, L. (1996). Automaticity of social behavior: Direct effects of trait construct and stereotype activation on action. *Journal of Personality and Social Psychology, 71*, 230-244.

Bargh, J. A., & Pietromonaco, P. (1982). Automatic information processing and social perception: The influence of trait information presented outside of conscious awareness on impression formation. *Journal of Personality and Social Psychology, 43*(3), 437-449.

Bargh, J. A., Schwader, K. L., Hailey, S. E., Dyer, R. L., & Boothby, E. J. (2012). Automaticity in social-cognitive processes. *Trends in Cognitive Sciences, 16*, 1-13. doi:10.1016/j.tics.2012.10.002

Carlin, S., & Standing, L. (2013). Is intelligence enhanced by letter priming? A failure to replicate the results of Ciani and Sheldon (2010). *Psychological Reports, 112*(2), 533-544.

Chartrand, T. L., Fitzsimons, G. M., & Fitzsimons, G. J. (2008). Automatic effects of anthropomorphized objects on behavior. *Social Cognition, 26*(2), 198-209.

Cheesman, J., & Merikle, P. M. (1986). Distinguishing conscious from unconscious perceptual processes. *Canadian Journal of Psychology/Revue canadienne de psychologie, 40*(4), 343-367.

Cleeremans, A. (2003). *The unity of consciousness: Binding, integration, and dissociation*. New York: Oxford University Press.

Cleeremans, A. (2011). The radical plasticity thesis: How the brain learns to be conscious. *Frontiers in Psychology, 2*. doi:10.3389/fpsyg.2011.00086

Cleeremans, A., Destrebecqz, A., & Boyer, M. (1998). Implicit learning: News from the front. *Trends in Cognitive Sciences, 2*(10), 406-416.

Collins, A. M., & Loftus, E. F. (1975). A spreading-activation theory of semantic processing. *Psychological Review, 82*(6), 407-428.

Dehaene, S. (2008). Conscious and nonconscious processes: Distinct forms of evidence accumulation? *Biological Physics, 60*, 141-168.

Dehaene, S., Naccache, L., Cohen, L., Le Bihan, D., Mangin, J., Poline, J., & Rivière, D. (2001). Cerebral mechanisms of word masking and unconscious repetition priming. *Nature Neuroscience, 4*(7), 752-758.

Desender, K., & Van den Bussche, E. (2012). Consciousness and cognition. *Consciousness and Cognition: An International Journal, 21*(3), 1571-1572. doi:10.1016/j.concog.2012.01.017

Devine, P. (1989). Stereotypes and prejudice: Their automatic and controlled components. *Journal of Personality and Social Psychology, 56*(1), 5-18.

Dijksterhuis, A., & Bargh, J. A. (2001). The perception-behavior expressway: Automatic effects of social perception on social behavior. *Advances in Experimental Social Psychology, 33*, 1-40.

Dijksterhuis, A., Preston, J., Wegner, D. M., & Aarts, H. (2008). Effects of subliminal priming of self and God on self-attribution of authorship for events. *Journal of Experimental Social Psychology, 44*(1), 2-9. doi:10.1016/j.jesp.2007.01.003

Dijksterhuis, A., & van Knippenberg, A. (1998). The relation between perception and behavior, or how to win a game of Trivial Pursuit. *Journal of Personality and Social Psychology, 74*(4), 865-877.

Doyen, S., Klein, O., Pichon, C. L., & Cleeremans, A. (2012). Behavioral priming: It's all in the mind, but whose mind? *PLOS ONE, 7*(1), e29081.

Draine, S. C., & Greenwald, A. G. (1998). Replicable unconscious semantic priming. *Journal of Experimental Psychology: General, 127*(3), 286-303.

Dulany, D. E. (2001). Inattentional awareness. *Psyche, 7*(5).

Gazzaniga, M. S. (2011). *Who's in charge?: Free will and the science of the brain.* New York: HarperCollins.

Gibson, B., & Zielaskowski, K. (2013). Subliminal priming of winning images prompts increased betting in slot machine play. *Journal of Applied Social Psychology, 43*(1), 106-115. doi:10.1111/j.1559-1816.2012.00985.x

Giner-Sorolla, R. (2012). Science or art? How aesthetic standards grease the way through the publication bottleneck but undermine science. *Perspectives on Psychological Science, 7*(6), 562-571. doi:10.1177/1745691612457576

Gray, K., & Wegner, D. M. (2013). Six guidelines for interesting research. *Perspectives on Psychological Science, 8*(5), 549-553.

Greenwald, A. G., Spangenberg, E. R., Pratkanis, A. R., & Eskenazi, J. (1991). Double-blind tests of subliminal self-help audiotapes. *Psychological Science, 2*(2), 119-122.

Hall, L., Johansson, P., Tärning, B., Sikström, S., & Deutgen, T. (2010). Magic at the marketplace: Choice blindness for the taste of jam and the smell of tea. *Cognition, 117*(1), 54-61. doi:10.1016/j.cognition.2010.06.010

Hannula, D. E., Simons, D. J., & Cohen, N. J. (2005). Imaging implicit perception: Promise and pitfalls. *Nature Reviews Neuroscience, 6*(3), 247-255.

Harris, C. R., Coburn, N., Rohrer, D., & Pashler, H. (2013). Two failures to replicate high-performance-goal priming effects. *PLOS ONE, 8*(8), e72467. doi:10.1371/journal.pone.0072467.g001

Hassin, R. R., Ferguson, M. J., Shidlovski, D., & Gross, T. (2007). Subliminal exposure to national flags affects political thought and behavior. *Proceedings of the National Academy of Sciences, 104*(50), 19757-19761.

Hepler, J., & Albarracin, D. (2013). Complete unconscious control: Using (in)action primes to demonstrate completely unconscious activation of inhibitory control mechanisms. *Cognition, 128*(3), 271-279. doi:10.1016/j.cognition.2013.04.012

Higgins, E. T. (1996). Knowledge activation: Accessibility, applicability and salience. In E. T. Higgins & A. E. Kruglanski (Eds.), *Social psychology: Handbook of basic principles* (pp. 133-168). New York: Guilford.

Higgins, T., Rholes, W., & Jones, C. (1977). Category accessibility and impression formation. *Journal of Experimental Social Psychology, 13*(2), 141-154.Hirschberger, G., Ein-Dor, T., Caspi, A., Arzouan, Y., & Zivotofsky, A. Z. (2010). Looking away from death: Defensive attention as a form of terror management. *Journal of Experimental Social Psychology, 46*(1), 172-178. doi:10.1016/j.jesp.2009.10.005

Holender, D. (1986). Semantic activation without conscious identification in dichotic listening, parafoveal vision, and visual masking: A survey and appraisal. *Behavioral and Brain Sciences, 9*(01), 1-23.

Jacoby, L. L. (1991). A process dissociation framework: Separating automatic from intentional uses of memory. *Journal of Memory and Language, 30*(5), 513-541.

John, L. K., Loewenstein, G., & Prelec, D. (2012). Measuring the prevalence of questionable research practices with incentives for truth telling. *Psychological Science, 23*(5), 524-532. doi:10.1177/0956797611430953

Jonas, K. J. (2013). Automatic behavior—Its social embedding and individual consequences. *Social and Personality Psychology Compass, 7*(9), 689-700. doi:10.1111/spc3.12060

Klein, O., Doyen, S., Magalhaes de Saldanha da Gama, P., Miller, S., Questienne, L., Leys, C., & Cleeremans, A. (2012). Low hopes, high expectations expectancy effects and the replicability of behavioral experiments. *Perspectives on Psychological Science, 7*(6), 572-584. doi:10.1177/1745691612463704

Kouider, S., & Dehaene, S. (2007). Levels of processing during non-conscious perception: A critical review of visual masking. *Philosophical Transactions of the Royal Society B: Biological Sciences, 362*(1481), 857-875. doi:10.1098/rstb.2007.2093

Lammers, J., Dubois, D., Rucker, D. D., & Galinsky, A. D. (2013). Power gets the job: Priming power improves interview outcomes. *Journal of Experimental Social Psychology, 49*(4), 776-779. doi:10.1016/j.jesp.2013.02.008

Loersch, C., & Payne, B. K. (2011). The situated inference model an integrative account of the effects of primes on perception, behavior, and motivation. *Perspectives on Psychological Science, 6*(3), 234-252.

Mandler, J. M., & Mandler, G. (1964). *Thinking: From association to Gestalt.* New York: Wiley.

Marcel, A. J. (1983). Conscious and unconscious perception: Experiments on visual masking and word recognition. *Cognitive Psychology, 15*(2), 197-237.

McNamara, T. P. (1992). Theories of priming: I. Associative distance and lag. *Journal of Experimental Psychology: Learning, Memory, and Cognition, 18*(6), 1173-1190.

Muscarella, C., Brintazzoli, G., Gordts, S., Soetens, E., & Van den Bussche, E. (2013). Short- and long-term effects of conscious, minimally conscious and unconscious brand logos. *PLOS ONE, 8*(5), e57738. doi:10.1371/journal.pone.0057738.s003

Naccache, L., & Dehaene, S. (2001). Unconscious semantic priming extends to novel unseen stimuli. *Cognition, 80*(3), 215-229.

Neely, J. H. (1977). Semantic priming and retrieval from lexical memory: Roles of inhibitionless spreading activation and limited-capacity attention. *Journal of Experimental Psychology: General, 106*(3), 226.

Newell, J., & Shanks, D. (2012). Unconscious influences on decision making: A critical review. *Behavioral and Brain Sciences*, 1-19.

Nisbett, R. E., & Wilson, T. D. (1977). Telling more than we can know: Verbal reports on mental processes. *Psychological Review, 84*(3), 231.

Pashler, H., Coburn, N., & Harris, C. R. (2012). Priming of social distance? Failure to replicate effects on social and food judgments. (J. Lauwereyns, Ed.). *PLOS ONE, 7*(8), e42510. doi:10.1371/journal.pone.0042510.t002

Pashler, H., & Harris, C. (2012). Is the replicability crisis overblown? Three arguments examined. *Perspectives on Psychological Science, 7*, 531-536.

Patterson, K., Nestor, P. J., & Rogers, T. T. (2007). Where do you know what you know? The representation of semantic knowledge in the human brain. *Nature Reviews Neuroscience, 8*(12), 976-987. doi:10.1038/nrn2277

Payne, B. K. (2001). Prejudice and perception: the role of automatic and controlled processes in misperceiving a weapon. *Journal of Personality and Social Psychology, 81*(2), 181-192.

Payne, B. K., Jacoby, L. L., & Lambert, A. J. (2004). Memory monitoring and the control of stereotype distortion. *Journal of Experimental Social Psychology, 40*, 52-64.

Payne, B. K., Lambert, A. J., & Jacoby, L. L. (2002). Best laid plans: Effects of goals on accessibility bias and cognitive control in race-based misperceptions of weapons. *Journal of Experimental Social Psychology, 38*, 384-396.

Reingold, E. M., & Merikle, P. M. (1988). Using direct and indirect measures to study perception without awareness. *Attention, Perception, & Psychophysics, 44*(6), 563-575.

Rosenthal, R. (2009). Interpersonal expectations: Effects of the experimenter's hypothesis. In R. Rosenthal & R. Rosnow (Eds.), *Artifacts in behavioral research* (pp. 138-210). New York: Oxford University Press.

Schacter, D. L., Dobbins, I. G., & Schnyer, D. M. (2004). Specificity of priming: A cognitive neuroscience perspective. *Nature Reviews Neuroscience, 5*(11), 853-862. doi:10.1038/nrn1534

Shanks, D., Newell, B. R., Lee, E. H., Balakrishnan, D., Ekelund, L., Cenac, Z., et al. (2013). Priming intelligent behavior: An elusive phenomenon. *PLOS ONE, 8*(4), e56515. doi:10.1371/journal.pone.0056515.s001

Shanks, D., & St John, M. (1994). Characteristics of dissociable human learning systems. *Behavioral and Brain Sciences, 17*(3), 367-395.

Shimizu, M., Sperry, J. J., & Pelham, B. W. (2013). The effect of subliminal priming on sleep duration. *Journal of Applied Social Psychology, 43*(9), 1777-1783. doi:10.1111/jasp.12123

Sidis, B. (1898). *The psychology of suggestion, a research into the subconscious nature of man and society.* New York: Appleton.

Simons, D. J. (2000). Attentional capture and inattentional blindness. *Trends in Cognitive Sciences, 4*(4), 147-155.

Simons, D. J. (2014). The value of direct replication. *Perspectives on*

Psychological Science, 9(1), 76-80. doi:10.1177/1745691613514755

Simons, D. J., & Chabris, C. F. (1999). Gorillas in our midst: Sustained inattentional blindness for dynamic events. *Perception-London, 28*(9), 1059-1074.

Simonsohn, U. (2014, 3 March). *No-way interactions.* Retrieved from http://datacolada.org/2014/03/12/17-no-way-interactions-2/

Snodgrass, M., Bernat, E., & Shevrin, H. (2004). Unconscious perception: A model-based approach to method and evidence. *Perception & Psychophysics, 66*(5), 846-867.

Srull, K., & Wyer, J. (1979). The role of category accessibility in the interpretation of information about persons: Some determinants and implications. *Journal of Personality and Social Psychology, 37*(10), 1660-1672.

Stewart, B. D., & Payne, B. K. (2008). Bringing automatic stereotyping under control: Implementation intentions as efficient means of thought control. *Personality and Social Psychology Bulletin, 34*(10), 1332-1345. doi:10.1177/0146167208321269

Strahan, E. J., Spencer, S. J., & Zanna, M. P. (2002). Subliminal priming and persuasion: Striking while the iron is hot. *Journal of Experimental Social Psychology, 38*(6), 556-568.

Stroebe, W., & Strack, F. (2014). The alleged crisis and the illusion of exact replication. *Perspectives on Psychological Science, 9*(1), 59-71. doi:10.1177/1745691613514450

Titchener, E. B. (1902). *Experimental psychology: A manual of laboratory practice* (Vol. 1). New York: Macmillan.

Van den Bussche, E., Van den Noortgate, W., & Reynvoet, B. (2009). Mechanisms of masked priming: A meta-analysis. *Psychological Bulletin, 135*(3), 452-477. doi:10.1037/a0015329

Van Opstal, F., Gevers, W., Osman, M., & Verguts, T. (2010). Unconscious task application. *Consiousness and Cognition, 19*, 999-1006.

Veltkamp, M., Custers, R., & Aarts, H. (2011). Motivating consumer behavior by subliminal conditioning in the absence of basic needs: Striking even while the iron is cold. *Journal of Consumer Psychology, 21*(1), 49-56. doi:10.1016/j.jcps.2010.09.011

Vermeiren, A., & Cleeremans, A. (2012). The validity of d' measures. *PLOS ONE, 7*(2), e31595. doi:10.1371/journal.pone.0031595.g003

Vohs, K. D., Redden, J. P., & Rahinel, R. (2013). Physical order produces healthy choices, generosity, conventionality, whereas disorder produces creativity. *Perspectives on Psychological Science, 24*(9), 1860-1867. doi:10.1177/0956797613480186

Wegner, D. M. (2002). *The illusion of conscious will.* Cambridge, MA: MIT Press.

Wheeler, S. C., & DeMarree, K. G. (2009). Multiple mechanisms of prime-to-behavior effects. *Social and Personality Psychology Compass, 3*(4), 566-581. doi:10.1111/j.1751-9004.2009.00187.x

Williams, L. E., & Bargh, J. A. (2008). Experiencing physical warmth promotes interpersonal warmth. *Science, 322*(5901), 606-607. doi:10.1126/science.1162548

Wolfe, J. M. (1999). Inattentional amnesia. In V. Coltheart (Ed.), *Fleeting memories* (pp. 71-94). Cambridge, MA: MIT Press.

Zhong, C. B., & DeVoe, S. E. (2010). You are how you eat: Fast food and impatience. *Psychological Science, 21*(5), 619-622. doi:10.1177/0956797610366090

EFFECTS OF EVALUATION: AN EXAMPLE OF ROBUST "SOCIAL" PRIMING

Melissa J. Ferguson and Thomas C. Mann
Cornell University

> Evaluation serves a fundamental role in human life, allowing us to safely and successfully interact with our world—much of which is in some way social. We review the vast literature in social psychology on the unintentional impact of evaluation on our mental processing, and locate these effects within longstanding and emerging research traditions. We argue that poorly specified critiques of "social" priming threaten to unfairly ostracize robust findings, stunt exciting new investigations into when and how unintentional influences occur (which we review), and are inconsistent with work in cognitive psychology and modern theory on the nature of information processing in the brain. Finally, we argue that full-hearted endorsement of the evaluative priming that we discuss likely cannot peacefully coexist with strong skepticism of all forms of behavior priming, sketching an argument for why the robustness of the former likely compels the existence of some amount of the latter.

Priming research in social psychology has made its way into the limelight in the last decade, its discoveries featured in mainstream as well as nontraditional media outlets. Amazingly, friends and family outside of academia may have even heard of social psychological research. This is largely seen as a positive development (cf., Ledgerwood & Sherman, 2012). In the United States, people's federal tax dollars are being used to better understand human behavior, and the findings are being communicated to the public in increasingly effective ways.

At the same time, over the last couple of years, the headlining star of social psychological research is having a hard time of it. Various reporters and even psychologists have made statements lately about a string of non-replications and the resulting potential demise of priming, and even social psychology itself (e.g., see Bartlett, 2012; Bower, 2012; Kahneman, 2012; Shanks, 2013; Yong, 2012, 2013).

This research was supported by a National Science Foundation Graduate Research Fellowship awarded to T. C. Mann.

Address correspondence to Melissa J. Ferguson, Department of Psychology, Cornell University, 230 Uris Hall, Ithaca, NY 14853. E-mail: mjf44@cornell.edu.

Does this crisis portend the end of priming research? Has social psychology gone astray? Should we ever trust psychological research?

In the current chapter, we address this controversy by making three theoretical arguments. The first is that the conceptual boundary of the area of "priming" is fuzzy. The difference between robust, established, and fairly well understood (and seemingly accepted) priming in cognitive psychology (e.g., semantic, lexical, associative) versus the "social priming" that has been targeted lately is theoretically unspecified. Second, in an attempt to demonstrate how the robustness of a kind of social priming is very similar to that of the priming found in the cognitive psychology literature, we present and review the evidence for evaluative priming. We show that priming that emerges from the evaluation of relatively abstract social stimuli is reliable and has been replicated many thousands of times. Finally, our third argument is that a meaningful distinction between semantic (and other kinds of) priming in cognitive psychology and "behavioral priming" is similarly underspecified. We consider the theoretical support for the possibility of behavioral priming.

DEFINITIONS MATTER

In the recent publicity frenzy surrounding priming, people have referred to the area of problematic research as *priming* (Yong, 2012), *social priming* (Kahneman, 2012), *goal priming* (Pashler, Coburn, & Harris, 2012), or *behavioral priming* (Doyen, Klein, Pichon, & Cleeremans, 2012). Because this area of research is reportedly in demise and endangering the enterprise of social psychology, we should know what area of research we are talking about. It turns out, however, that even though some of these terms reference different bodies of empirical findings and theory, non-superficial distinctions between them are hard to identify. As such, it is difficult to determine whether critiques are targeting specific findings or underlying mechanisms that probably apply broadly in various priming domains and are quite well established.

The term *priming* originally referred to how the processing of a stimulus makes the person more "perceptually ready" (Bruner, 1957) to recognize or respond to that *same* stimulus some time after. For example, as you read the word **ridiculous** now, versus do not, you will be able to read the same word faster later in this paper. The consequence of a prolonged activation is that if the same stimulus is seen again, the mind is already geared up to recognize/process it, allowing us to learn connections among stimuli (e.g., Hebb, 1949; Lashley, 1951; see also Bargh, 2006). The evidence for this kind of *repetition* priming is solid (e.g., Tulving & Schacter, 1990). Exposure to a given stimulus *also* affects the processing of subsequent stimuli that are related but not identical. So, reading **ridiculous** will also allow you to later recognize **lunacy** faster, for example. Stimuli that are semantically, lexically, or perceptually similar to the initial prime will be more readily processed and responded to. Here too, the evidence across decades of research and areas of psychology is robust (e.g., for reviews, see Förster, Liberman, & Friedman, 2007; McNamara, 2005; Neely, 1991; Ratcliff & McKoon, 1997).

We do not think recent criticisms are leveled against any of these types of priming, but the use of the term *priming* obscures the true target of the criticism and unfairly characterizes robust findings. In particular for those outside of the field, the conflation threatens to fuel warrantless skepticism of work foundational to cognitive science.

Instead, the criticism is aimed at "social" or "behavioral" or "goal" priming. But what do these terms mean? Starting with the adjective of social, we argue that it is problematic to draw a definitive line between social versus non-social concepts. More precisely, it is difficult to know what concepts would qualify as clearly non-social. For example, all of language itself is embedded within a social context where social others are real, imagined, or hypothesized (e.g., Clark, 1996). We are not aware of any research that suggests a difference *in kind* between social and non-social priming (even though these topics fall into different areas within psychology), and thus we assume that the term *social priming* is probably some fusion of social psychology with the broad term of *priming*.

We suspect that what some people mean when they talk about social priming is *behavioral* or *goal* priming. Behavioral priming occurs when the incidental processing of a cue changes behavior (e.g., Bargh, Chen, & Burrows, 1996; Dijksterhuis & van Knippenberg, 1998), whereas goal priming occurs when exposure to some cue shifts one's goal-pursuit (which is usually measured via behavior; see Bargh, 1990). For the purposes of this paper, we assume that goal priming is just one type of behavior priming (though with meaningful differences; see Förster et al., 2007). But, what kind of dependent measures qualify as behavior, exactly? This is a famously difficult question, with debate about whether completing a self-report survey or pressing a key on a computer, for example, qualifies as behavior (e.g., Baumeister, Vohs, & Funder, 2007). The studies that have been mentioned in articles or blogs all involve behavior at a relatively macro level of description, where behavior is coded in terms of personality traits (e.g., as more or less aggressive, or social). So, perhaps behavior that is relatively abstract is at the center of the scrutiny, but the boundaries of what qualifies behavior as sufficiently abstract or macro to meet this definition are not defined by critics.

Another component of priming definitions that seems relevant to recent controversy is intentionality. In cognitive psychology, priming is sometimes assumed to emerge even when the person does not (and cannot) explicitly recall the prime (Tulving & Schacter, 1990). In somewhat of a contrast, in social psychology, priming usually refers to the *unintentional* influence of some prime on some target, even if the person can explicitly remember the prime itself (see Greenwald & Banaji, 1995). Note that an assumption of a lack of intention refers to a characteristic of the process of how the prime influences the target, and such an assumption is not strictly needed for the basic phenomenon of a prime affecting the processing of a target. And yet, almost all of the priming work in social psychology assumes, and tests, that the influence of the prime is unintentional (e.g., see Bargh & Ferguson, 2000). This may be due to the long history of interest in social psychology in whether people act in "knowing" versus unknowing ways (e.g., Bargh & Chartrand, 1999; Nisbett & Wilson, 1977; Wilson, 2002), and thus there has been great emphasis on whether people *realize* that a prime affected their judgment, attitude, or behavior. However, there is great variability in social psychological research in the way in which intentionality is conceptualized and measured (Ferguson & Cone, 2013; Uhlmann, Pizarro, & Bloom, 2008), and it remains unclear what aspects of intentionality are implicated in the priming research under scrutiny.

We think the ambiguity surrounding the definitional terms is a serious issue that almost completely prohibits any clear discussion of the problems, because it precludes inducing the commonalities among the examples. But, in the remainder of this chapter, we put these definitional issues aside. Given that there appears to be a solid foundation for semantic priming, we present and review a type of semantic priming that could easily be deemed "social," both in terms of being a topic studied almost exclusively by social psychologists and also involving stimuli that might often be deemed social-like (e.g., social groups). In this way, we present one example of a type of social priming that is robust and reliable.

EFFECTS OF EVALUATION

In the attitudes literature, *evaluative priming* usually refers to when the evaluation of some stimulus unintentionally influences subsequent processing, such as the evaluation of another stimulus (e.g., see Herring et al., 2013). Evaluative priming can be thought of as a type of semantic priming (Osgood, Suci, & Tannenbaum, 1957). The first critical issue to note is that researchers in this area take for granted that evaluative priming *occurs*, and thus many demonstrations of it take place in the course of examining other questions. For example, many researchers are interested in whether evaluation can proceed unintentionally, and to test this they employ evaluative priming paradigms. Thus, they assume that if a stimulus is evaluated, then the evaluative information will (unintentionally) influence the processing of a subsequently encountered stimulus.

For example, Fazio and colleagues were the first to demonstrate an evaluative priming effect in the attitudes literature (e.g., Fazio, Sanbonmatsu, Powell, & Kardes, 1986). They were trying to test whether attitudes (positivity versus negativity) toward stimuli are activated upon the mere presentation of those stimuli, without the perceiver's intent to evaluate those stimuli (see also Bargh, Chaiken, Govender, & Pratto, 1992). To test this, they developed an evaluative priming task (EPT) similar to semantic priming tasks (Meyer & Schvaneveldt, 1971) as well as response conflict tasks (Eriksen & Eriksen, 1974; Rosenbaum & Kornblum, 1982; Stroop, 1935). In brief, pairs of stimuli (primes and evaluative targets) are presented sequentially on a computer monitor (for more details, see Wentura & Degner, 2010). The prime is typically presented briefly (300 ms) and followed by the target, which must be categorized quickly as positive or negative. The usual and robust EPT finding is that people are faster to respond to targets when the targets and primes match versus mismatch in valence (see Herring et al., 2013, for a meta-analysis). This shows that upon exposure to some stimulus, whatever is activated then unintentionally interferes with the processing of subsequent target stimuli, along evaluative dimensions.

The Affective Misattribution Procedure (AMP; Payne, Cheng, Govorun, & Stewart, 2005) is another type of sequential priming paradigm. After the brief presentation of a prime stimulus, an ideograph appears that participants have to explicitly evaluate as more or less pleasant than average. When primes are stimuli that are normatively evaluated (explicitly) as positive (vs. negative), participants are likely to evaluate the (unfamiliar) ideographs as more (vs. less) pleasant. Just as with the EPT, the theoretical assumption is that the unintentional evaluation of the prime stimuli triggers information that then interferes with the explicit evaluation of the target stimuli. Although work is ongoing concerning the degree to which priming on the AMP reflects relatively "cold," semantic evaluative knowledge or relatively "hot" affective feelings (Blaison, Imhoff, Hühnel, Hess, & Banse, 2012; Gawronski & Ye, 2013), it seems reasonably clear (to us, at this point) that priming occurs regardless of intention to avoid this influence (Payne et al., 2005; Payne, Burkley, & Stokes, 2008; Payne et al., 2013; cf. Bar-Anan & Nosek, 2012).

Another option to study unintentional evaluation is the Implicit Association Test (IAT; Greenwald, McGhee, & Schwartz, 1998). Instead of being a sequential priming paradigm, participants have to categorize each of a series of stimuli into one of 4 potential categories. Two of the categories are "good" and "bad" and the other two categories represent the stimulus of interest (e.g., racial groups). The trick is that participants have to use only 2 response keys for these 4 categories, so the categories are combined in different ways. The main assessment is relative, in terms of whether it is easier for someone to combine (via using the same response key) good with White (and bad with Black) compared with the reverse, for example. Some have argued that the IAT can be interpreted as a measure of evaluative priming (see De Houwer, 2001, 2003; De Houwer, Teige-Mocigemba, Spruyt, & Moors, 2009) and we agree. Even though participants are not instructed to categorize Black or White faces (for instance) as good or bad, evaluative information about them is nevertheless activated in memory as soon as those stimuli are processed. This activates the response of pressing the key that has become associated with that evaluation through the IAT task. And, this response may be compatible or incompatible with the correct response (depending on the category assignments of the response keys). When the response triggered by an evaluation conflicts with the correct response, this presents a response conflict, which slows the person down. Under this conception, IAT effects illustrate that unintentional evaluations of stimuli occur and then prime congruent evaluative responses, and thus qualify as evidence for evaluative priming. Other mechanisms also likely contribute to IAT effects, such as task switching (e.g., Klauer & Mierke, 2005), salience asymmetries (e.g., Rothermund & Wentura, 2004), and potentially strategic recoding (e.g., Mierke & Klauer, 2003; Wentura & Rothermund, 2007; see De Houwer et al., 2009), and these may or may not be consistent with an evaluative priming interpretation.

UNINTENTIONAL PRIME EVALUATION VERSUS INFLUENCE

All three of the most commonly used implicit attitude measures, then, are designed with the assumption that if respondents evaluate the prime stimuli, then priming will emerge. This in and of itself speaks to the presumed strength of evaluative priming. Rather than this area of work primarily being about whether evaluative priming emerges once the prime has been evaluated, a considerable amount of it focuses on whether the *evaluation of the prime* is unintentional (for reviews, see Gawronski & Payne, 2010; Herring et al., 2013; Petty, Fazio, & Briñol, 2009). As such, this area of research demonstrates that evaluative priming can be a useful tool for gathering evidence of unintentional evaluations by looking for the *effects* of those evaluations on evaluating subsequent stimuli (EPT and AMP) or categorizing the same stimulus on a non-evaluative dimension (IAT).

And yet, note that whether or not the prime stimuli are evaluated intentionally is conceptually orthogonal to the question of whether priming, in our sense of *unintentional influence*, occurs. From our definition, evaluative priming occurs any time an evaluation has an unintended effect on subsequent processing, regardless of whether that initial evaluation was itself intentional or unintentional. If the intentional nature of the prime *evaluation* is orthogonal to the intentional nature of the prime *influence*, then why are we reviewing research on unintentional prime evaluation in order to demonstrate unintentional prime influence? Even though the two are conceptually orthogonal, they are practically related. Researchers interested in studying unintentional evaluations have to use methods in which participants do not realize they are evaluating stimuli. The best way to do that is to use a paradigm where the influence of that evaluation is also not intentional. This way, it is possible to gather evidence of evaluation indirectly. Thus, evaluative priming paradigms provide direct evidence of evaluative priming, and indirect evidence of prime evaluation. But how solid is the evidence that the priming in these paradigms is unintentional?

TASK PARAMETERS FOR UNINTENTIONAL INFLUENCE

Timing. The evaluative priming paradigm developed by Fazio and colleagues was designed specifically to minimize any intentional influence of the primes on the targets. The primes and targets are presented so close together in time (and space) that people are assumed to be unlikely to be able to strategically modify their responses to the target according to their responses to the prime (Neely, 1977). The stimulus onset asynchrony (SOA) used in most EPT work is assumed to effectively guard against an intentional influence, though recent work suggests that participants can control their responses when given clear instructions and response deadlines (e.g., Teige-Mocigemba & Klauer, 2013; see also Teige-Mocigemba & Klauer, 2008; cf. Degner, 2009).

Similarly, in the AMP, the prime and target stimuli are presented so close together that people are assumed to be unable to use their reaction to the prime to influence their reaction to the target. Recent work shows that when the SOA is increased to 1000 ms (Hofmann, van Koningsbruggen, Stroebe, Ramanathan, & Aarts, 2010), the nature of the evaluative priming changes. Specifically, with this kind of longer duration, the primes are still significantly influencing the targets (and thus this could be considered priming without the assumption of intentionality), but in a different way than when the SOA is 100 ms. It is not clear whether there is more intentionality in this kind of SOA condition.

The IAT does not test the average influence of a prime on an immediately subsequently presented target across trials (like in the EPT and AMP). Instead, it measures the average interference across trials in response mapping. But, timing here is still important. Participants are asked to categorize the target stimuli as quickly as possible, and are sometimes given strict response deadlines. Imposing fast responding undoubtedly increases the response conflict when the stimulus (e.g., a flower) is assigned to the same key as the incongruent evaluation (i.e., bad). Presumably, this also increases the tendency to evaluate such stimuli even when it is not germane to the categorization. The EPT and the AMP also require respondents to respond as quickly as possible, in order to decrease controlled processing of target stimuli.

Instructions. Implicit attitude measures are also typically described in such a way as to minimize any inferred relation between the primes and targets. In the EPT, instructions usually consist of asking participants to ignore the primes altogether or to just focus on responding to the targets, which minimizes the likelihood that they would try to use their response from the prime to react to the target. However, we do not know of any systematic attempt to analyze the differences among results, if any, according to the degree to which the primes are attended. Thus, this strategy seems designed to minimize influence, but we do not know whether it does.

A different strategy is used in the AMP. Here, participants are actually told that the primes might influence their responses to the ideographs and are told to try to prevent that from happening (see Payne et al., 2005). Thus, any priming effect that emerges is unintentional, as long as we believe that participants were paying attention and trying to follow instructions. Bar-Anan and Nosek (2012) recently questioned this assumption, claiming that effects on the AMP may be driven by a small subset of participants explicitly evaluating the primes (going against the instructions). Supporting this, they found that participants who were more likely to agree that they had done so showed the strongest effects on the AMP. Payne and colleagues (2013), however, found that this might instead reflect post-hoc rationalizations on the part of participants who had some sense of being influenced by the primes, and that on a trial-by-trial basis participants did not tend to think that their judgments of the ideographs were meaningfully affected by the primes (even though analysis of the data revealed reliable priming).

In the IAT, participants are simply told of the two different categorization tasks. Some work suggests that even minimal changes in instruction can produce differences in IAT scores by encouraging participants to plan strategies for altering their scores (especially if they have prior IAT experience; Fiedler & Bluemke, 2005). The possibility of respondents trying to intentionally control the interference from response mapping seems potentially bigger with the IAT (than with the EPT and AMP), such as through strategic recoding (e.g., Wentura & Rothermund, 2007; see also Payne, 2005). However, evidence suggests that IAT effects still emerge when features of the task discourage strategies like strategic recoding (e.g., De Houwer, 2001).

Despite the above data, we suggest that when considering their utility in exploring the possibility of unintended evaluation and unintended priming, the pertinent question is not *can these measures be controlled under any circumstances*, but rather *are they controlled under typical task circumstances*? Take, for instance, the AMP: Though it is possible for participants to explicitly evaluate the primes rather than the targets, a circumstance which removes the "implicitness" of the AMP, this is apparently not what participants generally do under normal task instructions (Payne et al., 2013). The same likely applies to the risk of faking on the EPT. Teige-Mocigemba and Klauer (2013) note that "the present findings will in all likelihood not pose a threat to the validity of evaluative-priming measures in most research situations in which participants are not motivated to fake, not given specific directions on how to do so, and/or in which the measurement purpose is often obscured on purpose" (p. 654).

SCOPE OF THE EVIDENCE

We have used findings in the attitudes literature as evidence for evaluative priming. In doing so, we have only looked at cases where the unintentional evaluation of a prime has unintentionally influenced target processing, setting aside cases where the intentional evaluation of a stimulus unintentionally influences target processing. Even with this limited slice of available evidence, the robustness of the evaluative priming effect is unmistakable. This effect, in its various measure-based variations (including the IAT), has been found many thousands of times over by participants in these studies. We conclude that evaluative priming in particular offers exceptionally strong evidence for the general phenomenon of priming, and in particular of "social" priming (see Herring et al., 2013). This robustness is not surprising, given the possible closeness in presumed process(es) between semantic priming and evaluative priming. That one type typically lives in the cognitive literature and the other in the social psychological literature would seem to be the only (superficial) difference.

HOW COULD THERE NOT BE BEHAVIORAL PRIMING?

In our final section, we make our third argument concerning the debate on social priming. Some have been skeptical not of the type of priming we describe above, but rather only of the type of priming that involves a certain type of behavior (again, the question of what qualifies as sufficiently behavioral is completely unspecified; we would maintain that key presses—such as those observed in evaluative priming research—are indeed behavior). Are there any reasons that the above type of priming (as well as semantic, associative, lexical, etc.) might be robust while behavioral priming is not? Are there important differences between these types of priming? We consider theory and findings that would argue strongly for the occurrence of behavior priming.

OVERLAP OF PERCEPTION, COGNITION, AND BEHAVIOR

Would it be possible for a stimulus to unintentionally prime semantic, evaluative, or other kinds of information related to that stimulus, but not behavioral representations? There are several lines of work that argue against this possibility. First, there is considerable overlap among the representations used to perceive an action, and those used to enact the action. Mirror neurons, for example, fire both when animals (including humans) see another individual performing an action and when they enact the same action (e.g., Rizzolatti & Craighero, 2004). This "common coding" (Hommel, Müsseler, Aschersleben, & Prinz, 2001) is highly suggestive that knowledge about an action could activate the representations involved in performing the action. If so, this suggests that processing words or images related to behavior could make the person more likely to enact that behavior (e.g., Dijksterhuis & Bargh, 2001).

Even more suggestive, the last two decades of work in cognitive science have shown that the field's traditional assumptions about how information flows through the brain from perception to cognition to behavior is outdated. Traditional perspectives suggest that motoric output is the end product of a serial, feed-forward process from perception, through cognition, and finally to action, but more recent work shows that motor movement is continuously updated by perceptual-cognitive processing over time (e.g., Gold & Shadlen, 2001; Song & Nakayama, 2008; Spivey, 2007). For example, when people have to reach for the object whose name is announced, they will reach toward the *candle* as soon as they hear the first phoneme of that word (*can-*) and then correct their reach once they have heard the full word (*candy*; see Spivey, 2007). This work suggests that the boundary between perception/cognition and action is relatively less strict than once assumed, and that action is an online product that is continuously updated, corrected, and changed depending on ongoing cognition (see also Freeman & Ambady, 2011, 2014). This perspective implies that once knowledge is made more accessible via analysis of a stimulus—if the person *can* behave in a way that is related to that stimulus (see Higgins, 1996)—it seems likely that the stimulus could unintentionally shape behavioral representations.

Evaluative priming research itself also directly reveals the tight link between cognition and action (e.g., Berntson, Boysen, & Cacioppo, 1993). The evaluation of a stimulus activates approach or avoidance response tendencies (e.g., Chen & Bargh, 1999; see Krieglmeyer, De Houwer, & Deutsch, 2013, for a review). For instance, Krieglmeyer, Deutsch, De Houwer, and De Raedt (2010) showed that even in the absence of an intention to approach, avoid, or even evaluate stimuli, positive stimuli facilitated approach and negative stimuli facilitated avoidance behaviors.

One might object that although it is possible to activate many different thoughts about something in parallel, behavior is necessarily more constrained. That is, in the end, one can only reach for one or the other target, not both. This suggests that there may be a restriction in range that emerges for behavior relative to perceptual-cognitive processing. Although this seems true at first glance, it may actually apply to fewer cases than assumed. Whereas many behaviors have to be precise (reaching for something), many others do not. In daily life, there would seem to exist many variants of a behavior that could complete any given task successfully (e.g., take notes on paper, type them, or jot comments in margins), many behaviors that would fit the overarching goal (e.g., succeed academically by taking notes, doing extra readings, or getting a good night's sleep), and many goals that could be pursued at a given time (e.g., academics, social life, or physical fitness). In these senses, behavior is relatively unconstrained. (This also reveals the importance of considering the level of analysis at which this question is posed.) In fact, the availability of a multitude of plausible behaviors at any time is precisely the kind of ambiguous situation that may be most conducive to priming effects, as they can "nudge" the decision one way or the other (e.g., see Higgins, 1996).

A second response is that this restriction in range may not matter. Whatever reduction in information (as the mind settles on an interpretation or decision; e.g., Spivey, 2007) occurs as behavior unfolds following perception of a stimulus, there is presumably still sufficient room for primes to influence such processing. In other words, if there is a bottleneck between perceptual-cognitive processing and behavior, whether it is early (e.g., Loersch & Payne, 2011, 2012, 2014) or late (e.g., Bargh, 2006) in processing, it does not imply on the face of it that primes would not be able to pass through this bottleneck, and thereby affect behavior. In fact, although Loersch and Payne (2011, 2014) argue that it may be rare for primes to have *direct* effects on behavior (though see Schröder & Thagard, 2013, 2014), their model by no means implies that priming effects on behavior will be trivial. They review evidence that when the effects of primes are misattributed to whatever is the focus of a participant's attention, be it an issue of perception, judgment, or behavior, the impact of the prime can be substantial. When any such impact on ongoing processing occurs, the amount of time and processing that intervenes between the presentation of the prime and the selection of behavior may not *dilute* the effect of the prime, but instead *magnify* it. This provides an explanation for subtle yet powerful effects, like the impact of a simple image on how we vote (Carter, Ferguson, & Hassin, 2011; Hassin, Ferguson, Shidlovski, & Gross, 2007), and bears similarities to recursive effects, like self-affirmation (Cohen, Garcia, Purdie-Vaughns, Apfel, & Brzustoski, 2009; Walton & Cohen, 2011). If subtle cues can affect perception and cognition, which in turn affect behavior, then it seems untenable to deny that primes can impact behavior, however directly or indirectly. Like spreading waves from a stone hitting the surface of a pond, the downstream consequences of a prime may far exceed the here and now.

CONCLUSIONS

We have argued that the current controversy surrounding social priming is suffering from a comprehensive lack of definitional precision. This limits the ability to accurately assess (and remedy) any issues or problems. We see no a priori difference in kind between the sort of priming reported in the cognitive psychology literature and evaluative priming reported in the social psychology literature. And, not surprisingly given the robustness of semantic priming, we review evaluative priming and conclude that it is an extremely reliable phenomenon. Finally, we argue that if one accepts the types of "non-behavioral" priming such as semantic and evaluative priming, it is very difficult to reject outright the possibility of other sorts of behavioral priming.

We offer a few final words on the "crisis" in social psychology. It may well turn out that many of the findings in the pages of psychology journals turn out to be non-replicable. The question is why, and we urge scholars to not assume the cart before the horse. First, some non-replications are to be expected (we as a field have to figure out how much is too much). If there is too much non-replication (though see Stanley & Spence, 2014), then we need to assess how much of it is due to poor methodological practices versus shoddy theory (or both). If the methods are sound (which seems unlikely given the plethora of between-participant designs in social psychological research; see also Simmons, Nelson, & Simonsohn, 2011), then the pertinent theories need to be revised. If the vast majority of the problem turns out to be methodological, however, then the theoretical assumptions related to the empirical results have yet to be tested properly. We are nowhere close to having to abandon the longstanding claim that we routinely, and unintentionally, "go beyond the information given" (Bruner, 1957).

REFERENCES

Bar-Anan, Y., & Nosek, B. A. (2012). Reporting intentional rating of the primes predicts priming effects in the affective misattribution procedure. *Personality and Social Psychology Bulletin, 38,* 1194-1208.

Bargh, J. A. (1990). Auto-motives: Preconscious determinants of social interaction. In E. T. Higgins & R. M. Sorrentino (Eds.), *Handbook of motivation and cognition* (Vol. 2, pp. 93-130). New York: Guilford.

Bargh, J. A. (2006). What have we been priming all these years? On the development, mechanisms, and ecology of nonconscious social behavior. *European Journal of Social Psychology, 36*(2), 147-168.

Bargh, J. A., Chaiken, S., Govender, R., & Pratto, F. (1992). The generality of the automatic attitude activation effect. *Journal of Personality & Social Psychology, 62*(6), 893-912.

Bargh, J. A., & Chartrand, T. L. (1999). The chameleon effect: The perception–behavior link and social interaction. *Journal of Personality and Social Psychology, 76*(6), 893-910.

Bargh, J. A., Chen, M., & Burrows, L. (1996). Automaticity of social behavior: Direct effects of trait construct and stereotype activation on action. *Journal of Personality and Social Psychology, 71*, 230-244.

Bargh, J. A., & Ferguson, M. J. (2000). Beyond behaviorism: On the automaticity of higher mental processes. *Psychological Bulletin, 126*(6), 925-945.

Bartlett, T. (2012, January 30). Power of suggestion: The amazing influence of unconscious cues is among the most fascinating discoveries of our time—that is, if it's true. *The Chronicle of Higher Education*. Retrieved from http://chronicle.com/article/Power-of-Suggestion/136907/.

Baumeister, R. F., Vohs, K. D., & Funder, D. C. (2007). Psychology as the science of self-reports and finger movements: Whatever happened to actual behavior? *Perspectives on Psychological Science, 2*, 396-403.

Berntson, G. G., Boysen, S. T., & Cacioppo, J. T. (1993). Neurobehavioral organization and the cardinal principle of evaluative bivalence. *Annals of the New York Academy of Sciences, 702*, 75-102.

Blaison, C., Imhoff, R., Hühnel, I., Hess, U., & Banse, R. (2012). The affect misattribution procedure: Hot or not? *Emotion, 12*(2), 403-412.

Bower, B. (2012, May 4). The hot and cold of priming: Psychologists are divided over whether unnoticed cues can influence behavior. *Science News*. Retrieved from https://www.sciencenews.org/article/hot-and-cold-priming.

Bruner, J. S. (1957). On perceptual readiness. *Psychological Review, 64*(2), 123-152.

Carter, T. J., Ferguson, M. J., & Hassin, R. R. (2011). A single exposure to the American flag shifts support toward republicanism up to 8 months later. *Psychological Science, 22*(8), 1011-1018.

Chen, M., & Bargh, J. A. (1999). Consequences of automatic evaluation: Immediate behavioral predispositions to approach or avoid the stimulus. *Personality and Social Psychology Bulletin, 25*, 215-224.

Clark, H. H. (1996). *Using language*. Cambridge: Cambridge University Press.

Cohen, G. L., Garcia, J., Purdie-Vaughns, V., Apfel, N., & Brzustoski, P. (2009). Recursive processes in self-affirmation: Intervening to close the minority achievement gap. *Science, 324*(5925), 400-403.

Degner, J. (2009). On the (un-)controllability of affective priming: Strategic manipulation is feasible but can possibly be prevented. *Cognition and Emotion, 23*, 327-354.

De Houwer, J. (2001). A structural and process analysis of the Implicit Association Test. *Journal of Experimental Social Psychology, 37*, 443-451.

De Houwer, J. (2003). A structural analysis of indirect measures of attitudes. In J. Musch & K. C. Klauer (Eds.), *The psychology of evaluation: Affective processes in cognition and emotion* (pp. 219-244). Mahwah, NJ: Erlbaum.

De Houwer, J., Teige-Mocigemba, S., Spruyt, A., & Moors, A. (2009). Implicit measures: A normative analysis and review. *Psychological Bulletin, 135*(3), 347-368.

Dijksterhuis, A., & Bargh, J. A. (2001). The perception-behavior expressway: The automatic effects of social perception on social behavior. In M. P. Zanna (Ed.), *Advances in experimental social psychology* (Vol. 33, pp. 1-40). San Diego, CA: Academic Press.

Dijksterhuis, A., & Knippenberg, A. V. (1998). The relation between perception and behavior, or how to win a game of trivial pursuit. *Journal of Personality and Social Psychology, 74*(4), 865-877.

Doyen, S., Klein, O., Pichon, C.-L., & Cleeremans, A. (2012). Behavioral priming: It's all in the mind, but whose mind? *PLOS ONE, 7*(1), e29081.

Eriksen, B. A., & Eriksen, C. W. (1974). Effects of noise letters upon the identification of a target letter in a nonsearch task. *Perception & Psychophysics, 16*(1), 143-149.

Fazio, R. H., Sanbonmatsu, D. M., Powell, M. C., & Kardes, F. R. (1986). On the automatic activation of attitudes. *Journal of Personality and Social Psychology, 50*, 229-238.

Ferguson, M. J., & Cone, J. (2013). The mind in motivation: A social cognitive perspective on the role of consciousness in goal pursuit. In D. Carlston (Ed.), *Handbook of social cognition* (pp. 476-496). New York: Oxford University Press.

Fiedler, K., & Bluemke, M. (2005). Faking the IAT: Aided and unaided response control on the implicit association tests. *Basic and Applied Social Psychology, 27*(4), 307-316.

Förster, J., Liberman, N., & Friedman, R. S. (2007). Seven principles of goal activation: A systematic approach to distinguishing goal priming from priming of non-goal constructs. *Personality and Social Psychology Review, 11*(3), 211-233.

Freeman, J. B., & Ambady, N. (2011). A dynamic interactive theory of person construal. *Psychological Review, 118*, 247-279.

Freeman, J. B., & Ambady, N. (2014). The dynamic interactive model of person construal: Coordinating sensory and social processes. In J. Sherman, B. Gawronski, & Y. Trope (Eds.), *Dual process theories of the social mind* (pp. 235-248). New York: Guilford.

Gawronski, B., & Payne, B. K. (Eds.). (2010). *Handbook of implicit social cognition: Measurement, theory, and applications.* New York: Guilford.

Gawronski, B., & Ye, Y. (2013). What drives priming effects in the Affect Misattribution Procedure. *Personality Social Psychology Bulletin, 40*(1), 3-15.

Gold, J. I., & Shadlen, M. N. (2001). Neural computations that underlie decisions about sensory stimuli. *Trends in Cognitive Sciences, 5*(1), 10-16.

Greenwald, A. G., & Banaji, M. R. (1995). Implicit social cognition: Attitudes, self-esteem, and stereotypes. *Psychological Review, 102*, 4-27.

Greenwald, A. G., McGhee, D. E., & Schwartz, J. K. L. (1998). Measuring individual differences in implicit cognition: The Implicit Association Test. *Journal of Personality and Social Psychology, 74*, 1464-1480.

Hassin, R. R., Ferguson, M. J., Shidlovski, D., & Gross, T. (2007). Subliminal exposure to national flags affects political thought and behavior. *Proceedings of the National Academy of Sciences, 104*(50), 19757-19761.

Hebb, D. O. (1949). *The organization of behavior: A neuropsychological theory.* New York: Wiley.

Herring, D. R., White, K. R., Jabeen, L. N., Hinojos, M., Terrazas, G., Reyes, S. M., et al. (2013). On the automatic activation of attitudes: A quarter century of evaluative priming research. *Psychological Bulletin, 139*(5), 1062-1089.

Higgins, E. T. (1996). Knowledge activation: Accessibility, applicability, and salience. In E. T. Higgins & A. W. Kruglanski (Eds.), *Social psychology: Handbook of basic principles* (pp. 133-168). New York: Guilford.

Hofmann, W., van Koningsbruggen, G. M., Stroebe, W., Ramanathan, S., & Aarts, H. (2010). As pleasure unfolds: Hedonic responses to tempting food. *Psychological Science, 21*(12), 1863-1870.

Hommel, B., Müsseler, J., Aschersleben, G., & Prinz, W. (2001). The theory of event coding (TEC): A framework for perception and action planning. *Behavioral and Brain Sciences, 24*(5), 849-937.

Kahneman, D. (2012, September 26). A proposal to deal with questions about priming effects. Open letter. Retrieved from http://www.nature.com/polopoly_fs/7.6716.1349271308!/suppinfoFile/Kahneman%20Letter.pdf.

Klauer, K. C., & Mierke, J. (2005). Task-set inertia, attitude accessibility, and compatibility-order effects: New evidence for a task-set switching account of the Implicit Association Test effect. *Personality and Social Psychology Bulletin, 31*, 208-217.

Krieglmeyer, R., De Houwer, J., & Deutsch, R. (2013). On the nature of automatically triggered approach-avoidance behavior. *Emotion Review, 5*(3), 280-284.

Krieglmeyer, R., Deutsch, R., De Houwer, J., & De Raedt, R. (2010). Being moved: Valence activates approach-avoidance behavior independently of evaluation and approach-avoidance intentions. *Psychological Science, 21*, 607-613.

Lashley, K. S. (1951). The problem of serial order in behavior. In L. A. Jeffress (Ed.), *Cerebral mechanisms in behavior: The Hi-*

xon symposium (pp. 112-136). New York: Wiley.

Ledgerwood, A., & Sherman, J. W. (2012). Short, sweet, and problematic? The rise of the short report in psychological science. *Perspectives on Psychological Science, 7*, 60-66.

Loersch, C., & Payne, B. K. (2011). The situated inference model: An integrative account of the effects of primes on perception, behavior, and motivation. *Perspectives on Psychological Science, 6*(3), 234-252.

Loersch, C., & Payne, B. K. (2012). On mental contamination: The role of (mis)attribution in behavior priming. *Social Cognition, 30*, 241-252.

Loersch, C., & Payne, B. K. (2014). Situated inferences and the what, who, and where of priming. This volume.

McNamara, T. P. (2005) *Semantic priming: Perspectives from memory and word recognition.* New York: Psychology Press.

Meyer, D. E., & Schvaneveldt, R. W. (1971). Facilitation in recognizing pairs of words: Evidence of a dependence between retrieval operations. *Journal of Experimental Psychology, 90*, 227-234.

Mierke, J., & Klauer, K. C. (2003). Method – specific variance in the implicit association test. *Journal of Personality and Social Psychology, 85*(6), 1180-1192.

Neely, J. H. (1977). Semantic priming and retrieval from lexical memory: Roles of inhibitionless spreading activation and limited-capacity attention. *Journal of Experimental Psychology: General, 106*, 225-254.

Neely, J. H. (1991). Semantic priming effects in visual word recognition: A selective review of current findings and theories. In D. Besener & G. W. Humphreys (Eds.), *Basic processes in reading: Visual word recognition* (pp. 264-336). Hillsdale, NJ: Erlbaum.

Nisbett, R. E., & Wilson, T. D. (1977). Telling more than we can know: Verbal reports on mental processes. *Psychological Review, 84*, 231-259.

Osgood, C. E., Suci, G. J., & Tannenbaum, P. H. (1957). *The measurement of meaning.* Urbana: University of Illinois Press.

Pashler, H., Coburn, N., and Harris, C. (2012). Priming of social distance? Failure to replicate effects on social and food judgements. *PLOS ONE, 7*(8), e42510.

Payne, B. K. (2005). Conceptualizing control in social cognition: How executive control modulates the expression of automatic stereotyping. *Journal of Personality and Social Psychology, 89*, 488-503.

Payne, B. K., Brown-Iannuzzi, J., Burkley, M., Arbuckle, N. L., Cooley, E., Cameron, C. D., & Lundberg, K. B. (2013). Intention invention and the affect misattribution procedure: Reply to Bar-Anan and Nosek (2012). *Personality and Social Psychology Bulletin, 39*(3), 375-386.

Payne, B. K., Burkley, M. A., & Stokes, M. B. (2008). Why do implicit and explicit attitude tests diverge? The role of structural fit. *Journal of Personality and Social Psychology, 94*(1), 16-31.

Payne, B. K., Cheng, S. M., Govorun, O., & Stewart, B. D. (2005). An inkblot for attitudes: Affect misattribution as implicit measurement. *Journal of Personality and Social Psychology, 89*, 277-293.

Petty, R. E., Fazio, R. H., & Briñol, P. (Eds.). (2009). *Attitudes: Insights from the new implicit measures.* New York: Psychology Press.

Ratcliff, R., & McKoon, G. (1997). A counter model for implicit priming in perceptual word identification. *Psychological Review, 104*, 319-343.

Rizzolatti, G., & Craighero, L. (2004). The mirror-neuron system. *Annual Review of Neuroscience, 27*(1), 169-192.

Rosenbaum, D. A., & Kornblum, S. (1982). A priming method for investigating the selection of motor responses. *Acta Psychologica, 51*, 223-243.

Rothermund, K., & Wentura, D. (2004). Underlying processes in the Implicit Association Test (IAT): Dissociating salience from associations. *Journal of Experimental Psychology: General, 133*, 139-165.

Schröder, T., & Thagard, P. (2013). The affective meanings of automatic social behaviors: Three mechanisms that explain priming. *Psychological Review, 120*(1), 255-280.

Schröder, T., & Thagard, P. (2014). Priming: Constraint satisfaction, competition, and creativity. This volume.

Shanks, D. R., Newell, B. R., Lee, E. H., Balakrishnan, D., Ekelund, L., et al. (2013). Priming intelligent behavior: An elusive phenomenon. *PLOS ONE, 8*(4), e56515.

Simmons, J. P., Nelson, L. D., & Simonsohn, U. (2011). False-Positive psychology: Undisclosed flexibility in data collection and analysis allow presenting anything as significant. *Psychological Science, 22*(11), 1359-1366.

Song, J. H., & Nakayama, K. (2008). Target selection in visual search as revealed by movement trajectories. *Vision Research, 48*, 853-861.

Spivey, M. J. (2007). *The continuity of mind*. New York: Oxford University Press.

Stanley, D. J., & Spence, J. R. (2014). Expectations for replications: Are yours realistic? Perspectives on *Psychological Science, 9*, 305-318.

Stroop, J. R. (1935). Studies of interference in serial verbal reactions. *Journal of Experimental Psychology, 18*, 643-662.

Teige-Mocigemba, S., & Klauer, K. C. (2008). Automatic' evaluation? Strategic effects on affective priming. *Journal of Experimental Social Psychology, 44*, 1414-1417.

Teige-Mocigemba, S., & Klauer, K. C. (2013). On the controllability of evaluative-priming effects: Some limits that are none. *Cognition & Emotion, 27*(4), 632-657.

Tulving, E., & Schacter, D. L. (1990). Priming and human memory systems. *Science, 247*, 301-306.

Uhlmann, E.L., Pizarro, D.A., & Bloom, P. (2008). Varieties of unconscious social cognition. *Journal for the Theory of Social Behaviour, 38*, 293-322.

Walton, G. M., & Cohen, G. L. (2011). A brief social-belonging intervention improves academic and health outcomes of minority students. *Science, 331*(6023), 1447-1451.

Wentura, D., & Degner, J. (2010). A practical guide to sequential priming and related tasks. In B. Gawronski & B. K. Payne (Eds.), *Handbook of implicit social cognition: Measurement, theory, and applications* (pp. 95-115). New York: Guilford.

Wentura, D., & Rothermund, K. (2007). Paradigms we live by: A plea for more basic research on the IAT. In B. Wittenbrink & N. Schwarz (Eds.), *Implicit measures of attitudes* (pp. 195-215). New York: Guilford.

Wilson, T. D. (2002). *Strangers to ourselves: Discovering the adaptive unconscious*. Cambridge: Belknap Press.

Yong, E. (2012). Replication studies: Bad copy. *Nature, 485*, 298-300.

Yong, E. (2013, November 26). Psychologists strike a blow for reproducibility: Thirty-six labs collaborate to check 13 earlier findings. *Nature*. Retrieved from http://www.nature.com/news/psychologists-strike-a-blow-for-reproducibility-1.14232.

PRIMING IS NOT PRIMING IS NOT PRIMING

Dirk Wentura
Saarland University, Saarbrücken, Germany

Klaus Rothermund
University of Jena, Germany

> We propose a taxonomy according to which priming studies in social cognition research can be classified. Long-term priming is characterized by a long delay between the prime and test situations (several minutes or more) whereas short-term priming studies investigate short-term consequences (occurring within hundreds of milliseconds) of primes on subsequent target processing and response activation. Within short-term priming, we distinguish between response priming and semantic priming designs, and discuss the underlying mechanisms that mediate priming effects in the different designs. On the basis of these distinctions, we discuss the role of short-term priming research for an understanding of long-term priming effects in social cognition.

Broadly speaking, priming research in the social cognition literature can be split into two-and-a-half branches by reference to prototypical designs. The most obvious differentiation (into the two dominant branches) can be made between what we will tentatively term *long-term* versus *short-term priming* designs. In *long-term priming* studies, the goal is almost always to activate some broad knowledge structure (a trait category, a stereotype, a goal, a mindset, an emotion). The aftermath of this activation is then tested in an appropriate context. Studies that aim at exploring what Molden (2014, this volume) generally described as *social priming* fall into the category of long-term priming, that is, studies that are concerned with effects related to standard categories of everyday behavior that are of evident practical or applied interest. What is most important for the remainder of the text is that long-term priming effects are on a time scale ranging from minutes to hours or even days and weeks.

Address correspondence to either Dirk Wentura, Department of Psychology, Saarland University, Campus A2 4, D-66123 Saarbrücken, Germany; E-mail: wentura@mx.uni-saarland.de, or to Klaus Rothermund, Department of Psychology, FSU Jena, Am Steiger 3, Haus 1, D-07743 Jena, Germany; E-mail: klaus.rothermund@uni-jena.de.

On the other hand, studies investigating rapid, short-lived, trial-by-trial priming effects in a time range from fractions of a second to maximally a few seconds are denoted as *short-term priming* studies. These studies are mostly conducted in order to investigate the cognitive architecture and mental representation of concepts and their interrelations, and of the basic processes that are operating on this structure, and thus are mostly of theoretical importance. As we will see, within short-term priming a further differentiation is of utmost important, that is, the distinction between *response priming designs* and *semantic priming designs* (hence the phrase "two-and-*a-half* branches").

Despite the apparent differences, the two types of priming are oftentimes treated as a single phenomenon. This chapter emphasizes the differences between long-term and short-term priming (but also between response priming and semantic priming), and aims at sensitizing social cognition researchers to take into account these important distinctions when discussing the implications of priming studies for an understanding of phenomena like stereotypes, attitudes, and social categorization (see also Bargh, 2014, this volume; Cesario & Jonas, 2014, this volume). Pointing out these differences is a prerequisite for analyzing the interrelations between the two broader types of priming (i.e., long-term and short-term), and also provides a basis for discussing long-term priming in terms of typical explanations for short-term priming effects, which are the topics that we address in a final section of our chapter.

TWO TYPES OF PRIMING

LONG-TERM PRIMING

Long-term priming studies usually employ between-participants designs. Participants are exposed to either an experimental priming condition or a control priming condition. In the experimental condition, stimuli have to be processed that belong to a certain knowledge structure. To prevent demand characteristics, processing is arranged in a way that prevents participants from noticing a relationship with part two of the experiment which includes the measurement of some behavioral outcome. A priming effect in long-term priming studies is defined as a mean difference in the outcome measure between the experimental and the control condition. Abstractly speaking, this difference has to be explained in terms of increased accessibility of the primed knowledge structure which is definitely not restricted to fractions of a second.

One of the first and most widely cited studies in social cognition exemplifying long-term priming was reported by Higgins, Rholes, and Jones (1977): In a first priming part (that was introduced as a study on perception), different groups of participants were told to maintain specific sets of trait concepts in memory while having to identify the background color of colored slides. In a purportedly unrelated second experiment, participants then read ambiguous behavioral descriptions of a person ("Donald") whom they had to characterize. The interpretation of Donald's behavior was influenced by the trait words that were memorized during the first, priming part of the study.

Since this seminal study, long-term priming has gone a long a way, and has become an immensely broad and diverse research field within the social cognition literature (see, e.g., Loersch & Payne, 2011; 2014, this volume; for an overview; see Molden, 2014, this volume). Long-term priming studies have provided an immensely rich set of provoking findings that have permeated most areas of social psychological research, and they constitute an indispensable research tool for a broad range of important research questions. Still, it is an open and interesting question what mediates these effects. There are several suggestions that focus on the question of how activated knowledge structures moderate judgments and behavior (e.g., Cesario & Jonas, 2014, this volume; Dijksterhuis & Bargh, 2001; Eitam & Higgins, 2010; Higgins & Eitam, 2014, this volume; Klatzky & Creswell, 2014; Loersch & Payne, 2011; 2014, this volume; Schröder & Thagard, 2014, this issAvue; Wheeler & DeMarree, 2009; Wheeler, DeMarree, & Petty, 2014, this volume). With regard to the first step, that is, the activation of knowledge, studies often refer to basic principles of cognitive psychology and studies on short-term priming. We have to see, however, whether explanations of short-term priming effects encompass the possibility that priming lasts for more than a second.

SHORT-TERM PRIMING

Short-term priming studies exclusively employ within-participants designs with a large number (usually three-figure) of trials, with the different conditions randomly distributed across the sequence of trials. Each trial consists of a prime and a target stimulus, usually (but not necessarily) presented in sequence; stimulus onset asynchronies (SOA) range from zero (in case of parallel presentation) to a second or so with a dominance of short SOAs (below 300 ms). The essential variation concerns the relationship between prime and target, that is, they either share features (e.g., valence, category-membership, co-occurrence, that is, they are associated) or not. For example, in evaluative priming (Fazio, Sanbonmatsu, Powell, & Kardes, 1986), primes and targets either share the evaluative category (i.e., they are both positive or negative) or not. The target has to be processed according to a task (e.g., lexical decision, evaluation, naming); response times (of correctly answered trials) or accuracies are the dependent variable. A priming effect in short-term studies is defined as a mean difference in these measures between the related and the unrelated condition.

Short-term priming studies also have been conducted for a broad range of research questions. Most prominent in social cognition research are studies that investigated the automatic activation of attitudes, in which stimuli representing attitude objects (e.g., social groups, political parties, individual persons) are presented as primes together with positive and negative targets (e.g., Dovidio, Evans, & Tyler, 1986; Fazio, Jackson, Dunton, & Williams, 1995; Gaertner & McLaughlin, 1983; see also Wittenbrink, 2007), and studies on stereotype activation using social categories and stereotypic attributes as primes and targets (e.g., Blair & Banaji, 1996). In some studies, self-related primes were presented to investigate either automatic self-evaluations or self-stereotyping (e.g., Casper & Rothermund, 2012; Latrofa, Vaes, Cadinu, & Carnaghi, 2010; Wentura, Kulfanek, & Greve, 2005).

In sum, short-term priming studies show some obvious similarities with long-term priming studies regarding the content of the materials that were used as primes, but also between the target materials of short-term priming studies and the effect indicators that were used in long-term priming studies (e.g., facilitated processing of words belonging to the elderly stereotype as a consequence of prime sentences with an old protagonist [Wentura & Brandtstädter, 2003] and slow walking as a consequence of processing age stereotypical material [Bargh, Chen, & Burrows, 1996]). Despite these apparent similarities, however, it is far from clear whether and how long-term and short-term priming effects are related. In the following, we first discuss issues regarding paradigms of short-term priming and underlying effects in these paradigms, before we turn back to an investigation of potential relations between the two basic forms of priming in a final section.

TWO CORE PARADIGMS OF SHORT-TERM PRIMING

A differentiation within short-term priming is of utmost importance for an adequate understanding of what a priming effect in a short-term priming study indicates, that is, the difference between response priming and semantic priming (see Wentura & Degner, 2010). With regard to social cognition research, both variants are well-known. Affective/evaluative priming in the tradition of Fazio and colleagues (1986) which is well-known as an "implicit attitude" measure is a version of response priming; experiments aiming at exploring the automaticity of stereotype activation by using, for example, the lexical decision task are versions of semantic priming. Wentura and Degner (2010) used the labels "response priming" and "semantic priming" with reference to different research traditions in cognitive psychology (see, e.g., Schmidt, Haberkamp, & Schmidt, 2011; Vorberg, Mattler, Heinecke, Schmidt, & Schwarzbach, 2003, for response priming; McNamara, 2005; McNamara, 2013, for semantic priming).[1]

RESPONSE PRIMING PARADIGMS

The basic characteristic of response priming designs can be best explained by reference to the most prominent exemplar of this category, the evaluative priming paradigm as introduced by Fazio and colleagues (Fazio et al., 1986). The usual description is that prime and target are varied orthogonally with regard to their valence. However, since the task is to categorize the target's valence, one can alternatively describe the basic manipulation as to whether the prime's category matches or mismatches the response that has to be given to the target. Thus, in the terminology of De Houwer (2003), the paradigm is characterized by a confound: Prime and target are compatible or incompatible with regard to stimulus features (i.e., both share or do not share valence; S-S compatibility) and they are compatible or incompatible with regard to response categories (i.e., although the prime is declared as task-irrelevant, it would elicit either the same or a different response as the target if it had to be categorized as well; S-R compatibility). It should be evident that—given this confound—process theories can either focus on S-S compatibility or S-R compatibility as the decisive feature (see also Spruyt, Gast, & Moors, 2011); we will soon return to this issue.

---

1. Note that detached from these traditions, the labels might sometimes cause a bit of confusion. We will clarify this by footnotes at appropriate places.

However, whatever theory will be used for the explanation of effects in response priming designs, it must include the processing of the task-relevant feature of the task-irrelevant prime (i.e., the valence of the prime in evaluative priming).[2] This characteristic is highly valued in social cognition research because this paradigm can thus be used to unobtrusively assess the valence of attitude objects (Fazio et al., 1995). One should keep in mind two points, however: First, the involuntary activation of the prime's valence might depend on the current goal context of evaluating stimuli that are presented on the display (Spruyt, De Houwer, Hermans, & Eelen, 2007). Second, the effect is not immune against strategic influences (see, e.g., Degner, 2009; Teige-Mocigemba & Klauer, 2008). In this regard, it is interesting to note that in basic cognitive psychology, response priming paradigms employing masked primes are especially well-known in the field of unconscious cognition (e.g., Dehaene et al., 1998; Vorberg et al., 2003). Obviously, masked effects are of utmost importance for social cognition researchers because the aim of the researcher is completely hidden if the attitude-related stimulus is never consciously seen by participants (Custers & Aarts, 2007; de Paula Couto & Wentura, 2012; Degner & Wentura, 2010; Frings & Wentura, 2003; Otten & Wentura, 1999; Spalding & Hardin, 1999; Wentura et al., 2005; see also Doyen, Klein, Simons, & Cleeremans, 2014, this volume, for an extensive discussion on subliminal priming).

Beside the evaluative priming paradigm, other response priming designs were used in social cognition research. For example, the weapon identification task (Correll, Park, Judd, & Wittenbrink, 2002; Payne, 2001) and the affect misattribution procedure (AMP; Payne, Cheng, Govorun, & Stewart, 2005) both have the structure of a response priming paradigm (see Wentura & Degner, 2010, for a brief discussion). Blair and Banaji (1996) used a gender categorization task (i.e., whether target names were male or female) in research on gender stereotyping.

SEMANTIC PRIMING

Semantic priming can be best explained by a demarcation to response priming: The confound that characterizes response priming is removed. Whereas the S-S compatibility is still varied, the S-R compatibility is avoided. This is done by using tasks that are completely independent of the essential stimulus variations, for example, the lexical decision task or the naming task. Take, for example, the classical "bread-primes-butter" example (see Neely, 1991, for an early review). Targets are either words (e.g., butter) or non-words (e.g., wutter). Participants have to categorize accordingly. Targets are always preceded by a prime word which is (in case of word targets) either semantically related or unrelated to the target.[3] There are

---

2. A problem of terminology (I): Response priming experiments in basic cognitive psychology often use very simple stimuli with the task-relevant feature being a perceptual one (e.g., arrows pointing to the right or left; e.g., Vorberg et al., 2003). In demarcation to this research, some authors *within* the field of response priming use the term "semantic priming" if a semantic feature is task-relevant (e.g., whether a number is smaller or larger than five; e.g., Dehaene et al., 1998).

3. A problem of terminology (II): Within the category "semantic priming" in a broader sense (as used here and, for example, in reviews of McNamara, 2005; Neely, 1991), associative priming and semantic priming (in a narrower sense) are distinguished. The former refers to the use of associatively related prime-target pairs, the latter refers to different types of pure semantic relationships (e.g., category coordinates; sub-ordinates; synonyms; Lucas, 2000; Hutchison, 2003).

two important uses of semantic priming in social cognition research. First, testing the assumption that processing social category information leads to an automatic activation of stereotypic attributes of the respective category requires a semantic priming design (that is, interpretations focus on S-S-compatibility; see above). Interestingly, some of the studies that are most frequently cited as support for automatic stereotype activation employed response priming designs (e.g., Blair & Banaji, 1996; Kawakami & Dovidio, 2001) and are therefore open for interpretation in terms of S-R-compatibility. Only a few short-term stereotype priming studies employed a semantic priming design, and these studies provided mixed results (stereotype priming effects were weak, Banaji & Hardin, 1996, or restricted to affectively congruent prime/target pairs, Chasteen, Schwarz, & Park, 2002; Wittenbrink, Judd, & Park, 1997; Wittenbrink, Judd, & Park, 2001). In a recent large-scale replication study, Müller and Rothermund (2014) failed to obtain any evidence for stereotype priming effects with a semantic priming design. Relatedly, recent stereotype priming studies employing semantic priming designs revealed that an activation of specific stereotypic attributes requires a combination of category and context primes—without such a matching context, category primes did not facilitate processing of stereotypic target words (Casper, Rothermund, & Wentura, 2010, 2011; see also, Casper & Rothermund, 2012).

Second, semantic priming paradigms have also been used to investigate whether S-S–based evaluative priming exists. That is, these studies specifically address the question whether a positive or negative prime facilitates processing of any affectively congruent targets (i.e., whether, for example, *murder* facilitates *cockroach*). Thus, while using the same variation of evaluatively congruent versus incongruent prime-target pairs as in response priming designs (i.e., by using the evaluation task), participants now had to classify targets with regard to their lexical or semantic category (word vs. non-word; person vs. object) or had to quickly pronounce the target. Numerous semantic priming studies have been conducted to answer this theoretically important question, but findings are quite mixed: Some studies found no or even a reversed evaluative congruency effect with semantic priming designs (De Houwer, Hermans, Rothermund, & Wentura, 2002; Glaser & Banaji, 1999; Klauer & Musch, 2001, 2002; Klinger, Burton, & Pitts, 2000; Rothermund & Wentura, 1998; Werner & Rothermund, 2013), whereas other studies reported significant evaluative priming effects with such designs under specific conditions (De Houwer & Randell, 2002, 2004; Hermans, De Houwer, & Eelen, 1994; Schmitz & Wentura, 2012; Spruyt, De Houwer et al., 2007; Spruyt, Hermans, De Houwer, & Eelen, 2002; Wentura & Frings, 2008). A cautious conclusion is that these effects can be observed and that they pose a challenge to current theories of semantic memory (see Schmitz & Wentura, 2012, for a discussion).

UNDERLYING MECHANISMS OF SHORT-TERM PRIMING

As is evident from the previous descriptions, response priming and semantic priming designs give rise to qualitatively different types of priming effects. These differences are closely related to differences in the underlying processes or mechanisms that can explain these effects. In the following discussion of these processes, we will emphasize how much temporal contiguity of prime and target is assumed in the different theories. This will finally help to discuss the similarities and dissimilarities of long-term and short-term priming. Note, due to length restrictions we constrain our discussion to theories that focus on simple mechanisms that plausibly have an automatic, non-strategic character (see, e.g., Wentura & Degner, 2010, for a discussion of strategy-based theories).

RESPONSE COMPETITION AS THE PROMINENT THEORY FOR RESPONSE PRIMING

As noted above, process theories to explain effects in response priming designs can in principle focus either on stimulus-stimulus (S-S) compatibility or on stimulus-response (S-R) compatibility as the decisive feature. However, there is undoubtedly an asymmetry: It is rather undisputed that S-R-compatibilities contribute to these priming effects whereas it is still a matter of debate whether part of the effects in response priming designs might be due to S-S compatibilities. It is therefore legitimate to discuss response competition as the prominent theory for the response priming paradigm (for attempts to disentangle the contributions of S-S compatibility and S-R compatibility within response priming designs, see Bartholow, Riordan, Saults, & Lust, 2009; Eder, Leuthold, Rothermund, & Schweinberger, 2012; Schmitz, Wentura, & Brinkmann, 2014; Voss, Rothermund, Gast, & Wentura, 2013; Zhang, Lawson, Guo, & Jiang, 2006).

Response competition is a mechanism that produces fast responses and high accuracy in responding to the target stimulus if the prime has already activated the same response that is also required for the target stimulus (response facilitation), and that produces slow responses and low accuracy in responding to the target stimulus if the prime has already activated a different response from the one that is required for the target stimulus (response interference). Needless to say that response competition can explain priming effects in response priming designs since (a) both primes and targets can be mapped onto the response set of the task and (b) prime-target pairs of the different conditions of the experimental design differ with regard to their response relation. For example, in an evaluative priming study with the evaluation task, both primes and targets can be mapped onto the (positive and negative) response alternatives of the task, and evaluatively congruent prime-target pairs are characterized by a compatible relation between their responses, whereas prime and target are associated with opposite responses for affectively incongruent pairs. By definition, response competition cannot explain priming effects in a semantic priming design because in such a design, prime-target pairs do not differ systematically with regard to their response relation.

Note that within the response competition account several sub-types can be differentiated that are of special importance in the discussion of masked effects (see, e.g., Klauer, Eder, Greenwald, & Abrams, 2007, for a discussion). On a related note, we want to mention a recent variant of response competition theory by Klauer, Teige-Mocigeba, and Spruyt (2009) that can specify experimental settings that are associated with *prima facie* surprising contrast effects.

With regard to our discussion of the longevity of priming, obviously response competition is based on a very close temporal contiguity of prime and target. Therefore, an application of the response competition explanation to long-term priming is not conceivable.

SHORT-TERM INCREASED ACCESSIBILITY AS THE PROMINENT PRINCIPLE FOR SEMANTIC PRIMING

Two classes of theories focus on short-term changes in memory caused by the prime to explain effects in semantic priming experiments (and, of course, those parts of effects in response priming experiments that are potentially caused by S-S compatibilities; see above). With regard to our discussion of whether close contiguity of prime and target are a precondition for priming effects, these theories are again more on the side of close contiguity. However, here—in contrast to the response competition theory—the prime-related process is clearly separated in time from the target-related process.

Spreading of Activation. A propagation of activation from the prime to the target in a semantic network is a mechanism that can explain why responding is faster and more accurate for targets that were preceded by a prime stimulus that is related to the target (e.g., Collins & Loftus, 1975). Although semantic network models can be criticized on theoretical grounds (e.g., Johnson-Laird, Herrmann, & Chaffin, 1984), the basic idea of a facilitation of target processing (encoding, identification, classification) by some preparatory process that is elicited by the prime is still prominent in recent models that try to capture the idea of semantic relatedness. For two reasons it is important to note that semantic network models must put severe constraints on the process of spreading activation to prevent a kind of "semantic epileptic seizure" (see, e.g., Anderson, 1983). First, the spread of activation that reaches a goal node must be a function of the number of links that radiate from the source node. Second, the decay rate must be rather fast. The first constraint is important for the discussion of evaluative priming effects found with semantic priming designs (see above). If they exist, this would mean that any positive (negative) prime facilitates any other positive (negative) concept in semantic memory. However, this conclusion makes immediately clear that spreading activation models cannot adequately capture the underlying process because the activation arriving at a target-related node is too small to be assessable. Of utmost importance in the present context is the second constraint. Again we are faced by short-lived processes that cannot be easily used as a principle of explanation for long-term priming. The only possibility to explain effects that are more far-reaching is to assume that the prime concept is still a source of activation even after the corresponding stimulus is no longer visible (see McNamara, 2005, for this argument).

Parallel Distributed Representations. Models of semantic memory assuming a parallel distributed representation of concepts explain semantic priming on the basis of overlap between mental representations of prime and target, so that processing a prime establishes an activation pattern that is similar to the target pattern. Thus, processing the target is facilitated because transition time from prime to target pattern is fast (Masson, 1995; see also Lerner, Bentin, & Shriki, 2012; McRae, de Sa, & Seidenberg, 1997; Plaut & Booth, 2000; Sharkey, 1990). On first sight, this model seems to be perfectly suited to explain evaluative priming in a semantic priming design. If we assume that a considerable amount of units represent valence, the transition from one positive (negative) pattern to another positive (negative) pattern is fast. However, Spruyt, Hermans, and colleagues (2007) reminded of the fact that in Masson's simulations, overlap of pattern must be very large to obtain priming effects. Schmitz and Wentura (2012) noted that the model does not allow for a parallel activation of prime and target patterns, which is an implausible constraint.

With regard to the longevity discussion, priming effects seem to be *prima facie* restricted to moment-to-moment transitions. In fact, however, Masson (1995) was able to predict lag-1 priming effects, that is, priming designs with one intervening item between prime and target because the pattern established by the prime was not completely eroded by the intervening item. Thus, one might speculate about versions with a very high dimensional complexity: Processing completely dissimilar information subsequently to the prime changes the pattern only for those parts of the multidimensional vector that are unrelated to the prime. These intervening items leave the prime pattern more or less intact and thus might allow for priming with longer lags. Notwithstanding these speculations, at the moment the theory is not well suited to explain long-lasting priming effects.

A LESS-FAMILIAR THEORY: A RETRIEVAL ACCOUNT OF PRIMING

The theories mentioned so far have the commonality that the essential process leading to a priming effect is located in the processing of the prime. The prime involuntarily triggers a response, activates related memory nodes, or shifts the activation pattern in distributed memory into a specific state. Other theories focus on memory retrieval processes. Rather well-known is the compound-cue theory by Ratcliff and McKoon (1988; see also Dosher & Rosedale, 1989) with the basic idea that prime and target build a compound cue to memory. Priming effects are explained by the assumption that semantically related compounds elicit a larger familiarity signal than unrelated ones. We will not elaborate further on this theory because it is again based on close temporal contiguity of prime and target and does therefore not help to elucidate long-term priming phenomena. More radical is the approach by Whittlesea and Jacoby (1990) who argue that priming is *induced* by processing the target. To elucidate the difference to other approaches of priming, they give a new interpretation to the degraded target effect. It is known that semantic priming is increased if the target is presented in a degraded form (e.g., pLAnT instead of plant). Of course, this phenomenon can easily be accommodated by other theories. For example, it can be assumed that shallow, "pure lexical" processing is prevented by degradation such that pre-activation of the semantic unit will be of help. Thus, the priming process (i.e., the prime has facilitated the access to the semantic unit associated with the target) has taken place anyway; it can, however, be better detected by presenting a degraded target. Instead, Whittlesea and Jacoby argued that the priming phenomenon is induced by the demands to process the degraded target: A non-degraded target is simply processed without reference to the context because the task is very easy. Due to the demands of processing a degraded target, however, it is likely that the prime episode is integrated in the process. This sounds like a variant of the compound cue model (see above; and indeed Whittlesea and Jacoby use the term compound cue). However, their approach is more flexible. More abstractly, they argue that "if the probe task is difficult (e.g., degraded presentation), then performance will rely more heavily on resources made available by other stimulus encounters" (Hughes & Whittlesea, 2003; p. 402). Thus, this approach includes the possibility that the prime does not precede the target in close temporal contiguity. It might be that starting to process the target will lead to a retrieval of a similar processing episode of the past (with similarity in operations and content). Thus, this account of priming is *a priori* not restricted to short-term effects. We will return to this issue.

A COMPARISON OF LONG-TERM AND SHORT-TERM PRIMING

At first sight, it is evident that long-term priming of social cognition research cannot be based on the mechanisms made responsible for short-term priming. However, we should explicitly discuss this issue with an example from the long-term priming field. Englich, Mussweiler, and Strack (2006) recruited legal professionals (i.e., judges, prosecutors), presented them with case material about a case of rape, asked them to put themselves into the role of a judge, and to give a sentencing decision. Before the decision, participants were instructed to mentally simulate their response to a journalist's query: "Do you think that the sentence for the defendant in this case will be higher or lower than 1 (3) year(s)," with the number of years in the question (the anchor value) randomly varied between participants. Participants who had been exposed to the high anchor gave significantly longer sentences than participants who were confronted with a low anchor. The authors (see also Strack and Mussweiler, 1997) proposed a theory of the anchor effect that is based on the accessibility of relevant knowledge. Participants answer the comparison question (i.e., the journalist's query) in a positive testing mode, that is, they retrieve relevant knowledge that is most compatible with the anchor. If they are then asked to answer the absolute question (i.e., their sentencing decision), the just retrieved knowledge is (unbeknownst to the participant) more accessible than knowledge that is in favor of the counter-anchor. Thus, the answer to the absolute question is biased towards the anchor. Is this a case of priming? Yes, according to the authors. Is this the same kind of priming that we have termed (short-term) semantic priming? Definitely not. Even in the most prototypical studies on anchoring, the delay between responding to the comparison question and the absolute question is not a matter of one or two seconds: Mussweiler (2001) found that even a one-week delay between the comparison question and absolute question does not diminish the anchoring effect. Thus, although Strack and Mussweiler referred to the (short-term) semantic priming tradition in their explanation of the anchor effect, the kind of priming that is effective in the anchoring process must be of a different type.

The question arises: Has cognitive psychology completely ignored the issue of long-term semantic priming? No. Interestingly, however, it has only recently gained more interest. Of course, long-term *repetition* priming has been known for a long time (e.g., the word fragment "_AR_ VA _ _ is completed by "AARDVARK" with a higher than baseline probability if one has processed "AARDVARK" one week before; Tulving, Schacter, & Stark, 1982) and has extensively been discussed in the field of implicit memory research. Yet, we do not think that this phenomenon is the adequate model case for standard long-term priming effects in social cognition because these effects have to do with processing the specific stimulus and not its semantic relatives. However, in recent years a number of studies in cognitive psychology explicitly addressed long-term semantic priming. We will briefly review this research and the explanations that were given for long-term priming effects. Finally, we will return to the issue whether this part of cognitive psychology might be helpful in understanding long-term priming in social cognition.

LONG-TERM SEMANTIC PRIMING

Under the header "long-term semantic priming," semantic priming phenomena are categorized with a delay (either expressed as the number of intervening trials or expressed on a time scale) that is considerably longer than the usual within-trial priming. Thereby they either challenge the view of semantic priming as a short-lived phenomenon or they shed light on a new phenomenon (that has *a priori* more similarity with long-term priming in social cognition).

Becker, Moscovitch, Behrmann, and Joordens (1997) as well as Hughes and Whittlesea (2003) made comparable attempts to find robust long-term semantic priming. Participants processed a list of prime words (prime phase) followed by a target list (probe phase) that consisted half of semantically related targets (primed targets) and half of targets with no relationship to the primes (unprimed targets). In both studies, long-term semantic priming effects were found. In the study by Becker and colleagues, the average trial lag between prime and target was 21.5 items; in the study by Hughes and Whittlesea (2003), the two lists were separated by a retention interval of five minutes. Interestingly, both found no facilitation effects if rather shallow tasks were used, like lexical decision or naming. Robust priming effects were obtained, however, for tasks that required deep processing (Becker et al., 1997, used an animacy decision; Hughes and Whittlesea, 2003, employed a semantic categorization task: e.g., animal – lion – vitamin; which category – left or right – does the middle word belong to?).[4]

Similar long-term facilitation effects for semantically related items were reported by Woltz and Was (2006; see also Woltz & Was, 2007) who presented their participants with a working memory task that included four items from two different semantic categories (i.e., two items per category). Then, participants were cued by one category label and had to retrieve the two items that belong to this category. The trial ended by a category comparison task (Do the two items belong to the same category?), employing *new* exemplars from the focused category, the ignored category, and a new category. Reaction times were faster for both the focused category and the ignored category compared to the new category. Recently, Was (2010) replicated this effect with a 24-hour delay. One might speculate that it is decisive for long-term priming that the same or, at least, similar operations (e.g., categorization) must be applied to prime and target. However, recently Woltz (2010) showed long-term effects in a design with different (but complex) tasks for primes and targets.

We want to briefly mention a further experimental approach to long-term semantic priming, that is, the use of the DRM paradigm (Roediger & McDermott, 1995). In the original paradigm, participants are presented with a list of words that are all associates of one missing word (the lure). (False) recall of the lure occurs with a remarkable probability. Assuming that massive spread of activation

---

4. For the sake the completeness, Joordens and Becker (1997) found lag effects in the lexical decision task, but only when they made the task harder by using homophone non-words.

from the list words to the lure is responsible for the effect, several authors have tried to find facilitated lexical decision times for the lure (see Tse & Neely, 2005, for a review). Recently Sherman and Jordan (2011) found replicable priming effects (see also Tse & Neely, 2005, 2007). However, they discuss the phenomenon as still reflecting a rather short-lived effect, because it is more robust if each DRM list is directly followed by lexical decision trials (including the lure) compared to a design with several DRM lists followed by lexical decision trials including all lures.

Thus, there is considerable evidence for long-term semantic priming. The most convincing results were found with rather complex semantic tasks that have to be applied to the prime and to the target. The target thus must be processed more deeply than is typically the case in standard short-term priming experiments. Finally, aside from the recent studies by Woltz (2010), it was mostly the case that prime-related and target-related operations strongly overlapped.

EXPLANATIONS OF LONG-TERM SEMANTIC PRIMING

How are long-term semantic priming effects explained? There are several suggestions. All of them rely—in one way or the other—on long-term changes in memory and therefore depart from most theories on short-term priming.

Learning in a Neural Network. Becker and colleagues (1997) suggested a neural network model with the assumption that each processing instance of a word (on a semantic level) will not only result in a specific attractor state but also in slight changes of the weights that will "deepen" this attractor state. Thus, presenting either the same stimulus again or another one with considerable feature overlap (i.e., a semantically related stimulus) will result in faster processing. Thus, in contrast to the parallel distributed models explained above, priming causes a long-term change of semantic memory. In addition to their own results, especially the recent experiments by Woltz (2010) are in favor of this position. However, we have to see whether such a model of permanent change can handle what Grossberg (1987) had termed the "stability-plasticity" dilemma: "How can a learning system be designed to remain plastic in response to significant new events, yet also remain stable in response to irrelevant events?" (p. 30).

Strengthening of Procedural Memory. Woltz and Was (2006; 2007; see also Was, 2010) as well as Hughes and Whittlesea (2003) found evidence that lead to the conclusion that long-term effects are more a matter of strengthening content-specific *procedures* than increased accessibility of the content itself. Thus, the authors interpreted their findings against some sort of long-term activated nodes in semantic memory.

Hughes and Whittlesea (2003), who relate their work on long-term priming to the retrieval theory proposed by Whittlesea and Jacoby (1990; see above), argue in a more principled way: "Every stimulus encounter is a learning event, which can have consequences for later processing; each experience is preserved, rather than being amalgamated into an abstract, monolithic representation. However, the central principle of these accounts is that each processing event consists of a particular combination of task, context, stimulus properties, and cued memory traces" (p. 409). Important for this kind of explanation is the focus on retrieval processes during the probe phase: Priming occurs just because the same content-specific procedures as in the prime phase are employed.

Long-Term Working Memory. Within their approach, Woltz and Was (2006) introduced the concept of *available long-term memory*, that is, the heightened availability of long-term memory structures for processing. Thereby, they refer to the embedded working memory concept by Cowan (1999) and the long-term working memory concept by Ericsson and Kintsch (1995). Although Woltz and Was finally integrated these concepts into their procedural account (see above), it might be worthwhile in the present context to devote an extra paragraph on this idea. Ericsson and Kintsch pointed out that traditional working memory models fell short of giving a satisfying answer to the question of how people maintain access to large amounts of information while performing complex cognitive tasks. For example, while reading a newspaper article, the reader can interrupt reading (e.g., to get another cup of coffee) without noteworthy losses in performance upon return. According to Ericsson and Kintsch, highly connected and integrated long-term memory structures are created with a very efficient retrieval structure. While reading (with only short interruptions), only retrieval cues to these structures have to be maintained in current short-term working memory. However, even longer interruptions do not pose a hard problem. A reader can easily continue to read a novel on the next day. In some sense, these long-term structures are in a special state because, given the correct cues, a complex structure is immediately in the focus. However, if the reader is interrupted, a different context is active and the novel-related long-term structures are no longer active and will not modulate other thoughts.

LONG-TERM SEMANTIC PRIMING AND LONG-TERM PRIMING

What does long-term semantic priming and its explanations tell us about long-term priming in social cognition? We think a lot. Whereas short-term priming is most often (but see Whittlesea & Jacoby, 1990) characterized by moment-to-moment transitions that are not actively triggered by the target processing, long-term semantic priming seems to be a phenomenon that is best characterized by long-term memory changes (induced by extensive semantic processing) and by complex retrieval operations that are elicited during the probe phase. How can this characterization be reconciled with what we know about long-term priming in social cognition?

Example 1: The Anchoring Effect. Let us take the anchoring effect as an example again. Priming with a high or low anchor fits easily into the discussion of long-term priming. In principle, the theoretical line of reasoning provided by Strack and Mussweiler (1997) remains the same, albeit with a slightly different nuance. Answering the comparative question leads to a retrieval of anchor-consistent knowledge. However, subsequently it is no longer the same memory trace that is, for a while, in a temporarily altered state of accessibility. Instead, a new episode is created and stored in long-term memory, which is retrieved if strong cues point to this episode. Of course, trying to answer the absolute question is a strong cue to this episode, with a large procedural overlap. What is the difference to an account in terms of temporarily altered accessibility? For example, the longevity of the anchor effect is not a matter of decay of activation but a matter of interference. If cues become ambiguous, the "comparative anchor episode" will no longer be retrieved and loses its impact on judgments. Arguing the other way around: Given this perspective, one can easily conceive that anchor effects can be obtained even with delays longer than a week (see Mussweiler, 2001) as long as no retroactive interference is introduced.

Example 2: Priming Elderly Behavior. How can we reconcile the famous slow-walking priming effect found by Bargh and colleagues (1996) with these considerations, taking into account the recent replication attempts by Doyen, Klein, Pichon, and Cleeremans (2012)? To remind: Participants in the experimental group created sentences out of scrambled lists of words that contained cues to the age stereotype; subsequently, they walked more slowly down the hallway compared to the control group. Doyen and colleagues did not replicate the effect with experimenters that were completely blind (i.e., blind even with regard to the purpose of the study and blind with regard to participant's condition) and with automated measurement of walking speed (i.e., there was no person sitting in hallway who—of course, unbeknownst to the participant—stopped the time). However, they replicated the effect with automated measurement if (a) experimenters were correctly informed about the experiment (i.e., they were informed that age stereotype priming would lead to slow walking), (b) experimenters were not blind with regard to the assigned condition of participants, and (c) if walking speed was additionally assessed manually (i.e., there was a person present who stopped the time). A condition with incorrectly informed experimenters (i.e., they were informed that age stereotype priming would lead to fast walking) did not yield a priming effect (with automated measurement). We do not know which role features (a), (b), and (c) play. We cannot rule out that (b) is the decisive feature. If so, we have to discuss the phenomenon in the tradition of Pygmalion effects, and here is not the right place. But since (b) has no symmetric effect (i.e., participants with incorrectly informed experimenters did not speed up in the priming condition), we can speculate about the role of (a) and (c). First of all, a kind of robot-like modulation of behavior by highly accessible semantic structures seems not to be the correct description if we take the failure to replicate seriously. Maybe the (correctly) informed experimenter as well as the presence of the experimenter who has to stop the time creates a social context that connects the scrambled sentence task to the walk in the hallway.

Example 3: Priming Intelligent Behavior. A further well-known priming study was published by Dijksterhuis and van Knippenberg (1998) who found that participants who extensively thought about the attributes of a typical professor showed higher performance in an (ostensibly unrelated) general knowledge test compared to a control group. Recently, there were several failures to replicate this effect, one published (Shanks et al., 2013) and two unpublished.[5] If our speculations above contain a grain of truth, we have to focus on features of the test situation that act

---

5. (1) Andreas Eder, Clarissa Leipert, Jochen Musch, & Karl-Christoph Klauer. Failed replication to prime intelligent behavior (2012, August 10). Retrieved January 30, 2014, from http://www.PsychFileDrawer.org/replication.php?attempt=MTI0 (with regard to the procedural detail mentioned in the text, Andreas Eder, personal communication, January 17, 2014); (2) Meigan S. Roberts, William Crooks, Tyler J. Kolody, Teodora Pavlovic, Kailey J. Rombola, and Lionel G. Standing. No effect on intelligence from priming (2013, January 1). Retrieved January 30, 2014, from http://www.PsychFileDrawer.org/replication.php?attempt=MTQz

as retrieval cues to the priming episode. Interestingly, in the original study procedure there was a detail that appeared in only one of three replication attempts (Dijksterhuis & van Knippenberg, 1998, p. 869): "Participants were told that the Personality Department was currently developing a 'general knowledge' scale. This scale consisted of five subscales, each containing 42 questions. The subscales ranged from very easy (1) to very difficult (5). At that time, we told participants, we were testing the differences in difficulty between the five subscales. *For ethical purposes we told all participants that they would receive the most difficult subscale*" (emphasis added). Thus, the instruction provides a strong cue to the most recent episode that dealt with "being intelligent" and "being erudite." However, we have to admit that Shanks and colleagues (2013) employed exactly these instructions and did not find the effect either.

Referring again to Ericsson and Kintsch (1995), understanding a situation is like comprehending a story: As long as I'm not interrupted, working memory contains strong retrieval cues to what I have learned so far about the situation. But when I'm interrupted, the consequences of reading the story are minimal until a strong cue reinstates the story context again. Let's connect this abstract logic to priming of behavior by a simple everyday example: As long as a boy is mentally "into" the western movie after "The End" has appeared on the screen, he will likely leave the theater in a rolling gait. But if he is interrupted by his best friend making him aware of the next sensation, we will not observe any aftermath of the western.

One might argue that this kind of explanation ignores one of the most intriguing features of typical long-term priming studies, that is, that the link between the prime and the behavior is non-conscious. That would be a misunderstanding. By writing about the possible importance of retrieval processes, we do not want to insinuate that priming effects are a kind of demand effect, that is, that participants consciously connect the behavior episode with the prime episode to infer how they should behave. For example, in the priming of intelligent behavior, study participants would surely agree with the statement that there are not many degrees of freedom for their behavior in a general knowledge test: one either knows the correct answer for a given question or not. Nevertheless, performance might be clearly dependent on subtleties of the subjective situation (e.g., whether one sees the test as an opportunity to excel or as a danger to make a fool of oneself). Those subtleties might be primed.

CONCLUSIONS

A comparison of long-term and short-term priming effects in social cognition research has revealed some obvious similarities and analogies (e.g., with regard to the content of materials that were used and the behaviors that were assessed) but also important differences. Due to the completely different time scale of the two paradigms, it is extremely unlikely that the mediating processes are similar for the two types of priming. Long-term and short-term priming thus are qualitatively distinct phenomena and also have to be interpreted differently: Short-term priming effects are indicative of structural associations in semantic memory that determine the ease of switching between mental representations or the likelihood of short-term response activations. Long-term priming, on the other hand, most likely reflects some kind of enduring and context-dependent *change* in long-term memory structures that is related to the retrieval or reenactment of previous processing episodes, as it is also involved in long-term semantic priming.

Given these fundamental differences between long-term and short-term priming, one is left wondering whether short-term priming studies are at all helpful and necessary for an understanding of long-term priming. Although our chapter makes a strong case for keeping relevant distinctions between different forms of priming in mind, we are nevertheless convinced that short-term priming is informative and indispensable also with regard to an understanding of long-term priming: In particular, all forms of short-term priming (and of long-term semantic priming as well) that go beyond mere repetition or identity priming have to assume that some kind of *semantic* relation exists between the prime and probe, which is a necessary condition for the emergence of these semantically mediated long-term priming effects. Long-term priming thus can be decomposed into two different kinds of processes: A fast-acting process prepares for transitions between semantically related elements (e.g., from a social category to stereotypic attributes, from an attitude object to its evaluation); these facilitative effects possibly play a role during the priming and testing phase of long-term priming studies. In addition, a more enduring process is involved in long-term priming that changes representational structures and leaves its traces in memory for later retrieval. Short-term priming studies typically investigate the structure and strengths of semantic relations and provide important information regarding which kind of transfer is to be expected from the prime to the test situation, and what kind of moderating effects one has to keep in mind regarding contextual circumstances (e.g., Doyen et al., 2012; Müller & Rothermund, 2012). In addition, however, long-term priming involves other processes that are responsible for the long-term effects of the priming episode on behavior that standard short-term priming studies do not provide an explanation for. Our chapter has reviewed recent research from cognitive psychology focusing on long-term semantic priming that might provide an interesting point of departure to more systematically investigate what is going on in long-term priming during temporally separated prime and testing episodes.

REFERENCES

Anderson, J. R. (1983). A spreading activation theory of memory. *Journal of Verbal Learning & Verbal Behavior, 22,* 261-295.

Banaji, M. R., & Hardin, C. D. (1996). Automatic stereotyping. *Psychological Science, 7,* 136-141.

Bargh, J. A. (2014). The historical origins of priming as the preparation of behavioral responses: Unconscious carry-over and contextual influences of real-world importance. This volume.

Bargh, J. A., Chen, M., & Burrows, L. (1996). Automaticity of social behavior: Direct effects of trait construct and stereotype activation on action. *Journal of Personality and Social Psychology, 71,* 230-244.

Bartholow, B. D., Riordan, M. A., Saults, J. S., & Lust, S. A. (2009). Psychophysiological evidence of response conflict and strategic control of responses in affective priming. *Journal of Experimental Social Psychology, 45,* 655-666.

Becker, S., Moscovitch, M., Behrmann, M., & Joordens, S. (1997). Long-term semantic priming: A computational account and empirical evidence. *Journal of Experimental Psychology: Learning, Memory, and Cognition, 23,* 1059-1082.

Blair, I. V., & Banaji, M. R. (1996). Automatic and controlled processes in stereotype priming. *Journal of Personality and Social Psychology, 70,* 1142-1163.

Casper, C., & Rothermund, K. (2012). Gender self-stereotyping is context dependent for men but not for women. *Basic and Applied Social Psychology, 34,* 434-442.

Casper, C., Rothermund, K., & Wentura, D. (2010). Automatic stereotype activation is context dependent. *Social Psychology, 41,* 131-136.

Casper, C., Rothermund, K., & Wentura, D. (2011). The activation of specific facets of age stereotypes depends on individuating information. *Social Cognition, 29,* 393-414.

Cesario, J., & Jonas, K. J. (2014). Replicability and models of priming: What a resource computation framework can tell us about expectations of replicability. This volume.

Chasteen, A. L., Schwarz, N., & Park, D. C. (2002). The activation of aging stereotypes in younger and older adults. *The Journals of Gerontology: Series B: Psychological Sciences and Social Sciences, 57B,* P540-P547.

Collins, A. M., & Loftus, E. F. (1975). A spreading-activation theory of semantic processing. *Psychological Review, 82,* 407-428.

Correll, J., Park, B., Judd, C. M., & Wittenbrink, B. (2002). The police officer's dilemma: Using ethnicity to disambiguate potentially threatening individuals. *Journal of Personality and Social Psychology, 83,* 1314-1329.

Cowan, N. (1999). An embedded-processes model of working memory. In A. Miyake & P. Shah (Eds.), *Models of working memory: Mechanisms of active maintenance and executive control* (pp. 62-101). New York: Cambridge University Press.

Custers, R., & Aarts, H. (2007). In search of the nonconscious sources of goal pursuit: Accessibility and positive affective valence of the goal state. *Journal of Experimental Social Psychology, 43,* 312-318.

De Houwer, J. (2003). On the role of stimulus-response and stimulus-stimulus compatibility in the Stroop effect. *Memory & Cognition, 31,* 353-359.

De Houwer, J., Hermans, D., Rothermund, K., & Wentura, D. (2002). Affective priming of semantic categorisation responses. *Cognition & Emotion, 16,* 643-666.

De Houwer, J., & Randell, T. (2002). Attention to primes modulates affective priming of pronunciation responses. *Experimental Psychology, 49,* 163-170.

De Houwer, J., & Randell, T. (2004). Robust affective priming effects in a conditional pronunciation task: Evidence for the semantic representation of evaluative information. *Cognition & Emotion, 18,* 251-264.

de Paula Couto, M. C. P., & Wentura, D. (2012). Automatically activated facets of ageism: Masked evaluative priming allows for a differentiation of age-related prejudice. *European Journal of Social Psychology, 42,* 852-863.

Degner, J. (2009). On the (un)controllability of affective priming: Strategic manipulation is feasible but can possibly be prevented. *Cognition & Emotion, 23,* 327-354.

Degner, J., & Wentura, D. (2010). Automatic prejudice in childhood and early adolescence. *Journal of Personality and Social Psychology, 98,* 356-374.

Dehaene, S., Naccache, L., Clec'H, L., G., Koechlin, E., Mueller, M., et al. (1998). Imaging unconscious semantic priming. *Nature, 395,* 597-600.

Dijksterhuis, A., & Bargh, J. A. (2001). The perception-behavior expressway: Automatic effects of social perception on social behavior. *Advances in Experimental Social Psychology, 33,* 1-40.

Dijksterhuis, A., & van Knippenberg, A. (1998). The relation between perception and behavior, or how to win a game of Trivial Pursuit. *Journal of Personality and Social Psychology, 74,* 865-877.

Dosher, B. A., & Rosedale, G. (1989). Integrated retrieval cues as a mechanism for priming in retrieval from memory. *Journal of Experimental Psychology: General, 118,* 191-211.

Dovidio, J. F., Evans, N., & Tyler, R. B. (1986). Racial stereotypes: The contents of their cognitive representations. *Journal of Experimental Social Psychology, 22,* 22-37.

Doyen, S., Klein, O., Pichon, C. L., & Cleeremans, A. (2012). Behavioral priming: It's all in the mind, but whose mind? *PLOS ONE, 7,* 7.

Doyen, S., Klein, O., Simons, D. J., & Cleeremans, A. (2014). On the other side of the mirror: Priming in cognitive and social psychology. This volume.

Eder, A. B., Leuthold, H., Rothermund, K., & Schweinberger, S. R. (2012). Automatic response activation in sequential affective priming: An ERP study. *Social Cognitive and Affective Neuroscience, 7,* 436-445.

Eitam, B., & Higgins, E. T. (2010). Motivation in mental accessibility: Relevance of a Representation (ROAR) as a new framework. *Social and Personality Psychology Compass, 4,* 951-967.

Englich, B., Mussweiler, T., & Strack, F. (2006). Playing dice with criminal sentences: The influence of irrelevant anchors on experts' judicial decision making. *Personality and Social Psychology Bulletin, 32,* 188-200.

Ericsson, K. A., & Kintsch, W. (1995). Long-term working memory. *Psychological Review, 102,* 211-245.

Fazio, R. H., Jackson, J. R., Dunton, B. C., & Williams, C. J. (1995). Variability in automatic activation as an unobtrusive measure of racial attitudes: A bona fide pipeline? *Journal of Personality and Social Psychology, 69,* 1013-1027.

Fazio, R. H., Sanbonmatsu, D. M., Powell, M. C., & Kardes, F. R. (1986). On the automatic activation of attitudes. *Journal of Personality and Social Psychology, 50,* 229-238.

Frings, C., & Wentura, D. (2003). Who is watching "Big Brother"? TV consumption predicted by masked affective Priming. *European Journal of Social Psychology, 33,* 779-791.

Gaertner, S. L., & McLaughlin, J. P. (1983). Racial stereotypes: Associations and ascriptions of positive and negative characteristics. *Social Psychology Quarterly, 46,* 23-30.

Glaser, J., & Banaji, M. R. (1999). When fair is foul and foul is fair: Reverse priming in automatic evaluation. *Journal of Personality and Social Psychology, 77,* 669-687.

Grossberg, S. (1987). Competitive learning: From interactive activation to adaptive resonance. *Cognitive Science, 11,* 23-63.

Hermans, D., De Houwer, J., & Eelen, P. (1994). The affective priming effect: Automatic activation of evaluative information in memory. *Cognition & Emotion, 8,* 515-533.

Higgins, E. T., & Eitam, B. (2014). Priming . . . shmiming: It's about knowing when and why stimulated memory representations become active. This volume.

Higgins, E. T., Rholes, W. S., & Jones, C. R. (1977). Category accessibility and impression formation. *Journal of Experimental Social Psychology, 13,* 141-154.

Hughes, A. D., & Whittlesea, B. W. A. (2003). Long-term semantic transfer: An overlapping-operations account. *Memory & Cognition, 31,* 401-411.

Hutchison, K. A. (2003). Is semantic priming due to association strength or feature overlap? A microanalytic review. *Psychonomic Bulletin & Review, 10,* 785-813.

Johnson-Laird, P. N., Herrmann, D. J., & Chaffin, R. (1984). Only connections: A critique of semantic networks. *Psychological Bulletin, 96,* 292-315.

Joordens, S., & Becker, S. (1997). The long and short of semantic priming effects in lexical decision. *Journal of Experimental Psychology: Learning, Memory, and Cognition, 23,* 1083-1105.

Kawakami, K., & Dovidio, J. F. (2001). The reliability of implicit stereotyping. *Personality and Social Psychology Bulletin, 27,* 212-225.

Klatzky, R. L., & Creswell, J. D. (2014). An intersensory interaction account of priming effects—and their absence. *Perspectives on Psychological Science, 9,* 49-58.

Klauer, K. C., Eder, A. B., Greenwald, A. G., & Abrams, R. L. (2007). Priming of semantic classifications by novel subliminal prime words. *Consciousness and Cognition, 16,* 63-83.

Klauer, K. C., & Musch, J. (2001). Does sunshine prime loyal? Affective priming in the naming task. *Quarterly Journal of Experimental Psychology, A54,* 727-751.

Klauer, K. C., & Musch, J. (2002). Goal-dependent and goal-independent effects of irrelevant evaluations. *Personality and Social Psychology Bulletin, 28,* 802-814.

Klauer, K. C., Teige-Mocigemba, S., & Spruyt, A. (2009). Contrast effects in spontaneous evaluations: A psychophysical account. *Journal of Personality and Social Psychology, 96,* 265-287.

Klinger, M. R., Burton, P. C., & Pitts, G. S. (2000). Mechanisms of unconscious priming: I. Response competition, not spreading activation. *Journal of Experi-*

mental Psychology: Learning, Memory, and Cognition, 26,* 441-455.

Latrofa, M., Vaes, J., Cadinu, M., & Carnaghi, A. (2010). The cognitive representation of self-stereotyping. *Personality and Social Psychology Bulletin, 36,* 911-922.

Lerner, I., Bentin, S., & Shriki, O. (2012). Spreading activation in an attractor network with latching dynamics: Automatic semantic priming revisited. *Cognitive Science, 36,* 1339-1382.

Loersch, C., & Payne, B. K. (2011). The situated inference model: An integrative account of the effects of primes on perception, behavior, and motivation. *Perspectives on Psychological Science, 6,* 234-252.

Loersch, C., & Payne, B. K. (2014). Situated inferences and the what, who, and where of priming. This volume.

Lucas, M. (2000). Semantic priming without association: A meta-analytic review. *Psychonomic Bulletin & Review, 7,* 618-630.

Masson, M. E. J. (1995). A distributed memory model of semantic priming. *Journal of Experimental Psychology: Learning, Memory, and Cognition, 21,* 3-23.

McNamara, T. P. (2005). *Semantic priming: Perspectives from memory and word recognition.* New York: Psychology Press.

McNamara, T. P. (2013). Semantic memory and priming. In A. F. Healy & R. W. Proctor (Eds.), *Handbook of psychology, Vol. 4: Experimental psychology* (2nd ed., pp. 449-471). Hoboken, NJ: Wiley.

McRae, K., de Sa, V. R., & Seidenberg, M. S. (1997). On the nature and scope of featural representations of word meaning. *Journal of Experimental Psychology: General, 126,* 99-130.

Molden, D. C. (2014). Understanding priming effects in social psychology: What is "social priming" and how does it occur? This volume.

Müller, F., & Rothermund, K. (2012). Talking loudly but lazing at work—Behavioral effects of stereotypes are context dependent. *European Journal of Social Psychology, 42,* 557-563.

Müller, F., & Rothermund, K. (2014). What does it take to activate stereotypes? Simple primes don't seem enough. *Social Psychology, 45,*(3), 187–193.

Mussweiler, T. (2001). The durability of anchoring effects. *European Journal of Social Psychology, 31,* 431-442.

Neely, J. H. (1991). Semantic priming effects in visual word recognition: A selective review of current findings and theories. In D. Besner & G. W. Humphreys (Eds.), *Basic processes in reading: Visual word recognition* (pp. 264-336). Hillsdale, NJ: Erlbaum.

Otten, S., & Wentura, D. (1999). About the impact of automaticity in the Minimal Group Paradigm: Evidence from affective priming tasks. *European Journal of Social Psychology, 29,* 1049-1071.

Payne, B. K. (2001). Prejudice and perception: The role of automatic and controlled processes in misperceiving a weapon. *Journal of Personality and Social Psychology, 81,* 181-192.

Payne, B. K., Cheng, C. M., Govorun, O., & Stewart, B. D. (2005). An inkblot for attitudes: Affect misattribution as implicit measurement. *Journal of Personality and Social Psychology, 89,* 277-293.

Plaut, D. C., & Booth, J. R. (2000). Individual and developmental differences in semantic priming: Empirical and computational support for a single-mechanism account of lexical processing. *Psychological Review, 107,* 786-823.

Ratcliff, R., & McKoon, G. (1988). A retrieval theory of priming in memory. *Psychological Review, 95,* 385-408.

Roediger, H. L., & McDermott, K. B. (1995). Creating false memories: Remembering words not presented in lists. *Journal of Experimental Psychology: Learning, Memory, and Cognition, 21,* 803-814.

Rothermund, K., & Wentura, D. (1998). Ein fairer Test für die Aktivationsausbreitungshypothese: Affektives Priming in der Stroop-Aufgabe [An unbiased test of a spreading activation account of affective priming: Analysis of affective congruency effects in the Stroop task]. *Zeitschrift für Experimentelle Psychologie, 45,* 120-135.

Schmidt, F., Haberkamp, A., & Schmidt, T. (2011). Dos and don'ts in response priming research. *Advances in Cognitive Psychology, 7,* 120-131.

Schmitz, M., & Wentura, D. (2012). Evaluative priming of naming and semantic categorization responses revisited: A mutual facilitation explanation. *Journal of Experimental Psychology: Learning Memory and Cognition, 38,* 984-1000.

Schmitz, M., Wentura, D., & Brinkmann, T. (2014). Evaluative priming in a semantic flanker task: ERP evidence for a mutual facilitation explanation. *Cognitive, Affective, and Behavioral Neuroscience, 14*, 426-442.

Schröder, T., & Thagard, P. (2013). The affective meanings of automatic social behaviors: Three mechanisms that explain priming. *Psychological Review, 120*, 255-280.

Schröder, T., & Thagard, P. (2014). Priming: Constraint satisfaction and interactive competition. This volume.

Shanks, D. R., Newell, B. R., Lee, E. H., Balakrishnan, D., Ekelund, L., Cenac, Z., et al. (2013). Priming intelligent behavior: An elusive phenomenon. *PLOS ONE, 8*, e56515.

Sharkey, N. E. (1990). A connectionist model of text comprehension. In D. A. Balota, G. B. Flores d'Arcais, & K. Rayner (Eds.), *Comprehension processes in reading* (pp. 487-514). Hillsdale, NJ: Erlbaum.

Sherman, S. M., & Jordan, T. R. (2011). Word-frequency effects in long-term semantic priming and false memory. *British Journal of Psychology, 102*, 559-568.

Spalding, L. R., & Hardin, C. D. (1999). Unconscious unease and self-handicapping: Behavioral consequences of individual differences in implicit and explicit self-esteem. *Psychological Science, 10*, 535-539.

Spruyt, A., De Houwer, J., Hermans, D., & Eelen, P. (2007). Affective priming of nonaffective semantic categorization responses. *Experimental Psychology, 54*, 44-53.

Spruyt, A., Gast, A., & Moors, A. (2011). The sequential priming paradigm: A primer. In K. C. Klauer, A. Voss, & C. Stahl (Eds.), *Cognitive methods in social psychology* (pp. 48-77). New York: Guilford.

Spruyt, A., Hermans, D., De Houwer, J., & Eelen, P. (2002). On the nature of the affective priming effect: Affective priming of naming responses. *Social Cognition, 20*, 227-256.

Spruyt, A., Hermans, D., De Houwer, J., Vandromme, H., & Eelen, P. (2007). On the nature of the affective priming effect: Effects of stimulus onset asynchrony and congruency proportion in naming and evaluative categorization. *Memory & Cognition, 35*, 95-106.

Strack, F., & Mussweiler, T. (1997). Explaining the enigmatic anchoring effect: Mechanisms of selective accessibility. *Journal of Personality and Social Psychology, 73*, 437-446.

Teige-Mocigemba, S., & Klauer, K. C. (2008). „Automatic" evaluation? Strategic effects on affective priming. *Journal of Experimental Social Psychology, 44*, 1414-1417.

Tse, C.-S., & Neely, J. H. (2005). Assessing activation without source monitoring in the DRM false memory paradigm. *Journal of Memory & Language, 53*, 532-550.

Tse, C.-S., & Neely, J. H. (2007). Semantic and repetition priming effects for Deese/Roediger-McDermott (DRM) critical items and associates produced by DRM and unrelated study lists. *Memory & Cognition, 35*, 1047-1066.

Tulving, E., Schacter, D. L., & Stark, H. A. (1982). Priming effects in word-fragment completion are independent of recognition memory. *Journal of Experimental Psychology: Learning, Memory, and Cognition, 8*, 336-342.

Vorberg, D., Mattler, U., Heinecke, A., Schmidt, T., & Schwarzbach, J. (2003). Different time courses for visual perception and action priming. *Proceedings of the National Academy of Sciences, 100*, 6275-6280.

Voss, A., Rothermund, K., Gast, A., & Wentura, D. (2013). Cognitive processes in associative and categorical priming: A diffusion model analysis. *Journal of Experimental Psychology: General, 142*, 536-559.

Was, C. A. (2010). The persistence of content-specific memory operations: Priming effects following a 24-h delay. *Psychonomic Bulletin & Review, 17*, 362-368.

Wentura, D., & Brandtstädter, J. (2003). Age stereotypes in younger and older women: Analyses of accommodative shifts with a sentence-priming task. *Experimental Psychology, 50*, 16-26.

Wentura, D., & Degner, J. (2010). Practical guide to sequential priming and related tasks. In B. Gawronski & B. K. Payne (Eds.), *Handbook of implicit social cognition: Measurement, theory, and applications* (pp. 95-116). New York: Guilford.

Wentura, D., & Frings, C. (2008). Response-bound primes diminish affective priming in the naming task. *Cognition and Emotion, 22*, 374-384.

Wentura, D., Kulfanek, M., & Greve, W. (2005). Masked affective priming by name letters: Evidence for a correspondence of explicit and implicit self-esteem. *Journal*

of *Experimental Social Psychology, 41,* 654-663.
Werner, B., & Rothermund, K. (2013). Attention please: No affective priming effects in a valent/neutral-categorisation task. *Cognition & Emotion, 27,* 119-132.
Wheeler, S. C., & DeMarree, K. G. (2009). Multiple mechanisms of prime-to-behavior effects. *Social and Personality Psychology Compass, 3,* 566-581.
Wheeler, S. C., DeMarree, K. G., & Petty, R. E. (2014). Understanding prime-to-behavior effects: Insights from the active-self account. This volume.
Whittlesea, B. W., & Jacoby, L. L. (1990). Interaction of prime repetition with visual degradation: Is priming a retrieval phenomenon? *Journal of Memory and Language, 29,* 546-565.
Wittenbrink, B. (2007). Measuring attitudes through priming. In B. Wittenbrink & N. Schwarz (Eds.), *Implicit measures of attitudes* (pp. 17-58). New York: Guilford.
Wittenbrink, B., Judd, C. M., & Park, B. (1997). Evidence for racial prejudice at the implicit level and its relationship with questionnaire measures. *Journal of Personality and Social Psychology, 72,* 262-274.
Wittenbrink, B., Judd, C. M., & Park, B. (2001). Evaluative versus conceptual judgments in automatic stereotyping and prejudice. *Journal of Experimental Social Psychology, 37,* 244-252.
Woltz, D. J. (2010). Long-term semantic priming of word meaning. *Journal of Experimental Psychology: Learning, Memory, and Cognition, 36,* 1510-1528.
Woltz, D. J., & Was, C. A. (2006). Availability of related long-term memory during and after attention focus in working memory. *Memory & Cognition, 34,* 668-684.
Woltz, D. J., & Was, C. A. (2007). Available but unattended conceptual information in working memory: Temporarily active semantic content or persistent memory for prior operations? *Journal of Experimental Psychology: Learning Memory and Cognition, 33,* 155-168.
Zhang, Q., Lawson, A., Guo, C., & Jiang, Y. (2006). Electrophysiological correlates of visual affective priming. *Brain Research Bulletin, 71,* 316-323.

STRUCTURED VERSUS UNSTRUCTURED REGULATION: ON PROCEDURAL MINDSETS AND THE MECHANISMS OF PRIMING EFFECTS

Kentaro Fujita
The Ohio State University

Yaacov Trope
New York University

> We propose that two distinct regulatory dynamics may produce social psychological priming effects, but under very different conditions. When engaged in structured regulation, people process information in light of their valued goals, responding to salient situational cues only to the extent that those cues are goal-relevant. By contrast, when engaged in unstructured regulation, people are more tuned to the demands of the present, tailoring their responses to the unique circumstances of the immediate context and evincing a greater openness to responding to salient cues in a cue-consistent manner. We explore construal level as one factor that dictates when people engage in one dynamic versus the other. We also discuss the distinction between traditional priming and mindset priming.

Priming represents one of the most studied judgmental and behavioral phenomena in social cognition research. "Priming effects" refer to the cognitive, motivational, affective, and behavioral consequences of subtly enhancing the accessibility of a given construct independent of either available cognitive resources, awareness of this influence, or control over this influence (see Molden, 2014, this volume). Accessibility is the ease and speed with which a cognitive construct or process is activated and comes to mind (e.g., Bruner, 1957; Higgins, 1996). Determinants of accessibility include the frequency and recency of activation as well as the goals and motives of the individual (Bruner, 1957). Priming research is based on the

---

This work was funded in part by a grant from the National Science Foundation (Award #BCS-1053128). We are grateful to members of our respective lab groups for feedback on an earlier version of this paper, as well as for comments from Dan Molden and an anonymous reviewer.

Address correspondence to Kentaro Fujita, The Ohio State University, 1827 Neil Avenue, Columbus, OH 43210; E-mail: fujita.5@osu.edu.

notion that exposure to a stimulus makes some constructs or processes temporarily more accessible, which in turn enhances their influence on thoughts, feelings, and behavior (e.g., Higgins, 1996). In the most dramatic demonstrations of priming, situational cues that make a construct more accessible (e.g., exposing people to stereotypes about the elderly) lead to changes in behavior (e.g., walking more slowly; Bargh, Chen, & Burrows, 1996; for reviews, see Dijksterhuis & Bargh, 2001; Wheeler & Petty, 2001).

Several recent highly publicized failures to replicate some priming effects—particularly those that demonstrate their impact on behavior—have led many to question their reliability (e.g., Doyen, Klein, Pichon, & Cleeremans, 2012; Shanks et al., 2013). Following the lead of others (e.g., Cesario, Plaks, & Higgins, 2006; Eitam & Higgins, 2010; Loersch & Payne, 2011, 2014, this volume; Wheeler, DeMarree, & Petty, 2007, 2014, this volume), we propose that more needs to be done to understand the active "ingredients" in priming effects and how these ingredients operate and interact. We suggest that researchers need to devote greater attention to the self-regulatory concerns participants have, and whether and how these concerns influence people's interpretation or construal of the priming context. When presented with priming stimuli, participants must ask themselves, implicitly or explicitly, "What is it?" and "How do I want to respond?" We propose that how people address these two questions determines the outcome of priming experiments.

We distinguish two regulatory dynamics that determine how people address these questions. These dynamics constitute the ends of a theoretical continuum. People may engage in more structured regulation whereby they impose interpretations of situations based on their valued goals in top-down fashion, striving to maintain goal-consistency in their judgments, decisions, and behavior (see also Fujita, Trope, Cunningham, & Liberman, 2014). Alternatively, people may engage in more unstructured regulation whereby they construct event construals in a bottom-up fashion, taking cues from and tailoring their psychological and behavioral responses to the immediate demands of the present. Both regulatory dynamics may produce priming effects, but under very different circumstances and for very different reasons. We suggest that understanding when and why one might expect to produce a priming effect in the lab (and presumably in the "wilds" outside the lab) requires appreciation of these two dynamics. Before delving into greater detail of our theoretical approach, however, we briefly review the priming literature.

TRADITIONAL PRIMING EFFECTS

Traditional social psychological priming studies expose participants to situational cues that are designed to make a construct more accessible, and then assess the effects of this exposure in subsequent, ostensibly unrelated tasks. For example, in the now classic Donald paradigm, participants perform a task that exposes them to a series of positive versus negative traits (e.g., "adventurous" vs. "reckless"). Next, in what is an ostensibly separate study, participants evaluate a target individual on the basis of ambiguous behaviors (e.g., "Donald was thinking, perhaps, he would do some skydiving"). The general finding is that people are more likely to disambiguate these behaviors in a positive direction when "primed" with relevant positive traits (i.e., "adventurous"), and more negative when primed with relevant negative traits (i.e., "reckless"; e.g., Higgins, Rholes, & Jones, 1977; Srull & Wyer, 1980). Similar paradigms are used in behavioral priming studies. For example, Bargh, Chen, and Burrows (1996) had participants complete a scrambled sentence task in which they attempted to create sentences from sets of words. Embedded within some of these sets were words that were either related to stereotypes about the elderly (e.g., "forgetful," "grey," "wrinkle") or stereotype-neutral (e.g., "thirsty," "clean," "private"). Those exposed to elderly stereotypes subsequently were observed to walk more slowly down a hallway than those exposed to stereotype-neutral content. This impact of enhanced accessibility of content is what is traditionally referred to as "priming effects."

PRIMING PROCESS RATHER THAN CONTENT

Anderson (1982, 1983) in his ACT* model of skill acquisition introduced the distinction between declarative and procedural knowledge. Whereas the activation of declarative knowledge made particular content more likely to be used to solve a given problem, the ACT* model also proposed that the activation of procedural knowledge could make particular cognitive operations more likely to be used. Thus, the ACT* model suggests that not only should one be able to prime content, but one should also be able to prime content-general cognitive procedures. Indeed, extensive research suggests that by having participants engage in a particular cognitive procedure in one task promotes the tendency for that same cognitive operation to be used in subsequently semantically unrelated tasks. For example, in one early example of such "procedural" or "mindset" priming, participants induced to use a heuristic versus algorithmic rule to solve a base-rate problem were more likely to use the same rule to solve subsequent problems that they encountered (Ginossar & Trope, 1987). In contrast to traditional priming which aims to make particular content more accessible, mindset priming attempts to activate a particular set of cognitive operations or procedures that may then carry over to subsequent unrelated tasks.

Procedural or mindset priming has been used to study a wide variety of psychological phenomena. One prominent example that has used such methodology is work examining the distinction between deliberative and implemental mindsets (e.g., Gollwitzer, 1990). Goal theorists posit that goal setting and goal striving are distinct phases of goal pursuit, with each activating distinct cognitive operations that help people address the challenges associated with each phase, namely, deliberative versus implemental mindsets, respectively (e.g., Gollwitzer, 1990; Heckhausen & Gollwitzer, 1987). In empirical demonstrations of this hypothesis, participants identify and elaborate on a goal they are considering but have not yet acted upon (goal setting) versus a goal they have committed to and are planning to execute in the near future (goal striving; e.g., Gollwitzer & Kinney, 1989; Taylor & Gollwitzer, 1995). The impact of this manipulation is assessed using measures that are unrelated in content to the goals that participants generate. For example, in one study, those who deliberated whether to commit to a personal goal (relative to those who generated the means by which to implement a decided-upon goal) were more likely to attend to distractor stimuli on a goal-irrelevant reaction time task (Fujita, Gollwitzer, & Oettingen, 1997). Findings such as these suggest that the deliberative mindset engages cognitive operations that render people more "open-minded" than the implemental mindset, and that these mindsets can carry over to tasks that are irrelevant to the context that initially induced them.

Mindset priming is also used to study regulatory focus theory, which proposes two distinct motivational orientations, namely, promotion versus prevention (e.g., Higgins, 1997, 1998). Promotion tunes people to concerns about nurturance and ideals, enhancing sensitivity to gains relative to non-gains. Prevention, by contrast, tunes people to concerns about security and obligations, enhancing sensitivity to losses relative to non-losses. To activate promotion (vs. prevention) as mindset, researchers ask participants to think about how their hopes and ideals (vs. duties and obligations) have changed over time (e.g., Higgins, Roney, Crowe, & Hymes, 1994). The impact of these manipulations is evident even on subsequent tasks that are irrelevant in content to the responses participants provide, such as people's willingness to take risky gambles (e.g., Scholer, Zou, Fujita, Stroessner, & Higgins, 2010).

Other areas of research that have incorporated the notion of mindsets include social power (Galinsky, Gruenfeld, & Magee, 2003; Smith & Trope, 2006), impression formation (Smith, 1984; Smith & Branscombe, 1987),[1] and construal level theory (e.g., Freitas, Gollwitzer, & Trope, 2004; Fujita, Trope, Liberman, & Levin-Sagi, 2006). Research on the latter is particularly relevant for the present paper and will be reviewed in more detail in subsequent sections. We note that for the sake of clarity, when discussing the priming of cognitive procedures, we will specifically use the term "mindset priming" to distinguish it from traditional "priming."

"THE BLOOMING, BUZZING CONFUSION"

Key to most priming studies is the lack of contingency awareness on the part of participants between the priming materials and the primary dependent behavior (e.g., Lombardi, Higgins, & Bargh, 1987). Once aware, participants may attempt to reduce the impact of the primed materials on their responses (e.g., Wegener & Petty, 1995). Another key is ambiguity. Accessibility is most likely to impact perception, judgment, decisions, and behavior when the accessible construct helps to disambiguate stimuli by "tipping" them in one direction or another (e.g., Bruner, 1957; Higgins, 1996). Given this, priming studies deliberately try to confuse participants, occluding the true purpose of various materials and procedures with little guidance on what constitutes an appropriate response. Borrowing a quote from James (1890), it is from this "blooming, buzzing confusion" that priming effects emerge.

---

1. We might note that these early procedural priming studies on impression formation suggest that what is primed in traditional priming effects is not specific content, as suggested by a number of priming researchers, but rather specific cognitive procedures (Smith, 1984; Smith & Branscombe, 1987). For reasons unclear to us, this alternative account of priming has been largely overlooked. We might observe that the account of priming that we present in this paper is agnostic as to whether traditional priming effects result from the activation of specific content versus procedures, and can incorporate both possibilities.

BEYOND ASSOCIATIONS: THE ROLE OF CONSTRUAL IN PRIMING EFFECTS

It is precisely because of the confusion and ambiguity that priming paradigms present that we argue it is critical to understand participants' subjective construal. To orient and organize a response, people must construct a mental representation of the circumstances in which they find themselves. They must interpret what it is that they are presented with ("what is it?") and determine what constitutes an appropriate response ("how do I want to respond"). Although early research recognized the need to understand such construal or interpretational processes (e.g., Higgins, 1996; Martin, 1986), it is surprising how little attention they have received in traditional accounts of priming effects.

Traditional theoretical accounts, particularly those concerned with behavioral priming effects, are grounded in passive associative models (e.g., Dijksterhuis & Bargh, 2001; Higgins, Bargh, & Lombardi, 1985; Srull & Wyer, 1980). Priming stimuli are believed to make accessible particular mental content, which then enhances the likelihood of a particular response. This is perhaps best captured in the ideomotor account of behavioral priming, which suggests that simply thinking of an act engages the same content and processes that are required to enact that act (James, 1890). Thus, making accessible cognitions relevant to an act may automatically activate the tendency to enact that behavior (e.g., Dijksterhuis & Bargh, 2001). Associative activation of mental constructs is also a component of the more recent active-self account (e.g., Wheeler et al., 2007, 2014, this volume), which suggests that one mechanism by which priming exerts its influence is by making more accessible a biased set of self-knowledge with judgmental and behavioral implications that are relevant to the focal task at hand. At the heart of many models of priming then is a focus on passive associative connections between prime and existing mental content.

By contrast, more recently proposed alternative models have instead adopted a constructionist perspective, emphasizing more active interpretation and meaning-making processes as key determinants of priming phenomena. For example, the motivated-preparation account suggests that people use the accessibility of primed concepts as input into a decision process that determines how best to respond to an environment given one's goals (e.g., Cesario et al., 2006; Cesario, Plaks, Hagiwara, Navarrete, & Higgins, 2010; Cesario & Jonas, 2014, this volume). Activated knowledge is interpreted in light of one's goals and one's environment to determine one's best response (see also the ROAR model proposed by Eitam & Higgins, 2010). When aggression is made accessible, for example, people may fight or flee depending on whether they believe they are capable of winning a fight, and whether the environment preferentially enables a fight or flight response (Cesario et al., 2010). The situated-inference model, another constructionist model, highlights one's attribution about the source of the accessibility of the primed concept as a key process in priming phenomena (Loersch & Payne, 2011, 2014, this volume). When the source of accessibility is attributed to internal factors such as one's goals and values, accessible knowledge then forms the basis of one's responses. By contrast, when the source of accessibility is attributed to external factors, such as features of one's social environment, accessible knowledge is more likely to be dismissed and have no impact on one's responses. The active-self account also proposes interpretational processes as a potential mechanism, suggesting that when accessible knowledge is mistaken for self-knowledge, priming effects are more likely to occur (Wheeler et al., 2007, 2014, this volume). Construal or interpretational processes, moreover, play a central role in more recent computational models of priming effects ("affective meaning" mechanisms; Schröder & Thagard, 2013, 2014, this volume). Thus, in contrast to traditional passive associative accounts, researchers increasingly recognize active meaning-making as an integral component in priming phenomena.

HOW STRUCTURED VERSUS UNSTRUCTURED REGULATION IMPACT PRIMING

Our approach extends these constructionist models of priming. Like many constructionist accounts, we propose that the meaning of stimuli in light of people's goals is central to understanding responses to priming stimuli. Under some conditions, however, people may not immediately recognize what personal goals should be or may be pursued in a given context. In such circumstances, people may be more susceptible to external influence, using salient cues to ascertain what their goals in that context should be. We propose that there may be two distinct regulatory dynamics. When engaged in more structured regulation, people bring their goals to the task at hand and actively strive to maintain goal consistency in their representations and their behavioral decisions. People use their goals as scaffolds with which to build mental representations of the present in a selective manner. When engaged in more unstructured regulation, people are more sensitive to the immediate demands of the present. People build representations "on the fly," attending to salient cues in an open, flexible manner to determine what constitutes an appropriate response to the immediate circumstances. Both dynamics play important functions. The former ensures people remain committed to their goals, whereas the latter ensures people are attuned to their immediate environment. We propose that each of these dynamics may produce a priming effect, but may do so under very different circumstances.

Our constructionist approach is inspired by our own work on the influence of subjective construal on self-regulation. Our goals can impact what we "see" in social environments. Research suggests, for example, that we perceive desired objects as closer, and undesired objects farther, than they objectively are (e.g., Balcetis & Dunning, 2010). When observing ambiguous stimuli, we tend to perceive that stimuli in a goal-consistent manner, and ignore goal-inconsistent interpretations (e.g., Balcetis & Dunning, 2006; Balcetis, Dunning, & Granot, 2012). If a situational cue is consistent with the goals that participants bring to a given situation, then it is more likely to be integrated into their subjective construal of that context and impact responses. If a cue is irrelevant to one's goals, then it may be ignored and dismissed. If cues suggest threats to one's goals, they may be summarily dismissed, or be actively attended to and provoke information processing, judgment, and behavior in the opposing direction suggested by the cue in an effort to protect those valued goals.[2]

Conversely, how people construe a given context may change what goals appear relevant, which then may impact behavior. Research suggests, for example, that providing extrinsic rewards can undermine motivation toward what was originally an intrinsically motivated task (Lepper, Greene, & Nisbett, 1973). The extrinsic rewards presumably changed people's construal of the task from one engaged in for fun to one that is engaged in to obtain the reward, which then in turn leads to decreases in motivation when rewards are no longer available. Similarly, whereas construing a flu shot as "immunization" may promote inoculation behavior, construing the same behavior as "injection" may inhibit inoculation behavior (Young & Fazio, 2013). Although both construals equally describe the act of getting a flu shot, they direct attention to features that reflect contrasting concerns (health vs. pain), and thus motivate very different behavior. In this way, salient situational cues that activate or "prime" one subjective construal over others can promote the pursuit of motivated behavior.

Our work in particular has focused on contexts which present situational cues that promote behavior that runs contrary to people's valued goals. A prototypical example of such a situation is a self-control dilemma in which the availability of some reward or outcome in one's immediate environment (e.g., a piece of cake) tempts people to engage in behaviors that endanger the attainment of more remote rewards or outcomes (e.g., weight loss; Ainslie, 1975; Fujita, 2011; Mischel, Shoda, & Rodriguez, 1989; Rachlin, 2000; Thaler & Shefrin, 1981). Whereas self-control failure entails advancing the attainment of the more immediate reward, self-control success entails advancing the attainment of the more remote reward. Self-control is particularly challenging because the immediate presence of the proximal rewards present numerous cues to indulge. In essence, people are "primed" by their environments to indulge in the proximal temptation. Sustaining motivation toward more remote yet valued rewards is difficult because of the lack of concrete cues in the here and now. Successful self-control requires ignoring salient cues to indulge in proximal temptation, and instead engage in processing that supports the attainment of more distal ends (e.g., Fujita, 2011; Mischel et al., 1989; Rachlin, 2000; Trope & Fishbach, 2005). That is, people must construe the context in a way that sustains and supports their long-term goals to be successful at self-control.

The parallels between priming and self-control research, respectively, are highlighted by numerous studies. For example, exposure to words related to palatable foods spontaneously activates positive hedonic thoughts among restrained eaters, distracting them from the focal task at hand (e.g., Papies, Stroebe, & Aarts, 2007). Similarly, smokers who have abstained from smoking report significantly more positive thoughts about smoking when exposed to a lit cigarette versus a roll of tape (e.g., Sayette & Hufford, 1997). Exposure to these situational cues can also im-

---

2. Schroeder & Thagard (2013) refer to the integration of inputs into a representation as "positive constraint satisfaction," and refer to the inhibition of inputs as "negative constraint satisfaction." Other computational neuroscientists have referred to these same processes as "foregrounding" and "backgrounding," respectively (Hazy, Frank, & O'Reilly, 2007; Zelazo & Cunningham, 2007). These models suggest that such processes can occur without requiring conscious intention or awareness.

pact behavior. Food cues, such as visual displays and smells, prompt restrained dieters to report greater hunger and cause them to eat greater quantities of indulgent foods (e.g., Federoff, Polivy, & Herman, 1997). This work collectively suggests that situational cues can make more accessible (and thus "prime") thoughts, feelings, and behaviors that promote indulgence in proximal temptation to the detriment of long-term goals.

Much of the work mentioned above describes people's more unstructured responses to goal-undermining temptations. Our work, along with others, by contrast, has focused on the structured regulatory mechanisms that people engage in to maintain goal-consistent construals in the face of goal-undermining cues (e.g., Fujita, 2011; Trope & Fishbach, 2005). Consider, for example, work by Fishbach, Friedman, and Kruglanski (2003). To defend against goal-undermining temptation, people may learn to associate temptation cues with goal-related cognition. This temptation-cued goal priming should promote goal success in the face of temptation by biasing information processing in favor of one's goals. Most associations, however, are bidirectional, which may create self-regulatory problems. A bidirectional association between temptation and goal could undermine goal pursuit by allowing goal cues to prime temptation-related cognition. To address this latter possibility, Fishbach and colleagues (2003) suggest that people develop asymmetric temptation-goal associations, whereby exposure to temptation cues prime overriding goal concepts, but exposure to goal cues does not reciprocally prime temptation concepts. Indeed, empirical evidence supports the assertion that asymmetric associative links enhance goal-directed behavior in the face of salient temptation cues, biasing thoughts in favor of goals over temptations (Fishbach et al., 2003; see also Papies, Stroebe, & Aarts, 2008). Likewise, people's evaluative associations appear to be sensitive to their goals. When engaged in goal pursuit, people evince an enhanced readiness to associate positivity to goal-relevant objects (e.g., Ferguson & Bargh, 2004). These changes in evaluation appear not to require conscious intention or monitoring. Similarly, goal-undermining temptations are associated automatically with negativity (e.g., Fishbach & Shah, 2006; Fishbach, Zhang, & Trope, 2010). These cognitive and evaluative associations appear to help sustain goal-consistent construal of events, even in the face of salient cues that may suggest alternative courses of behavior.

Although people have available to them a number of regulatory mechanisms for sustaining goal-consistent construals, and thereby enhancing goal-directed behavior in the face of tempting alternatives, they do not always engage them (e.g., Fishbach et al., 2010; Fujita & Han, 2009; Fujita & Roberts, 2010; Fujita & Sasota, 2011; Myrseth & Fishbach, 2009). When people fail to engage these mechanisms, they are more vulnerable to the influence of salient local rewards. The goal of our research has been to understand when and why people evoke versus fail to evoke these mechanisms. This work has highlighted the central role that structured versus unstructured regulation plays in people's responses to situational cues.

In essence, we are proposing that participants in a priming experiment context are posed with a self-regulatory challenge. Like those presented with self-control dilemmas, participants in priming experiments must understand what goals are relevant in a particular context, and construct representations around those goals by making implicit or explicit decisions about the goal relevance of various cues. Determining what relevance various cues have for their goals, however, can be a difficult, given that experimenters purposely occlude the purpose of the tasks at hand with the hope that participants will decide, implicitly or explicitly, that priming stimuli are relevant and informative. Participants may or may not appreciate the relevance of the task at hand for the goals that they themselves bring to the experiment. From our perspective, key to understanding when priming is likely to be evident depends on whether the mental representation that people construct reflects their goals and what, if any, relationship those goals have to the salient cues in the immediate environment.

When engaged in structured regulation, the primary determination of what, if any, impact priming stimuli may have depends on goal relevance of the stimuli. People should be more responsive to goal-relevant stimuli and less responsive to goal-irrelevant stimuli. However, priming stimuli may also impact people through an alternative mechanism. When engaged in unstructured regulation, people may be more likely to use priming stimuli as cues to what their goals should be. As such, they may become more likely to act in a manner consistent with priming stimuli, even when such judgments, decisions, and behavior are inconsistent with valued goals. Thus, to understand priming phenomena, we propose that researchers need to appreciate the potential operation of two distinct dynamics by understanding what goals people are pursing, whether people use these goals to frame their construals of the priming context, and what relevance the priming stimuli have to these goals.

LEVEL OF CONSTRUAL

Drawing from construal level theory (CLT; e.g., Trope & Liberman, 2003; 2010), our work focuses on level of construal as an important determinant of whether people engage in structured versus unstructured regulation (Fujita, 2008; Fujita & Carnevale, 2012; Fujita et al., 2014). Central to CLT is the notion of psychological distance—any removal of objects and events from direct experience. An event that is to occur next year, for example, is more psychologically distant than an event that occurs next week. When events are psychologically distant, we generally lack reliable information about their specifics. To be able to think about such events in the absence of detailed specifics, we engage in cognitive abstraction, or high-level construal—constructing mental representations that capture the core, essential, goal-relevant features that are likely to be apparent in any possible manifestations of the events. For example, a distant beach vacation may conjure thoughts about sitting on sandy shore with a drink in hand feeling the warmth of the sun. We may not know which beach, what drink, or how warm, but every beach vacation will have these elements. As events become more proximal and detailed specifics become more available and reliable, we use this information to create more idiosyncratic representations via a process of low-level construal. Functionally, low-level construal allows us to tailor our thoughts, feelings, and actions to the unique demands of the present context. We can thus represent the present beach vacation as enjoying *this* stretch of beach, drinking *this* mojito made at *that* drink stand. Whereas high-level construal allows us to transcend the particulars of the here and now to consider remote time, places, people, and possibilities, low-level construal immerses us into them (see also Ledgerwood, Trope, & Liberman, 2010).

An extensive literature supports the proposition that people construe psychologically distant (vs. near) events by engaging in high-level (vs. low-level) construal. For example, when actions are to be performed next year versus tomorrow, people are more likely to identify those actions in terms of the general ends they can achieve than in terms of the specific means by which those actions are executed (Liberman & Trope, 1998). When asked to categorize objects associated with events to occur next year versus next week, people are more likely to sort these objects into fewer, broader categories, suggesting more abstract, superordinate categorization (Liberman, Sagristano, & Trope, 2002). Similar findings have been found when manipulating other dimensions of psychological distance, including spatial distance (e.g., Fujita, Henderson, Eng, Trope, & Liberman, 2006; Henderson, Fujita, Trope & Liberman, 2006), social distance (e.g., Liviatan, Trope, & Liberman, 2008; Smith & Trope, 2006), and hypotheticality (e.g., Todorov, Goren, & Trope, 2007; Wakslak, Trope, Liberman, & Alony, 2006). Thus, information about the psychological distance of an event can impact how people construe that event.

Research suggests that construal levels can also be primed as procedural mindsets in the absence of any information about psychological distance. For example, one commonly used manipulation presents participants with a behavior ("maintain good relationships") and asks them to generate responses as to "why" versus "how" they perform that action (e.g., Freitas et al., 2004). Whereas questions about "why" prompt participants to consider the general ends achieved by the behavior, questions about "how" prompt them to consider the specific means by which to enact that behavior (e.g., Liberman & Trope, 1998; Vallacher & Wegner, 1987; 1989). Not only does this procedure promote high-level versus low-level construal of the target behavior, respectively, but it also impacts how participants construe ostensibly unrelated events (e.g., Freitas et al., 2004; Fujita, Trope, et al., 2006). Another commonly used manipulation is the categories vs. exemplar task (Fujita, Trope et al., 2006). In this task, participants are presented with a series of objects ("dog") and asked to generate either superordinate category labels or subordinate exemplars (e.g., "animal" vs. "poodle"). This too promotes a tendency to construe ostensibly unrelated events in high-level versus low-level terms, such as identifying subsequent actions in terms of ends versus means (Fujita, Trope et al., 2006). Note that neither task is designed to activate any particular content, but rather is designed to prompt participants to rehearse the processes of abstraction and concretization that are at the heart of the distinction between high-level and low-level construal. The ability to prime construal level as a procedural mindset is a useful methodological tool with which to examine the impact of high-level versus low-level construal on various psychological phenomena, including self-regulation and goal pursuit.

STRUCTURED VERSUS UNSTRUCTURED REGULATION: THE ROLE OF CONSTRUAL LEVEL

CLT may be relevant to understanding the mechanisms that underlie traditional priming effects in that high-level and low-level construal differentially impact people's sensitivity to their goals and values, and recognizing the goal and value relevance of objects and events. The expanded "forest beyond the trees" perspective of high-level construal should enhance appreciation of the broader implications of one's behavior. This more expansive perspective should help heighten the relevance of one's goals and values to specific behaviors in specific contexts and therefore promote structured regulation. By contrast, the more focused "leaves and branches" perspective of low-level construal should heighten sensitivity to the idiosyncratic demands of the here and now. This narrowed perspective allows one to tailor behavior to capitalize on unique opportunities in current context, but potentially at the cost of losing sight of the big picture. Low-level construal may therefore be associated with unstructured regulation. Following this reasoning, construal level may be an important determinant in whether people respond to stimuli (including priming cues) in a structured versus unstructured regulatory manner.

Supporting this assertion, research suggests that high-level relative to low-level construal makes people more sensitive to their goals and values. As noted earlier, inducing high-level construal by temporally distancing an event promotes identifying actions in terms of the broader goals and values expressed by the acts rather than in terms of the specific means by which to carry out those actions (Liberman & Trope, 1998; see also Fujita, Henderson et al., 2006; Liviatan et al., 2008; Smith & Trope, 2006; Wakslak et al., 2006). This coding of events in terms of ends versus means appears to influence to what degree people make decisions and act in accordance with their goals and values. Research indicates that people are more likely to behave concordantly with their goals and values when they are engaged in high-level rather than low-level construal (e.g., Eyal, Sagristano, Trope, Liberman & Chaiken, 2009; Torelli & Kaikati, 2009; Trope & Liberman, 2000). For example, when given an opportunity to volunteer to help refugees, those participants who endorsed universalism values were more likely to volunteer their time when induced to construe events in high-level, rather than low-level, construal (Torelli & Kaikati, 2009). Thus, high-level relative to low-level construal appears to highlight the goal or value relevance of objects and events, and thus promotes structured rather than unstructured regulation.

Our research on self-control also suggests that whereas high-level construal promotes structured regulation, low-level construal promotes unstructured regulation. When presented with salient alluring temptations, those engaged in high-level rather than low-level construal are more likely to exhibit self-control, making behavioral decisions that are consistent with distal goals (for reviews, see Fujita, 2008; Fujita & Carnevale, 2012). In one study, for example, those concerned about weight loss preferred to eat an apple over a candy bar when engaged in high-level rather than low-level construal (Fujita & Han, 2009). This suggests that despite their immediate salience, people who are engaged in high-level relative to low-level construal are more likely to recognize temptations as inconsistent with their goals. Those engaged in low-level construal, by contrast, appeared to be more sensitive to the behavioral implications of salient cues, engaging in behavior that was inconsistent with their goals. People's behavior thus appears to be characterized by structured rather than unstructured regulation when induced to engage in high-level rather than low-level construal.

Research has also indicated that high-level relative to low-level construal promotes cognitive processes that are consistent with structured versus unstructured regulation, respectively. Most psychological models of self-control emphasize deliberate and effortful inhibition of impulses that are activated (or in some sense "primed") by salient temptations (for a review and critique, see Fujita, 2011). By contrast, our constructionist account suggests that self-control can be achieved by changing the construal or meaning of the temptation stimulus. A dieter may perceive a piece of chocolate cake as a "diet-buster" rather than a "tasty snack." These two interpretations of the same chocolate cake have very different evaluative connotations, which in turn should promote very different behaviors. To the extent that high-level (vs. low-level) construal promotes more goal-consistent construals of events, it should lead people to construct representations of temptations that emphasize their negative rather than positive features. Indeed, research suggests that temptations are evaluated more negatively by those engaged in high-level rather than low-level construal (e.g., Fujita & Han, 2009; Fujita, Trope et al., 2006). These changes in evaluation are evident even when assessed with implicit attitude measures—assessments that do not require conscious deliberation by participants (Fujita & Han, 2009). This latter finding indicates that these changes in evaluation are not likely due to some effortful or deliberative corrective mechanism, but rather to a change in the subjective interpretation or construal of the temptation (for similar distinctions between construal and inhibition, see e.g., Fucito, Juliano, & Toll, 2010; Goldin, McRae, Ramel, & Gross, 2008). High-level relative to low-level construal promotes representations that direct people's attention to the negative goal-relevant features of temptations, which in turn impacts behavioral decisions (Fujita & Han, 2009). Thus, in addition to behavior, high-level relative to low-level construal appears to impact people's evaluative processing in a manner that reflects structured rather than unstructured regulation.

Changes to the associative connections between various constructs in the mind also suggest that high-level (vs. low-level) construal promotes structured (vs. unstructured) regulation. As noted earlier, research suggests that self-control benefits from an asymmetric pattern of associations between temptation and goal concepts, such that temptation cues prime goal cognition, but goal cues do not reciprocally prime temptation cognition (Fishbach et al., 2003; Papies et al., 2008). Supporting the idea that construal level impacts whether people's self-regulation is characterized by structure, our work suggests that these functional asymmetric temptation-goal associations are evident only when people are engaged in high-level rather than low-level construal (Fujita & Sasota, 2011). It is important to note here that assessing temptation-goal associations fundamentally depends on priming methodology. That is, participants are first presented with a temptation or goal stimulus (i.e., the prime) and then with a target stimulus about which they must make a lexical decision (i.e., word vs. non-word). On critical trials, the target stimulus is either a goal or temptation stimulus. When primes and targets are cognitively associated, participants are faster to respond in making their lexical decisions (e.g., Neely, 1977). Our work suggests that whereas temptations and goals can reciprocally prime each other at low-level construal, these associative connections are much more selective and goal relevant at high-level construal: Temptations can prime goals, but goals do not prime temptations (Fujita & Sasota, 2011). This provides initial evidence that construal levels can impact whether and when priming effects are likely to appear. When induced to high-level construal, people's cognitive and behavioral responses to priming stimuli reflect a structured regulatory dynamic that systematizes cognitive associations around valued long-term goals. By contrast when induced to low-level construal, people's reactions appear less structured (and thus bi-directional), leading to behavior that is more confused and open to the influence of contextual cues irrespective of goal relevance—an indication of unstructured regulatory dynamic.[3]

CONSTRUAL LEVELS AND TRADITIONAL PRIMING EFFECTS

Research on the effects of construal level on traditional priming effects on social judgment has revealed inconsistent results. Research by Förster, Liberman, and Kuschel (2008) suggests that high-level, not low-level, construal promotes the assimilation of primed content into social judgment. Thus, when primed with the concept of aggressiveness, perceivers engaged in high-level construal were more likely to judge an ambiguous target as more aggressive than those engaged in low-level construal. In contrast, research by Henderson and Wakslak (2010) suggests that it is low-level, not high-level, construal that promotes assimilation of primed content. They find that when presented with ambiguous behavior, those primed with "reckless" are more likely to evaluate the target negatively than those primed with "adventurous" when engaged in low-level rather than high-level construal. We suggest that this apparent discrepancy in findings reflects the operation of the two dynamics that we propose. High-level construal, by enhancing one's recognition of the relevant goals, promotes priming effects when people perceive priming stimuli to be goal relevant. Low-level construal, by contrast, promotes priming effects via a different mechanism: taking cues from one's environment to determine what one's goals should be. Thus, Förster and colleagues (2008) may document priming effects via structured regulation, whereas Henderson and Wakslak (2010) may document priming effects via unstructured regulation.

Indeed, Henderson and Wakslak (2010) highlight important methodological differences that are consistent with this suggestion. Specifically, Förster and colleagues (2008) presented participants with priming stimuli after manipulating construal level, whereas Henderson and Wakslak (2010) presented priming stimuli before manipulating construal level. The ordering of the construal level and priming manipulations may have altered to what extent priming materials were seen as relevant to the goals of the subsequent judgment task. The greater temporal contiguity between priming manipulation and judgment task in the Förster and colleagues' (2008) work may have led participants to code the primed stimuli as relevant to the goals of the judgment task. Those induced to high-level relative to low-level construal may have thus been more ready to incorporate these goal-relevant cues into their judgments. By contrast, the temporal discontiguity between priming stimuli and judgment task in Henderson and Wakslak's (2010) work may have led participants to code the primed stimuli as irrelevant to the

---

3. Research in computational neuroscience suggests that changes in evaluative associations and asymmetric temptation-goal associations are examples of "gating" (e.g., Hazy, Frank & O'Reilly, 2007). Similar to our construal level argument, this work suggests that there are regions of the brain that represent abstract constructs such as goals, which exert a top-down influence on more basic neural and cognitive networks by biasing specific associations. We extend this work by suggesting situational variables may moderate the degree of top-down influence (see also Fujita et al., 2014; Zelazo & Cunningham, 2007).

goals of the judgment task. Whereas those engaged in high-level construal may have dismissed priming materials as goal irrelevant, those engaged in low-level construal may have been more open to using them as guides to how to respond in the judgment task. Although empirical support for these speculations is still wanting, our approach may help to resolve apparent inconsistencies in the literature.

CONSTRUAL LEVELS AND THE INFLUENCE OF SITUATIONAL CUES: EMBODIMENT AND FLUENCY

Studies examining the impact of construal level on embodiment also support our theoretical framework. Research suggests that people's sensorimotor experiences can exert a powerful contextual influence on people's evaluations and judgments. Research by Wells and Petty (1980), for example, demonstrates that the physical experience of nodding (vs. shaking) one's head enhances people's agreement with concurrently presented persuasive messages. Similarly, wearing a heavy backpack can make distances that must be traversed appear longer (Profitt, Stefannuci, Banton, & Epstein, 2003). Conceptually, embodiment is similar to priming in that it represents an incidental and contextual variable that leads people to think, feel, and act in a cue-consistent manner (e.g., Belding, Brinol, & Petty, 2014; Williams, Huang, & Bargh, 2009). Our framework suggests that the structured regulatory dynamic promoted by high-level construal should lead people to dismiss such cues to the extent that they are perceived as secondary and goal irrelevant to the task at hand. The unstructured regulatory dynamic promoted by low-level construal, by contrast, might be expected to enhance sensitivity to such cues. Indeed, research by Maglio and Trope (2012) supports these predictions. Wearing a heavy backpack had less impact on people's estimations of distances when they were engaged in high-level rather than low-level construal. We might note, too, that our approach suggests that to the extent that sensorimotor experiences are perceived as central rather than incidental to the task at hand, high-level over low-level construal should enhance rather than reduce embodiment effects. No work has yet manipulated the goal relevance of embodied cues to test this hypothesis.

Additional support for our theoretical framework can be found in research on fluency. People use fluency—the subjective ease or difficulty of processing stimuli—as a source of information in evaluating stimuli. Research suggests, for example, that fluent information is judged to be more truthful, inspires greater confidence, and generally promotes more positive evaluations (for review, see Alter & Oppenheimer, 2009). Like embodiment, fluency may also be viewed as an incidental and contextual cue that influences thoughts, feelings, and behavior. Our theoretical framework suggests, then, that the structured regulatory dynamic promoted by high-level construal should lead people to be less sensitive to the effects of fluency as compared to the unstructured regulatory dynamic promoted by low-level construal. Indeed, research by Tsai and Thomas (2011) confirms that high-level construal mitigates the effects of fluency on judgment. Whether an advertisement was clear versus blurry had less impact on participants' evaluation of the product when engaged in high-level versus low-level construal. However, our approach also suggests that high-level relative to low-level construal may at times enhance rather than reduce the effects of fluency, particularly when fluency is perceived as goal relevant to the judgment at hand. In a test of this hypothesis, Tsai and Thomas (2011) manipulated the goal relevance of their participants' fluency experience by having participants base their evaluations either on their subjective feelings (fluency as goal relevant) versus on the information presented by the advertisement (fluency as goal irrelevant). They found that high-level relative to low-level construal increased fluency effects when fluency was goal relevant, but reduced those effects when fluency was goal irrelevant. This work highlights the importance of understanding the distinction between structured versus unstructured regulatory dynamics, and various mechanisms by which incidental and contextual cues can impact judgment, decisions, and behavior.

SUMMARY AND CONCLUSIONS

Prominent non-replications of social psychological priming effects, particularly those related to behavior, highlight the need to understand better the "active ingredients" that produce these effects. Although a great deal of research has been done to understand the ingredients necessary to produce priming effects (i.e., the specific boundary conditions or moderators), we argue that we must also appreciate that there may be different "recipes." In this paper, we have proposed two regulatory dynamics (i.e., recipes) that may foster priming effects via different mechanisms. When engaged in structured regulation, people will be particularly sensitive to the goal relevance of salient stimuli, attending to and responding to goal-relevant stimuli, and ignoring or perhaps even acting in the opposing direction of goal-irrelevant or goal-undermining stimuli. When engaged in unstructured regulation, people may look to cues in their environment as suggestions for what goals to pursue, leading them to be more susceptible to priming effects in general. Although we have suggested construal level as one critical factor that determines which of these two dynamics is more likely, full empirical support for our speculations is still wanting.

Traditional models of priming have at times suggested priming as an example of psychological phenomena in which people are out of control and at the mercy of their environments (e.g., Bargh, 1999). By contrast, our model, like other constructionist models of priming (e.g., Cesario et al., 2006, 2010; Eitam & Higgins, 2010), suggests that priming results from very sophisticated self-regulation processes. Thus, whether people are affected by the priming stimuli presented by stimuli fundamentally depends on understanding the relationship between those materials, the goals the participants have, and the type of regulation dynamic in which those participants are engaged. Understanding priming as reflecting an agentic act of self-regulation, rather than of passive reaction, may provide deeper insight into when and why priming effects occur (or do not occur). We encourage and look forward to future research exploring these possibilities.

REFERENCES

Ainslie, G. (1975). Specious reward: A behavioral theory of impulsiveness and impulse control. *Psychological Bulletin, 82,* 463-496.

Alter, A. L., & Oppenheimer, D. M. (2009). Uniting the tribes of fluency to form a metacognitive nation. *Personality and Social Psychology Review, 13*(3), 219-235.

Anderson, J. R. (1982). The acquisition of cognitive skill. *Psychological Review, 89,* 369-406.

Anderson, J. R. (1983). *The architecture of cognition.* Cambridge, MA: Harvard University Press.

Balcetis, E., & Dunning, D. (2006). See what you want to see: Motivational influences on visual perception. *Journal of Personality and Social Psychology, 91,* 612-625.

Balcetis, E., & Dunning, D. (2010). Wishful seeing: Desired objects are seen as closer. *Psychological Science, 21,* 147-152.

Balcetis, E., Dunning, D., & Granot, Y. (2012). Subjective value determines initial dominance in binocular rivalry. *Journal of Experimental Social Psychology, 48,* 122-129.

Bargh, J. A. (1999). The cognitive monster: The case against the controllability of automatic stereotype effects. In S. Chaiken & Y. Trope (Eds.), *Dual-process theories in social psychology* (pp. 361-382). New York: Guilford.

Bargh, J. A., Chen, M., & Burrows, L. (1996). Automaticity of social behavior: Direct effects of trait construct and stereotype activation on action. *Journal of Personality and Social Psychology, 71*(2), 230-244.

Belding, J. N., Brinol, P., & Petty, R. E. (2014). Wearing unfamiliar objects can influence information processing and evaluation. Manuscript in preparation, The Ohio State University.

Bruner, J. S. (1957). On perceptual readiness. *Psychological Review, 64*(2), 123-152.

Cesario, J., & Jonas, K. J. (2014). Replicability and models of priming: What a resource computation framework can tell us about expectations of replicability. This volume.

Cesario, J., Plaks, J. E., & Higgins, E. T. (2006). Automatic social behavior as motivated preparation to interact. *Journal of Personality and Social Psychology, 90,* 893-910.

Cesario, J., Plaks, J. E., Hagiwara, N., Navarrete, C. D., & Higgins, E. T. (2010). The ecology of automaticity: How situational contingencies shape action semantics and social behavior. *Psychological Science, 21,* 1311-1317

Dijksterhuis, A., & Bargh, J. A. (2001). The perception-behavior expressway: Automatic effects of social perception on social behavior. In M. P. Zanna (Ed.), *Advances in experimental social psychology* (Vol. 33; pp. 1-40). San Diego, CA: Academic Press.

Doyen, S., Klein, O., Pichon, C. L., & Cleeremans, A. (2012). Behavioral priming: It's all in the mind, but whose mind? *PLOS ONE, 7*(1), e29081.

Eitam, B., & Higgins, E. T. (2010). Motivation in mental accessibility: Relevance of a representation (ROAR) as a new framework. *Social and Personality Psychology Compass, 4*(10), 951-967.

Eyal, T. Sagristano, M. D., Trope, Y., Liberman, N., & Chaiken, S. (2009). When values matter: Expressing values in behavioral intentions for the near vs. distant future. *Journal of Experimental Social Psychology, 45,* 35-43.

Fedoroff, I. C., Polivy, J., & Herman, C. P. (1997). The effect of pre-exposure to food cues on the eating behavior of restrained and unrestrained eaters. *Appetite, 28,* 33-47.

Ferguson, M. J., & Bargh, J. A. (2004). Liking is for doing: The effects of goal pursuit on automatic evaluation. *Journal of Personality and Social Psychology, 87*(5), 557-572.

Fishbach, A., Friedman, R. S., & Kruglanski, A. W. (2003). Leading us not into temptation: Momentary allurements elicit overriding goal activation. *Journal of Personality and Social Psychology, 84,* 296-309.

Fishbach, A., & Shah, J. Y. (2006). Self-control in action: Implicit dispositions toward goals and away from temptations. *Journal of Personality and Social Psychology, 90,* 820-832.

Fishbach, A., Zhang, Y., & Trope, Y. (2010). Counteractive evaluation: Asymmetric shifts in the implicit value of conflicting motivations. *Journal of Experimental Social Psychology, 46,* 29-38.

Förster, J., Liberman, N., & Kuschel, S. (2008). The effect of global versus local processing styles on assimilation versus contrast in social judgment. *Journal of Personality and Social Psychology, 94*(4), 579-599.

Freitas, A. L., Gollwitzer, P., & Trope, Y. (2004). The influence of abstract and concrete mindsets on anticipating and guiding others' self-regulatory efforts. *Journal of Experimental Social Psychology, 40*(6), 739-752.

Fucito, L. M., Juliano, L. M., & Toll, B. A. (2010). Cognitive reappraisal and expressive suppression emotion regulation strategies in cigarette smokers. *Nicotine & Tobacco Research, 12*(11), 1156-1161.

Fujita, K. (2008). Seeing the forest beyond the trees: A construal-level approach to self-control. *Social and Personality Psychology Compass, 2*, 1475-1496.

Fujita, K. (2011). On conceptualizing self-control as more than the effortful inhibition of impulses. *Personality and Social Psychology Review, 15*(4), 352-366.

Fujita, K., & Carnevale, J. J. (2012). Transcending temptation through abstraction: The role of construal level in self-control. *Current Directions in Psychological Science, 21*, 248-252.

Fujita, K., Gollwitzer, P. M., & Oettingen, G. (2007). Mindsets and pre-conscious open-mindedness to incidental information. *Journal of Experimental Social Psychology, 43*, 48-61.

Fujita, K., & Han, H. A. (2009). Moving beyond deliberative control of impulses: The effect of construal levels on evaluative associations in self-control conflicts. *Psychological Science, 20*, 799-804.

Fujita, K., Henderson, M., Eng, J., Trope, Y., & Liberman, N. (2006). Spatial distance and mental construal of social events. *Psychological Science, 17*, 278-282.

Fujita, K., & Roberts, J. C. (2010). Promoting prospective self-control through abstraction. *Journal of Experimental Social Psychology, 46*, 1049-1054.

Fujita, K., & Sasota, J. A. (2011). The effect of construal levels on asymmetric temptation-goal cognitive associations. *Social Cognition, 29*, 125-146.

Fujita, K., Trope, Y., Cunningham, W. A., & Liberman, N. (2014). What is control? A conceptual analysis. In J. W. Sherman, B. Gawronski, & Y. Trope (Eds.), *Dual-process theories of the social mind* (pp. 50-68). New York: Guilford.

Fujita, K., Trope, Y., Liberman, N., & Levin-Sagi, M. (2006). Construal levels and self-control. *Journal of Personality and Social Psychology, 90*, 351-367.

Galinsky, A. D., Gruenfeld, D. H., & Magee, J. C. (2003). From power to action. *Journal of Personality and Social Psychology, 85*(3), 453-466.

Ginossar, Z., & Trope, Y. (1987). Problem solving in judgment under uncertainty. *Journal of Personality and Social Psychology, 52*(3), 464-474.

Goldin, P. R., McRae, K., Ramel, W., & Gross, J. J. (2008). The neural bases of emotion regulation: Reappraisal and suppression of negative emotion. *Biological Psychiatry, 63*(6), 577-586.

Gollwitzer, P. M. (1990). Action phases and mind-sets. In E. T. Higgins & R. M. Sorrentino (Eds.), *Handbook of motivation and cognition* (Vol. 2; pp. 53-92). New York: Guilford.

Gollwitzer, P. M., & Kinney, R. F. (1989). Effects of deliberative and implemental mind-sets on illusion of control. *Journal of Personality and Social Psychology, 56*(4), 531-421.

Hazy, T. E., Frank, M. J., & O'Reilly, R. C. (2007). Towards an executive without a homunculus: Computational models of the prefrontal cortex/basal ganglia system. *Philosophical Transactions of the Royal Society B: Biological Sciences, 362*(1485), 1601-1613.

Heckhausen, H., & Gollwitzer, P. (1987). Thought contents and cognitive functioning in motivational versus volitional states of mind. *Motivation and Emotion, 11*(2), 101-120.

Henderson, M. D., Fujita, K., Trope, Y., & Liberman, N. (2006). Transcending the "here": The effect of spatial distance on social judgment. *Journal of Personality and Social Psychology, 91*, 845-856.

Henderson, M. D., & Wakslak, C. J. (2010). Psychological distance and priming: When do semantic primes impact social evaluations? *Personality and Social Psychology Bulletin, 36*(7), 975-985.

Higgins, E. T. (1996). Knowledge activation: Accessibility, applicability, and salience. In E. T. Higgins & A. W. Kruglanski (Eds.), *Social psychology: Handbook of basic principles* (pp. 133-168). New York: Guilford.

Higgins, E. T. (1997). Beyond pleasure and pain. *American Psychologist, 52*(12), 1280-1300.

Higgins, E. T. (1998). Promotion and prevention: Regulatory focus as a motivational principle. In M. P. Zanna (Ed.), *Advances in experimental social psychology* (Vol. 30; pp. 1-46). New York: Academic Press.

Higgins, E. T., Bargh, J. A., & Lombardi, W. J. (1985). Nature of priming effects on categorization. *Journal of Experimental Psychology, 11*(1), 59-69.

Higgins, E. T., Rholes, W. S., & Jones, C. R. (1977). Category accessibility and impression formation. *Journal of Experimental Social Psychology, 13*(2), 141-154.

Higgins, E. T., Roney, C. J. R., Crowe, E., & Hymes, C. (1994). Ideal versus ought predilections for approach and avoidance distinct self-regulatory systems. *Journal of Personality and Social Psychology, 66*(2), 276-286. James, W. (1890). *Principles of psychology*. New York: Henry Holt.

Ledgerwood, A., & Trope, Y., & Liberman, N. (2010). Flexibility and consistency in evaluative responding: The function of construal level. In M. P. Zanna & J. M. Olson (Eds.), *Advances in experimental social psychology* (Vol. 43; pp. 257-295). San Diego, CA: Academic Press.

Lepper, M. R., Greene, D., & Nisbett, R. E. (1973). Undermining children's intrinsic interest with extrinsic reward: A test of the "overjustification" hypothesis. *Journal of Personality and Social Psychology, 26*(1), 123-137.

Liberman, N., Sagristano, M. D., & Trope, Y. (2002). The effect of temporal distance on level of mental construal. *Journal of Experimental Social Psychology, 38*, 523-534.

Liberman, N., & Trope, Y. (1998). The role of feasibility and desirability considerations in near and distant future decisions: A test of temporal construal theory. *Journal of Personality and Social Psychology, 75*(1), 5-18.

Liviatan, I., Trope, Y., & Liberman, N. (2008). Interpersonal similarity as a social distance dimension: Implications for perception of others' actions. *Journal of Experimental Social Psychology, 44*, 1256-1269.

Loersch, C., & Payne, B. K. (2011). The situated inference model: An integrative account of the effects of primes on perception, behavior, and motivation. *Perspectives on Psychological Science, 6*(3), 234-252.

Loersch, C., & Payne, B. K. (2014). Situated inference and the what, who, and where of priming. This volume.

Lombardi, W. J., Higgins, E. T., & Bargh, J. A. (1987). The role of consciousness in priming effects on categorization assimilation versus contrast as a function of awareness of the priming task. *Personality and Social Psychology Bulletin, 13*(3), 411-429.

Maglio, S. J., & Trope, Y. (2012). Disembodiment: Abstract construal attenuates the influence of contextual bodily state in judgment. *Journal of Experimental Psychology: General, 141*(2), 211-216.

Martin, L. L. (1986). Set/reset: Use and disuse of concepts in impression formation. *Journal of Personality and Social Psychology, 51*(3), 493-504.

Mischel, W., Shoda, Y., & Rodriguez, M. L. (1989). Delay of gratification in children. *Science, 244*, 933-938.

Molden, D. C. (2014). Understanding priming effects in social psychology: What is "social priming" and how does it occur? This volume.

Myrseth, K. O. R., & Fishbach, A. (2009): Self-control: A function of knowing when and how to exercise restraint. *Current Directions in Psychological Science, 8*, 247-252.

Neely, J. H. (1977). Semantic priming and retrieval from lexical memory: Roles of inhibitionless spreading activation and limited-capacity attention. *Journal of Experimental Psychology: General, 106*(3), 226-254.

Papies, E., Stroebe, W., & Aarts, H. (2007). Pleasure in the mind: Restrained eating and spontaneous hedonic thoughts about food. *Journal of Experimental Social Psychology, 43*, 810-817.

Papies, E., Stroebe, W., & Aarts, H. (2008). Healthy cognition: Processes of self-regulatory success in restrained eating. *Personality and Social Psychology Bulletin, 34*, 1290-1300.

Proffitt, D. R., Stefanucci, J. K., Banton, T., & Epstein, W. (2003). The role of effort in perceiving distance. *Psychological Science, 14,* 106-112.

Rachlin, H. (2000). *The science of self-control.* Cambridge, MA: Harvard University Press.

Sayette, M. A., & Hufford, M. R. (1997). Effects of smoking urge on generation of smoking-related information. *Journal of Applied Social Psychology, 27,* 1395-1405.

Scholer, A. A., Zou, X., Fujita, K., Stroessner, S. J., & Higgins, E. T. (2010). When risk-seeking becomes a motivational necessity. *Journal of Personality and Social Psychology, 99,* 215-231.

Schröder, T., & Thagard, P. (2013). The affective meanings of automatic social behaviors: Three mechanisms that explain priming. *Psychological Review, 120*(1), 255-280.

Schröder, T., & Thagard, P. (2014). Priming: Constraint satisfaction and interactive competition. This volume.

Shanks, D. R., Newell, B. R., Lee, E. H., Balakrishnan, D., Ekelund, L., Cenac, Z., Kawadia, K., & Moore, C. (2013). Priming intelligent behavior: An elusive phenomenon. *PLOS ONE, 8*(4), e56515.

Smith, E. R. (1984). Model of social inference processes. *Psychological Review, 91*(3), 392-413.

Smith, E. R., & Branscombe, N. R. (1987). Procedurally mediated social inferences: The case of category accessibility effects. *Journal of Experimental Social Psychology, 23*(5), 361-382.

Smith, P. K., & Trope, Y. (2006). You focus on the forest when you're in charge of the trees: Power priming and abstract information processing. *Journal of Personality and Social Psychology, 90,* 578-596.

Srull, T. K., & Wyer, R. S. (1980). Category accessibility and social perception: Some implications for the study of person memory and interpersonal judgments. *Journal of Personality and Social Psychology, 38*(6), 841-856.

Taylor, S., & Gollwitzer, P. (1995). Effects of mindset on positive illusions. *Journal of Personality and Social Psychology, 69*(2), 213-226.

Thaler, R. H., & Shefrin, H. M. (1981). An economic theory of self-control. *Journal of Political Economy, 89,* 392-406.

Todorov, A., Goren, A., & Trope, Y. (2007). Probability as a psychological distance: Construal and preference. *Journal of Experimental Social Psychology, 43,* 473-482.

Torelli, C. J. & Kaikati, A. M. (2009). Values as predictors of judgments and behaviors: The role of abstract and concrete mindsets. *Journal of Personality and Social Psychology, 96,* 231-247.

Trope, Y., & Fishbach, A. (2005). Going beyond the motivation given: Self-control and situational control over behavior. In R. R. Hassin, J. Uleman, & J. A. Bargh (Eds.), *The new unconscious* (pp. 537-565), New York: Oxford University Press.

Trope, Y., & Liberman, N. (2000). Temporal construal and time-dependent changes in preference. *Journal of Personality and Social Psychology, 79,* 876-889.

Trope, Y., & Liberman, N. (2003). Temporal construal. *Psychological Review, 110,* 403-421.

Trope, Y., & Liberman, N. (2010). Construal-level theory of psychological distance. *Psychological Review, 117,* 440-463.

Tsai, C. I., & Thomas, M. (2011). When does feeling of fluency matter? How abstract and concrete thinking influence fluency effects. *Psychological Science, 22*(3), 348-354.

Vallacher, R. R., & Wegner, D. M. (1987). What do people think they're doing? Action identification and human behavior. *Psychological Review, 94,* 3-15.

Vallacher, R. R., & Wegner, D. M. (1989). Levels of personal agency: Individual variation in action identification. *Journal of Personality and Social Psychology, 57*(4), 660-671.

Wakslak, C. J., Trope, Y., Liberman, N., & Alony, R. (2006). Seeing the forest when entry is unlikely: Probability and the mental representation of events. *Journal of Experimental Psychology: General, 135,* 641-653.

Wegener, D. T., & Petty, R. E. (1995). Flexible correction processes in social judgment: The role of naive theories in corrections for perceived bias. *Journal of Personality and Social Psychology, 68*(1), 36-51.

Wells, G. L., & Petty, R. E. (1980). The effects of overt head movements on persuasion: Compatibility and incompatibility of responses. *Basic and Applied Social Psychology, 1,* 219-230.

Wheeler, S. C., DeMarree, K. G., & Petty, R. E. (2007). Understanding the role of the self in prime-to-behavior effects: The active-self account. *Personality and Social Psychology Review, 11*(3), 234-261.

Wheeler, S. C., DeMarree, K. G., & Petty, R. E. (2014). Understanding prime-to-behavior effects: Insights from the active-self account. This volume.

Wheeler, S. C., & Petty, R. E. (2001). The effects of stereotype activation on behavior: A review of possible mechanisms. *Psychological Bulletin, 127*(6), 797-826.

Williams, L. E., Huang, J. Y., & Bargh, J. A. (2009). The scaffolded mind: Higher mental processes are grounded in early experience of the physical world. *European Journal of Social Psychology, 39*, 1257-1267.

Young, A. I., & Fazio, R. H. (2013). Attitude accessibility as a determinant of object construal and evaluation. *Journal of Experimental Social Psychology, 49*(3), 404-418.

Zelazo, P. D., & Cunningham, W. (2007). Executive function: Mechanisms underlying emotion regulation. In J. Gross (Ed.), *Handbook of emotion regulation* (pp. 135-158). New York: Guilford.

WHEN AND HOW SOCIAL PRIMING OCCURS

PRIME NUMBERS: ANCHORING AND ITS IMPLICATIONS FOR THEORIES OF BEHAVIOR PRIMING

Ben R. Newell
University of New South Wales, Sydney, Australia

David R. Shanks
University College London, London, United Kingdom

>Subtle primes can influence behavior, often in ways that seem irrational. Anchoring provides a compelling illustration of this: judgments can be influenced by anchors even when the anchors are known to be irrelevant and uninformative. In this chapter, we selectively examine the anchoring literature in order to evaluate a theoretical framework which has been employed to interpret many social and other priming effects. In this framework, primes are assumed to have broad effects, influencing a wide range of possible downstream behaviors, and these influences are largely automatic. The anchoring literature supports neither of these hypotheses. Anchors have narrow effects on behavior with little transfer across judgments, these effects can be controlled, and deliberate engagement with the anchor is a prerequisite for obtaining influences on later judgments. We question whether priming studies reveal evidence for the sort of automatic and consequential mental processes that are commonly proposed.

Can behavior be influenced by subtle cues in the environment? Can such influences occur when the cues are in some normative or informational sense irrelevant to the behavior in question? And if the answer to these questions is "yes," what are the psychological mechanisms that mediate these influences? We take it that these questions lie at the heart of recent debates about "social" and "behavior" priming (henceforth "priming").

We thank Adam Harris, Magda Osman, Danny Oppenheimer, and Piotr Winkielman for many helpful discussions. Preparation of this paper was supported in part by an Australian Research Council Future Fellowship (FT110100151) awarded to Ben Newell.

Address correspondence to David R. Shanks, Division of Psychology and Language Sciences, University College London, 26 Bedford Way, London WC1H 0AP, United Kingdom. E-mail: d.shanks@ucl.ac.uk.

Although much of the recent controversy in this field has centered on the reality of some particularly eye-catching priming effects, the existence of subtle priming effects in general can hardly be disputed. Whether or not people can be primed to behave more or less intelligently by thinking about professors or soccer hooligans (Dijksterhuis & van Knippenberg, 1998; Shanks et al., 2013) or think differently about their emotional closeness to their family members after graphing a pair of points close or far apart on paper (Pashler, Coburn, & Harris, 2012; Williams & Bargh, 2008), no one seriously doubts that many behaviors can be subtly influenced. There are over 1,600 articles on Web of Science (WoS) on the priming of lexical decisions, for instance, where the speed to decide whether a letter string is a word or not is influenced by a preceding prime event, often the brief presentation of another letter string. Nor can it be doubted that long-lasting influences can occur. There are over 2,000 WoS articles on repetition priming, in which some response to the second presentation of a word, picture, or other item is altered as a result of an earlier presentation of the same item, often a long time (hours or days) previously. A striking illustration (reprinted in Gregory, 2005) shows a Dalmatian dog in a dappled image. Successful identification of this dog in the image can induce one-shot learning (priming) and affect perception of the same image years later.

In that case, why are priming effects so controversial? Why have many investigators been so unwilling to concede that asking participants to read sentences containing words related to the concept "old age" can induce them to walk more slowly down a corridor (Bargh, Chen, & Burrows, 1996; Doyen, Klein, Pichon, & Cleeremans, 2012)? Of course, one answer to this question is that behavior priming studies have focused attention on a range of dubious research practices that probably pervade the whole of psychology. Many priming studies have been underpowered, employed questionable statistical methods, or are simply unreplicable (excellent discussions of these issues in relation to experimental psychology generally can be found in Asendorpf et al., 2013; Bakker & Wicherts, 2011; Bertamini & Munafò, 2012; Francis, 2012; Klein et al., 2012; Kruschke, 2013; Pashler & Harris, 2012; Rouder, Speckman, Sun, Morey, & Iverson, 2009; Schimmack, 2012; Simmons, Nelson, & Simonsohn, 2011).

Another possible answer is that whereas standard priming effects such as lexical and repetition priming seem in some sense to be rational, many other behavior priming effects seem distinctly irrational. If one were designing a system for the rapid decoding of letter strings, then it might make sense for it to be biased by what was perceived a few tens or hundreds of milliseconds previously. If one were designing a system for identifying hidden objects, it might make sense to allow it to access and be influenced by memories of similar objects seen in the past. But how can it be rational for judgments about our emotional closeness to our family members to be affected by the proximity of a pair of points we have connected on a sheet of paper, or for our judgments of risk to be influenced by the activation of romantic thoughts (Greitemeyer, Kastenmüller, & Fischer, 2013)? Although it might be hard to reconcile such findings with rationalistic views of mind and behavior, we do not believe this provides reasonable grounds for doubting the reality of these priming effects themselves. In the present chapter, our focus will be on one particular priming effect, namely anchoring, and there is abundant evidence that this effect can often be profoundly irrational. For example, people's judgments can be influenced by an anchor even when they have seen that the anchor was randomly generated (Chapman & Johnson, 2002).

If the seeming irrationality of some priming effects is not a good reason to doubt their reality, then how else can we explain the persistent doubts that researchers have expressed? The answer that we explore here is that priming effects have tended to be couched in a theoretical framework which many researchers find unconvincing and that resistance to the framework has led to doubts about the experimental findings on which that framework is based. In brief, priming effects have been taken as evidence for the idea that primes automatically trigger mental processes, and that this triggering can have widespread consequences (e.g., Bargh, 2006). For instance, in reviewing the literature, Bargh and Huang (2009, p. 128) asserted that:

> [T]his priming research has shown that the mere, passive perception of environmental events directly triggers higher mental processes in the absence of any involvement by conscious, intentional processes

while Loersch and Payne (2011, p. 235) suggested that:

> If, for example, people were exposed to words related to the concept of hostility (e.g., "hit," "punch," "aggress"), it could reasonably be predicted that they would subsequently (a) be faster to identify a gun (semantic priming; Meyer & Schvaneveldt, 1971); (b) perceive another individual as more hostile (construal priming; Higgins, Rholes, & Jones, 1977; Srull & Wyer, 1979); (c) behave in a more hostile manner themselves (behavior priming; Carver, Ganellen, Froming, & Chambers, 1983); and (d) become motivated to actively seek out an opportunity to aggress against some other person or object (goal priming; Todorov & Bargh, 2002).

Thus, priming effects are viewed as arising unconsciously and automatically, beyond the individual's control, and with wide-ranging consequences on behavior. By comparison to typical theoretical models for lexical and repetition priming (Lachter, Forster, & Ruthruff, 2004; McNamara, 1992; Tenpenny, 1995), these are striking assertions because decades of research have raised more questions than answers concerning automatic and unconscious effects generally (Newell & Shanks, 2014), and a wealth of research in cognitive psychology has shown that far from being broad in their consequences, primes tend to have very narrow effects on judgments and behavior.

ANCHORING AS PRIMING

In the present chapter, we analyze these claims in the context of anchoring. Thus, we take as our domain a priming effect which is both beyond dispute in terms of replicability and which undoubtedly has all the hallmarks of the sort of irrationality that makes many of the headline priming effects so eye-catching. We ask whether the evidence supports the idea that anchors can have automatic and unconscious influences on judgments and whether their effects are narrow or broad. We assume a relatively broad definition of priming as simply reflecting any influence on later behavior (be it reports of judgments, impressions, attitudes, choices, or any other overt and observable act) of prior stimuli or events without deliberate intent to be influenced by them. Whereas some authors (e.g., Molden, this volume) prefer to include automaticity in their definition, we regard the question of whether examples of priming are or are not automatic as an empirical, not a definitional, matter.

A typical anchoring experiment employs a two-step procedure. In the first step, participants are asked whether the target attribute is higher or lower than the anchor, and in the second step, they give a numerical estimate of the target attribute. Thus, the first step might involve deciding whether John Kennedy first became president before or after 1962, and the second stating in which year he first became president. Anchoring is obtained if the estimate is drawn towards the anchor. Although anchoring effects might seem at first glance entirely consistent with deliberative thinking (and indeed it has been argued that anchoring in many circumstances may be a rational response by the individual to the implied communicative intent of the experimenter to transmit useful information—see Mussweiler & Strack, 1999), they are pervasive even in situations where the individual knows that the anchor value is uninformative, for instance when the person generates it by reading the last two digits of their social security number (Ariely, Loewenstein, & Prelec, 2003). Equally striking is Critcher and Gilovich's (2008) demonstration that incidental anchors can bias judgments: they found that participants' estimates of how much they would pay for a meal in a restaurant depicted in a photograph were higher if it was called Studio 97 than Studio 17, even though they were not explicitly required to think about the restaurant's name (we return to this study later).

Although our focus on anchoring will inevitably restrict the generality of the conclusions we can draw, we contend that anchoring serves as a prototypical example of the sorts of priming effects that have been the subject of so much recent controversy. If priming is defined as an incidental influence of stimuli or events on subsequent behavior, then clearly anchoring is an instance of priming (see Kahneman, 2011). Moreover, the significance of anchoring is probably considerably greater than for some other priming effects. Even if people think differently about their emotional closeness to their family members after graphing a pair of points close or far apart on paper (a questionable claim: Pashler et al., 2012), the wider consequences of such priming would be fairly modest. In contrast, anchors have been shown to influence buying and selling prices, purchasing decisions, credit card repayments, negotiation outcomes, jury verdicts, and so forth. As with repetition priming (Roediger & McDermott, 1993), anchoring can be long-lasting: anchors can bias judgments made even a week later (Mussweiler, 2001).

It is fundamental to emphasize that anchoring typically involves much more than simply priming numbers. First, it involves magnitudes rather than numerical concepts, and second, it is often mediated by priming of semantic features of the target object. When, as a result of some anchoring induction, participants give a larger estimate of the number of calories in a cheeseburger, this is not simply because a particular number has become more mentally accessible: they actually conceptualize the cheeseburger as being located at a different point on the calorie scale. Frederick and Mochon (2012) showed participants a list of 13 food items in ascending order from least caloric (hard-boiled egg) to most caloric (Burger King Whopper with cheese) and asked them to choose the item they judged closest to 400 calories. When participants had previously estimated an average apple's calories, they chose a more calorific item from the set. As this example illustrates, anchoring effects occur even when no numerical estimation is required. They also occur when the anchor is entirely non-numerical, and hence when no number processing is involved at all. For example, LeBoeuf and Shafir (2006) asked participants in one condition to add pennies to an empty cup, while those in another condition removed pennies from a cup which initially weighed 12 ounces, until the cup weighed the same as another cup they had held and subjectively weighed earlier and which actually weighed 6 ounces. The starting weight of the cup acted as an anchor such that final cup weights were larger in the group adjusting downwards from a high anchor (12 ounces) than in the group adjusting upwards from an empty cup (0 ounces). In other such physical, non-numerical anchoring studies, LeBoeuf and Shafir used lines of different length or music clips of different loudness as anchors.

Moreover, in many instances anchoring is mediated by selective semantic priming of the target's features. A compelling illustration of this was provided by Mussweiler and Strack (2000). They first asked participants to judge whether the annual mean temperature in Germany is higher or lower than 20°C. As a result of this standard high anchoring induction, participants decided more quickly that letter strings like *swim* and *beach* were valid words compared to *frost* and *winter*, while the converse pattern was found for other participants for whom the anchor was low, 5°C. Thus, the anchor changed the way in which participants conceptualized the target, Germany, selectively making some of its features more accessible than others. These demonstrations that anchoring extends beyond just the mental accessibility of numbers are important because if anchoring simply pertained to numerical concepts, one might legitimately wonder whether it has any implications for priming in general, given the obvious difference between the narrow conceptual representations primed by exposure to discrete numbers and the broader representations involved in other forms of semantic, trait, stereotype, goal, or behavior priming.

To what extent is anchoring an automatic process which transfers broadly across a range of judgments and behaviors? Automaticity is of course a complex concept, but here we adopt the standard viewpoint (Bargh, 1994; Moors & De Houwer, 2006) that it is characterized by (some or all of) four key features, which in the context of priming are: (1) absence of awareness of the prime, (2) absence of awareness of the prime's effect on behavior, (3) uncontrollability of the prime's influence, and (4) persistence of the prime's influence even when cognitive resources are diminished. We evaluate anchoring against the first three of these features. The fourth criterion has not been the subject of much research in the anchoring literature (though see footnote 3). To be clear, we do not assume that any one of these features is more important than the others, nor do we assume that anchoring would have to meet all of the criteria to be recognized as (at least in some sense) an automatic and unconscious process.

PROCESSING ACCOUNTS OF ANCHORING

To set the scene for our assessment of whether anchoring is an automatic process which transfers broadly, it is important to briefly discuss the range of information-processing accounts of anchoring that have been developed, as a way of introducing key explanatory constructs. A considerable body of research has explored two general classes of explanation. In the anchoring-and-adjustment account, which was first proposed by Tversky and Kahneman (1974), individuals are assumed to take the anchor as a reasonable starting point for their judgment and then move away from it as they retrieve relevant information from memory. However, these adjustments are assumed to be conservative and insufficient. In the selective accessibility model (Strack & Mussweiler, 1997), in contrast, the anchor is assumed to render anchor-consistent features of the target of judgment accessible via a process of semantic activation. These activated features then bias subsequent judgments. For example, if participants in the first step are asked to decide whether a typical Mercedes-Benz car costs more or less than €40,000, they might access the knowledge that they are usually classified as luxury cars. When asked in the second step to estimate the cost of a typical Mercedes-Benz car, participants rely heavily on whatever knowledge is most accessible, and the activated knowledge (luxury car) therefore plays a larger role in judgment formation than it would if it had not been activated by the anchor.

A large number of studies (see Chapman & Johnson, 2002) have sought to test these and other accounts of anchoring. A common viewpoint is that some forms of anchoring are best explained by anchoring-and-adjustment and others by selective accessibility. For instance, Kahneman (2011) interprets the former as a System 2 capacity (effortful, slow, conscious) and the latter as a System 1 capacity (automatic, fast, unconscious), each being evoked under different circumstances. Similarly, the attitudinal model of Wegener and colleagues (2010) distinguishes thoughtful from non-thoughtful routes to anchoring. These models share the assumption that anchoring, at least under some circumstances, can be a non-deliberative, automatic process. What is the evidence for this key claim?

SUBLIMINAL PRIMING

One way of demonstrating that anchoring can occur automatically is to show that anchors influence judgments even when they are barely attended to and are not deliberately processed as part of the task. Critcher and Gilovich (2008) examined this possibility by asking participants to make judgments about scenarios that were accompanied by photographs incorporating incidental anchors. In one experiment, for instance, a fictitious college linebacker, Stan Fischer, was described alongside a photograph of him wearing a jersey with either the number 54 (low anchor) or 94 (high anchor). Despite the fact that participants were not required to make any explicit judgment about the jersey number (as they would in a conventional anchoring task)—and indeed may have barely registered it—participants nevertheless judged Fischer more likely to register a sack in the conference playoff game in the high than in the low anchor condition.

It is nevertheless possible that at least some participants did think about the jersey number and that conscious reflection is a prerequisite for anchoring even in situations like this. A more compelling, though controversial, technique for demonstrating the automaticity of priming effects is to present the anchor prime subliminally, outside awareness. It is intriguing that in the wake of a comprehensive methodological debate nearly 30 years ago (Holender, 1986), subliminal processing was afforded a rather modest role in most theoretical debates about the causation of behavior. Yet in recent years there has been a wealth of claims concerning the importance of the unconscious in behavior, including some striking reports of subliminal priming effects, among them anchoring. Here, we do not attempt to review this extensive literature. We do, however, briefly comment on the pervasive methodological problems that plague interpretation of results in this field (Holender, 1986; J. Miller, 2000; Pratte & Rouder, 2009), and we illustrate these problems with reference to claims about subliminal influences on anchoring.

Adaval and Wyer (2011) asked participants to estimate how much they would be willing to pay for a DVD player or a pair of shoes. Beforehand, prime anchors that were either low (e.g., HK$112) or high (e.g., HK$9,779) were flashed for 16 msec on the computer display and masked to render them invisible. Adaval and Wyer found a typical anchoring effect in that participants were willing to pay more after a high than a low anchor (though the effect was only significant for the DVD player question and not for the shoes question). How did Adaval and Wyer confirm that the anchors were truly invisible? After making their judgments, participants were shown a further masked prime sequence, but this time were asked to write down whatever they saw after each trial. Twenty such trials were presented. No participant reported seeing any of the subliminal primes.

There are substantial problems with the inference that unconscious anchors exerted an influence on judgments in this study. For instance, the form of awareness check employed by Adaval and Wyer is susceptible to bias if participants' confidence about seeing the anchor prime is low. Even if they can actually see the prime occasionally, they may nonetheless give a negative report because their judgment is uncertain and they adopt a conservative response criterion. Bias can easily be reduced or eliminated by employing a procedure in which participants have to make a forced choice, such as "Was the briefly flashed number HK$112 or HK$9,779?"

In one of their experiments, Mussweiler and Englich (2005) asked participants to judge the annual mean temperature in Germany after thinking about this question for 1 minute, during which a briefly presented anchor was flashed 10 times. The anchor value was either high (20) or low (5) and was flashed for 15 msec every 6 seconds during the thinking period and masked by a consonant string. Judgments assimilated towards the anchor value: the temperature was estimated as higher after a high than after a low anchor. To evaluate whether the primes were consciously perceived, Mussweiler and Englich used a funnel debriefing in which a series of more and more specific questions was asked about the priming stage. They reported that 2 of 37 participants indicated some awareness, whereas the remainder did not. These 2 participants were excluded from the analysis. Many commentators have noted the limitations of such recall-based awareness assessments, however (Dawson & Reardon, 1973; Newell & Shanks, 2014), and have pointed out that their retrospective nature means that they are evaluating awareness for events that happened some time previously and that low confidence knowledge may be withheld. We thus need to examine evidence from alternative and more sensitive awareness checks.

In a further experiment (Study 2), Mussweiler and Englich (2005) used a more comprehensive awareness check. In this study, participants judged the average price of a mid-sized car while high (30,000) or low (10,000) anchors were flashed during the thinking period. After making their judgments (which again showed a reliable anchoring effect), participants were presented with a prime phase once again but this time were told that briefly presented numbers were being flashed and were asked to judge whether 10,000 or 30,000 was the flashed digit string. Ten such prime identification trials were presented. Mussweiler and Englich found that performance in this test was virtually at chance (50% correct) and concluded that the primes were indeed invisible.

A prime identification test such as this is methodologically far more sound and permits stronger inferences than a funnel debriefing or the type of test used by Adaval and Wyer (2011). It is not susceptible to the complaint that it relies on retrospective recall or to the objection that it might be contaminated by response bias: Since the test demands a forced choice between the two anchor values, participants should select the string they saw regardless of their confidence. But despite these advantages, such a test can still contribute towards the reporting of false positive subliminal perception results. One reason for this is that forced-choice tests with few trials are underpowered for detecting what is likely to be weak awareness. For example, imagine that a participant has a "true" long-run probability of 0.6 to discriminate the high and low anchors. This participant may consciously see enough of the anchors to show an entirely standard and supraliminal anchoring effect. But with only 10 binary choice trials, there is a high probability (almost .4) that this participant will be misclassified by the forced-choice awareness test (that is, will make 5 or fewer correct identifications and hence be judged to lack any awareness of the prime). This problem persists even when data are aggregated across participants. A typical statistical test based on only a small number of binary observations per participant is likely to have only low or moderate power to reject the hypothesis that discrimination is weakly but truly above chance (e.g., 0.6) (Rouder, Morey, Speckman, & Pratte, 2007). To eliminate or at least ameliorate this problem, the awareness test needs to employ far more than 10 trials (say 50).

Worse still, Pratte and Rouder (2009) have shown that typical forced-choice tests used to measure awareness in subliminal perception experiments (such as that used by Mussweiler and Englich) may significantly underestimate conscious perception as a result of task difficulty. Because tests assessing perception of near-threshold stimuli are very difficult, participants may lose motivation. In their experiments, Pratte and Rouder maintained participants' motivation by intermixing above-threshold and near-threshold stimuli and found that identification of the near-threshold stimuli increased reliably. Thus, brief stimulus presentations that would have been regarded as subliminal in a conventional awareness test were found to be supraliminal in a modified test designed to be more closely equated to the main priming test in terms of difficulty. Until subliminal priming experiments are able to rule out such artifacts, their conclusions will remain in doubt. Recent methodological advances (e.g., Rouder et al., 2007) offer the promise of more clear-cut tests of subliminal perception in the future.

Even if these subliminal priming experiments fail to provide compelling evidence that anchoring can occur automatically,[1] isn't the type of demonstration provided by Critcher and Gilovich (that incidental and irrelevant numbers can anchor judgments) sufficient to persuade us that anchoring can nevertheless occur automatically? It is common to think of automaticity as a continuum, so doesn't the effect of a jersey number on a judgment establish that anchoring extends up

---

1. Reitsma-van Rooijen and Daamen (2006) were unable to obtain a subliminal anchoring effect under normal conditions but did obtain an effect when judgments were made under time pressure.

to the automatic end of this continuum? The problem with this conclusion is that the effects documented by Critcher and Gilovich (2008) were remarkably fragile. From a Bayesian statistical perspective, the evidence they reported actually provides more support for the null hypothesis (no anchoring) than for the experimental hypothesis. As Matthews (2011) has noted, a study with a very large sample size and a test statistic that is only just significant provides evidence that should, if anything, persuade us more firmly to believe the null hypothesis. Further studies of incidental anchoring are much needed.

The studies reviewed in this section assess whether the simple presentation of a number can induce anchoring, and thus employ a "basic" anchoring method that is rather different from the standard method in which an explicit comparative judgment is made in relation to the anchor. Basic anchoring effects are extremely fragile though even when some degree of deliberate processing of the anchor is required, a finding which must cast further doubt on the subliminal effects discussed above. Wilson, Houston, Etling, and Brekke (1996) found that numbers influenced judgments if participants had copied 5 pages of these numbers, not if they had copied only one. Brewer and Chapman (2002) found that even this effect was weak and restricted to some very specific circumstances. It is certainly not the case that numbers randomly and incidentally encountered in the environment inevitably induce anchoring effects.

AWARENESS OF THE INFLUENCE OF AN ANCHOR

Studies employing supposedly subliminal stimuli seek to evaluate the effect of anchors when the individual is unaware of the anchor's presence. A related question, which focuses on a different criterion for automaticity, is whether individuals show anchoring even when they are unaware of the influence of the anchor. Even when the anchor is consciously perceived and processed, as it is in a typical anchoring situation, its influence may not be consciously registered, and in that case we would have to conclude that anchoring can be an automatic and unintentional process.

In Wilson and colleagues' (1996) study, participants were asked to estimate the number of physicians in the local phone book after processing an irrelevant numerical anchor, and were subsequently asked to assess the influence that the anchor had had on their physician estimates on a 9-point scale ranging from 1 ("decreased it a great deal") to 9 ("increased it a great deal"). Wilson and colleagues did not report the group mean estimate on this scale, so it is not known whether participants on average believed their physician estimates were affected by the anchor. Wilson and colleagues did state, however, that about three-quarters of the participants gave a rating of 5, labeled "have no effect," and despite believing there was no influence, these participants showed a robust anchoring effect. On the other hand, when evaluated across all participants, estimates of how much they were influenced did correlate significantly with their physician estimates, and as Wilson and colleagues concluded (p. 393), "the higher people's estimates of the number of doctors, the more they believed they were influenced by the anchor value." Thus, the conclusion of this study is not clear-cut: The average participant reported an influence of the anchor, while at the same time many participants who reported that it had no influence on them were affected by the anchor.

In an applied setting, Northcraft and Neale (1987) found that anchors (suggested listing prices) influenced the pricing decisions that both non-experts (students) and professional real estate agents made when they spent 20 minutes viewing a residential property. On a debriefing questionnaire, about half the non-experts reported that they had given consideration to the anchor in deriving their pricing decisions. Rather fewer (around a quarter) of the real estate agents did so. Thus, sizable numbers of participants (especially experts) did not report an influence of the anchor on their judgments. Interpretation of this pattern is not straightforward, however. First of all, the experts were rather less (though nonsignificantly) affected by the anchor,[2] so reports of an influence of the anchor correlated overall with anchoring itself. Second, it is possible that the anchoring effect was entirely borne by those participants who reported incorporating the anchor into their estimates. This may be unlikely, given how robust anchoring effects tend to be, but future research could usefully separate anchoring effects in aware and unaware individuals. Third, it is notoriously difficult to assess awareness exhaustively (e.g., Ericsson & Simon, 1984; Newell & Shanks, 2014) and experts may have avoided reporting use of the anchor because of the situational demands. As Northcraft and Neale (1987, p. 95) themselves put it, "[I]t remains an open question whether experts' denial of the use of listing price as a consideration in valuing property reflects a lack of awareness of their use of listing price as a consideration, or simply an unwillingness to acknowledge publicly their dependence on an admittedly inappropriate piece of information."

One methodological issue that future studies might address is that in order to accurately report the causal effect of an anchor, participants normatively need to experience both what their estimates would be with and without the anchor, and of course this is unfeasible in what is necessarily a between-subjects design in which different groups receiving different anchors are compared. As Hogarth (2014) has noted, mismatches may occur between verbal reports about causal influences and the reality of those influences as a result of experimenters and participants adopting different perspectives on the "causal field." An experimental participant might deny that an anchor influenced her behavior, whereas an experimenter able to compare behavior between subjects in conditions of low or high anchors might conclude in contrast that there was an influence. Such differences in conceptualization of the causal field might lead to erroneous conclusions, as the participant is surely right that (from her perspective) she only experienced one value of the anchor and therefore does not have the evidence necessary to assign it a causal role.

CAN THE INFLUENCE OF ANCHORS BE INTENTIONALLY AVOIDED?

We argue that it is a misconception to view priming effects as low level, unconscious, and automatic. A powerful reason why early studies of anchoring have been taken as providing some encouragement to this viewpoint is that they ap-

---

2. Combining all 4 pricing estimates participants made in Experiment 2, the lowest and highest anchors induced a 12% influence on experts' estimates, while the effect was more than twice as large, 27%, in the non-experts.

peared to show that people find it very hard to avoid being influenced by anchors. Of course, if subliminal anchoring can occur, or if anchors can bias judgments even when individuals are unaware of this influence, then it would follow that anchoring effects cannot always be avoided: If you don't believe the anchor has affected you, then there is subjectively no influence that you believe needs avoiding. Yet the preceding sections have highlighted that the evidence for these effects is rather weak. The controllability of the influence of anchors thus relates to a different aspect of the standard multi-faceted conception of automaticity.

Early studies examining avoidance more directly revealed that the bias is undiminished by forewarning participants about the potential influence of anchors (Wilson et al., 1996) and that increased motivation to be accurate (induced for instance by financial incentives) is usually ineffective (see Chapman & Johnson, 2002). But more recently it has become apparent that considerable control can be exerted over the bias, at variance with the automaticity view. Epley and Gilovich (2005) showed that the effect of self-generated anchors was influenced by financial incentives. For instance, when participants are asked to estimate the freezing point of vodka, they tend to generate the freezing point of water (0°C) and use this as an anchor, an effect that was attenuated by an explicit incentive designed to encourage participants to think more deeply.

Although this result suggests that the proposed automaticity of anchoring has been overstated, Epley and Gilovich also found that incentives had no effect on the size of the bias induced by externally generated anchors. Thus, in a standard situation in which participants first judged whether Mt. Everest is higher than 45,500 feet and then judged its height, the influence of the anchor was unaffected by incentives. Epley and Gilovich proposed that there are multiple (or at least two) forms of anchoring bias, one of which depends on controlled deliberate thought (self-generated anchors) and one of which depends on automatic semantic priming (externally generated anchors), but even this viewpoint may overstate the role of automatic processes. Simmons, LeBoeuf, and Nelson (2010) found that they could attenuate both forms of anchoring with incentives for accuracy. Their key insight was that even if participants are highly motivated and have the deliberative capacity to overcome an anchor's influence, they may have little ability to do so if they are uncertain about which way to adjust from the anchor. Imagine that you are asked to estimate the year in which the actor Jack Nicholson was born (the correct answer is 1937) and are given 1945 as an anchor. In other words, you first decide whether he was born before or after 1945, and then estimate the correct year. Under conditions of high motivation, you are aware that you need to adjust sufficiently from the anchor, but the problem is that you don't know whether the anchor is pulling your estimate up or down. You don't know what your estimate would have been counterfactually in the absence of the anchor, and hence do not know whether the 1945 anchor is pulling a low counterfactual estimate upwards or a high counterfactual estimate downwards. If you believe that the anchor is pulling your estimate upwards, then you will adjust downwards. If you believe that the anchor is pulling your estimate downwards, then you will adjust upwards. But one of these influences will result in a greater, not weaker, influence of the anchor on your answer. It is easy to see that by aggregating across items for some of which the motivated adjustment is in the correct direction and for some of which it is in the incorrect direction, a null effect of motivation can be obtained.

Simmons and colleagues tested this account in a number of ways. For example, they showed that motivation does reduce the anchoring effect when the anchor value is implausible (such as a date of 1977 for Jack Nicholson's birth). Under such circumstances, where the anchor value is so extreme that it can immediately be recognized as being too high, participants were unlikely to be in any doubt about the required direction of adjustment.

The fact that the influence of an anchor on judgments can be attenuated under conditions of heightened motivation (through financial incentives) speaks directly against the hypothesis that anchors affect judgments automatically. Rather, the anchor is one piece of evidence taken into account in the individual's deliberative thinking. Further support for this alternative viewpoint comes from two sources. First, Epley and Gilovich (2006) found that overcoming the effects of self-generated anchors was impaired under conditions of cognitive load. Thus deliberative System 2 capacity is required by whatever process attenuates anchoring.[3] Second, it has been demonstrated that the effects of anchors can be diluted by adopting deliberative reasoning strategies such as "consider the opposite." As Larrick (2004) notes, this strategy simply amounts to asking oneself, "What are some of the reasons that my initial judgment might be wrong?" Mussweiler, Strack, and Pfeiffer (2000) provide an experimental example of the strategy in the context of anchoring by demonstrating that the magnitude of the anchoring effect can be reduced simply by asking people to list anchor-inconsistent arguments. Mussweiler and colleagues presented car experts with an actual car and an anchor estimate, either high (5000 German Marks) or low (2800 German Marks). Following the standard procedure in anchoring experiments, the expert first decided whether the anchor was too high or too low, and then provided his own estimate. The novel manipulation was that before providing an estimate, some of the experts were instructed to consider possible reasons why the anchor value might be inappropriate. The results indicated a clear effect of this manipulation: When the experts were instructed to generate anchor-inconsistent arguments, the anchoring effect was attenuated. For example, experts provided a mean estimate of 3563 German Marks when given the high anchor and not asked to generate opposite arguments, compared to an estimate of only 3130 German Marks when required to generate anchor-inconsistent arguments beforehand.

A related question is whether anchoring effects can be attenuated in experts who have knowledge of the judgment domain, as compared to non-experts who do not. If deliberative processes such as intentional memory retrieval play a role, then an expert who knows a great deal about German cars ought to be able to dilute the effect of an anchor by accessing relevant knowledge. Conversely, if anchoring is as strong in experts as in non-experts, this would imply that it is driven by automatic (System 1) processes. Just as with studies on incentives, several early reports (e.g., Northcraft & Neale, 1987; but see footnote 2) suggested no effect of knowledge level, but more recent research challenges this conclusion. Smith, Windschitl, and Bruchmann (2013) reported 4 studies in each of which anchoring was attenuated (though not eliminated) in individuals with greater expertise. For example, when

---

3. As with the Epley and Gilovich (2005) work on incentives, Epley and Gilovich (2006) found that cognitive load did not affect anchoring with externally provided anchors. But Simmons and colleagues' (2010) results suggest that this latter failure again may be an artefact of uncertainty about the required direction of adjustment. The same point applies to results reported by Blankenship and colleagues (2008).

asked the questions, "How many US states are west of the Mississippi River?" and "How many states in India have a population of more than 25 million people," anchoring was weaker in US participants for the question about the US and weaker in Indian participants for the question about India.

Plainly, much if not all of the influence of an anchor is mediated by deliberative thinking. We acknowledge the possibility that anchoring effects are not completely controllable and that there may in principle be residual effects that are immune to deliberative processes. It must remain an important question for future research whether or not unequivocal evidence for this can be obtained (see Englich, Mussweiler, & Strack, 2006, for a striking example).

BREADTH OF TRANSFER

As the quotation from Loersch and Payne (2011) above highlights, a common assertion in the priming field is that a prime can have a broad influence on behavior. If true, this would be a surprising finding and would require an account of priming which is very different from the sorts of explanations typically put forward to explain effects such as repetition and lexical priming. These effects are usually assumed to arise from some process in which specific perceptual or semantic features of the prime are activated and can influence responses to a target to the extent that the target shares those features. Lexical decision and repetition priming effects tend to be extremely narrow in the extent to which they show transfer. What gets activated in most situations is a specific representation that is stimulus- and response-bound. For instance, making a man-made (yes/no) judgment of a visual object in the first stage does not prime making a bigger-than-a-shoe-box (yes/no) decision in the test (Horner & Henson, 2009), and other research shows that almost any change in the processing engaged by the target relative to that engaged by the prime dilutes the magnitude of repetition priming (Franks, Bilbrey, Lien, & McNamara, 2000). A large literature documents the dilution of cross-modal compared to intra-modal priming: Whereas responding to the written word *knife* will typically be primed by reading the word previously, this influence will typically be much reduced or even absent if the prime (*knife*) is heard rather than read (Roediger & McDermott, 1993).

This narrowness of transfer applies to many instances of anchoring as well. Frederick and Mochon (2012) reported that while judging the weight of a raccoon or a whale in pounds influenced later estimates of the weight of a giraffe in pounds, no such anchoring influence was obtained when the weight of the raccoon was estimated on a 7-point heaviness scale or if the weight of the whale was estimated in tons. Frederick and Mochon concluded that anchoring effects only occur on the specific scale on which the object has been judged and not on other scales, even if they are related, such as weight in pounds and weight in tons. They explained this narrowness by a scale distortion mechanism in which the initial decision concerning the anchor distorts the psychological scale and hence biases the subsequent judgment. A similar failure to find transfer across scales was reported by Chapman and Johnson (1994) who found that dollar anchors did not influence life-expectancy estimates.

Even more strikingly, anchoring effects can be very narrow even within the same judgment dimension. Strack and Mussweiler (1997) found that asking participants to make a comparative judgment with respect to one attribute of an object (such as the height of the Brandenburg Gate) had little effect on their absolute judgments of this object with respect to a different attribute (e.g., the width of the Brandenburg Gate), even though both are on the same scale.

Adaval and Wyer (2011), in the study discussed previously, reported a somewhat more nuanced (and complex) pattern of transfer across attributes. In an experiment using supraliminal price anchors, participants were asked to judge whether the average price of an electronics product (e.g., a DVD player) or an article of clothing (e.g., running shoes) was higher or lower than a high (or low) price anchor. The product category (clothing/electronic) and the anchors (high/low) were both manipulated between subjects. Participants were then asked a willingness-to-pay (WTP) judgment about a target product which was the same, related, or unrelated to the product about which they had made the original anchor judgment. The results revealed an asymmetry whereby anchoring on an electronics product led to raised WTP for the *same* target item, but had no effect on related (i.e., another electronics product) or unrelated (i.e., an article of clothing) products. In contrast, anchoring on an item of clothing led to higher (lower) WTP for all three target types (same piece of clothing, another clothing item, and an electronics product) as a function of the originally presented price anchor value.

Adaval and Wyer (2011) suggest that this asymmetric transfer arises because electronics products tend to be evaluated on the basis of product-specific features (e.g., laser quality in a DVD player), whereas clothing is evaluated on the basis of more generic attributes such as style, attractiveness, and so forth. Thus, comparing the price of a piece of clothing with a high or low anchor value will prime price estimates for electronics products because the generic activated attributes will readily transfer across product categories. However, thinking about prices of electronics products will not prime estimates for clothes because the specific activated attributes are largely inapplicable to clothing.

While there might be some limitations to this account—for example, presumably brand status is an activated attribute in both clothing and electronics price comparisons—the findings nonetheless highlight the relatively narrow nature of transfer. It is clearly not the case here that activation of the concept "high (low) value" via a price anchor has general effects on downstream behavior. Rather, the activated attributes have a specific or selective (cf. Strack & Forster, 1995) influence on particular subsequent judgments.

In contrast to these examples of relatively narrow transfer, Oppenheimer, LeBoeuf, and Brewer (2008) reported four experiments in which they found a variety of much broader *cross-modal* anchoring effects. How compelling is their evidence? In their first experiment, Oppenheimer and colleagues gave participants a piece of paper with either three short (1-inch) or three long (3.5-inch) lines and asked them to copy the lines (without using a ruler). In a subsequent (apparently unrelated task), they were then asked to estimate the length of the Mississippi River in miles. Surprisingly, participants who had drawn the short lines estimated on average that the river was shorter ($M = 720$ miles) than those who had drawn long lines ($M = 1,224$ miles) (the correct answer is 2,320 miles). Even more surprisingly, in a follow-up experiment (Experiment 2), participants primed with the longer lines estimated the average temperature in Hawaii in July to be higher ($M = 87.5F$) than those primed with short lines ($M = 84.0F$). Oppenheimer and colleagues explained these results by arguing that the line-drawing task primed or activated a general notion of magnitude (largeness or smallness) that then transferred to subsequently encountered stimuli and questions. They say:

> We propose that large or small anchors may prime the notion of their general magnitudes (e.g., "largeness" or "smallness") and that the activated sense of magnitude may be influential when judges next form an estimate, leading to an anchoring effect. That is, merely activating a sense of size, unattached even to a rating scale, may bias subsequent judgments to be consistent with that activated size, regardless of the modality of judgment. Hence, cross-modal effects of anchors may arise, with a large anchor in any one modality leading to a large judgment in any other (or the same) modality. (p. 15)

Thus, we see again the claim that primes can activate very general concepts which can have multiple and widespread downstream effects on behavior. Further evidence for this viewpoint came from their final study in which drawing longer lines led participants to be more likely to complete the word fragments B_G, _ONG, and _ALL with their magnitude-related-synonyms (BIG, LONG, and TALL) than if they had drawn shorter lines.

Oppenheimer and colleagues' (2008) explanation of their results bears a striking similarity to those offered in other examples of behavior priming. The activation of a concept (e.g., "largeness") is observed to have widespread consequences for judgments about stimuli across scales, domains, and modalities. Moreover, although the effects were not automatic—attention had to be drawn to the anchors initially—they did appear to be unintentional because participants did not have to be asked to draw explicit comparisons between line lengths and the quantities to be estimated for the effects to obtain.

It is not easy to reconcile these examples of broad transfer across modality with the much narrower, within-modality (and scale) effects reviewed earlier. Why in the line-length examples does a transferable general notion of "largeness" or "smallness" become activated, when in other arguably more plausible situations (such as the Brandenburg Gate, or whale-weight examples) it does not?

The results raise important questions about the boundary conditions of such transfer effects. For example, would line-drawing also transfer to estimates about weights and sizes of objects? Frederick and Mochon's (2012) account suggests that it would not, whereas Oppenheimer and colleagues have to predict that it would. Is it possible to obtain bi-directional cross-modal priming—such that estimating a numeric quantity would influence a physical task? Oppenheimer and colleagues tested the latter prediction in a follow-up experiment briefly reported in their general discussion. Participants answered a question about the length of the Mississippi River, anchored with either a short (15 miles) or long (4,800 miles) anchor and were then asked to draw a toothpick. Oppenheimer and colleagues argued that the mean lengths of 2.19 inches (long anchor) and 2.08 inches (short anchor) of the sketched toothpicks provide suggestive evidence in support of a bi-directional transfer effect, and thus evidence of a general magnitude priming mechanism. However, with an N of 82 and a reported t-value of 1.7 in that study, the evidence, in fact, weakly favors the null hypothesis under a Bayesian analysis (cf. Matthews, 2011).[4]

---

4. The effect Oppenheimer and colleagues obtained in their Experiment 2, where lines of different lengths affected estimates of the average temperature in Hawaii, is also judged by a Bayesian t-test to be inconclusive.

The reason for dwelling on Oppenheimer and colleagues' study is that it represents an important challenge to the notion that anchoring effects are typically narrow. The narrowness argument is crucial to many researchers' resistance toward the theoretical framework underpinning priming, and thus if anchoring effects can indeed cross modalities and scales, then the types of transfer highlighted in the Loersch and Payne quotation seem less controversial. However, as far as we can tell, the Oppenheimer and colleagues' study is an outlier in the anchoring literature. The effects in each of their studies, although reliable, were small (as the authors freely admit, e.g., p. 22) and thus would benefit from replication; likewise, many of the predictions of their general activation account await much needed empirical testing.

ANCHORING AS AN EXAMPLE OF A SITUATED INFERENCE?

Our review[5] suggests that (1) subliminal or incidental effects of anchors are difficult to confirm and/or rather fragile; (2) anchoring effects can be intentionally avoided when (additional) deliberative thinking is encouraged; and (3) anchors tend to result in the activation of specific rather than general features (i.e., narrow transfer appears to be the norm). This pattern of effects seems readily reconcilable with widely held views about the nature of priming in other domains, and it can also be accommodated by at least some popular models of priming.

Consider the situated-inference model of Loersch and Payne (2011), developed in an attempt to explain the diverse impacts primes are claimed to have on a range of downstream behaviors (e.g., the *hostility* prime described in the quote above). The emphasis in their model is on a person's ability to assess the content of their own thoughts and to determine the relevance of these thoughts for the task at hand. For example, they write:

> [T]he situated-inference model predicts that metacognitive judgments about the meaning and validity of thoughts are critical... If one's thoughts are viewed as invalid, nondiagnostic, or otherwise inappropriate for use in the inference process, then priming will have no effect on subsequent judgment, behavior, or motivation. (p. 215)

Such a view seems to fit well with the effects of anchoring reviewed here. First, when participants are sufficiently incentivized or induced to think differently, non-diagnostic information is discounted (Larrick, 2004; Simmons et al. 2010). There is no automatic effect of accessible thoughts on behavior: Instead, thoughts are only instrumental if they are interpreted as valid reasons for behavior. Second, in situations involving broader transfer, information that could be activated is, presumably, either assessed as inappropriate or does not enter into consideration because of the distance between the prime and the target. The attribution process at the heart of the model is likely to be highly sensitive to implausible influences of a prime, in the same way that attributions of fluent processing are known to be constrained (J. K. Miller, Lloyd, & Westerman, 2008).

---

5. Notwithstanding the admittedly selective nature of our review, we think these conclusions are representative of the wider anchoring literature.

A similar notion is discussed by Klatzky and Creswell (2014) in their application of an intersensory interaction model to the priming literature. In essence, Klatzky and Creswell argue that priming effects might result from competition between multiple mechanisms—memory retrieval, associative chaining, heuristic inference—all of which "bid" to influence an outcome. The model explains when and why different types of priming are observed by assuming that these mechanisms are subject to different sources of variability (e.g., cognitive control, semantic context, cue reliability) that can affect the strength of each bid. For example, the influence of an elderly prime on walking speed might have differential effects on US and European participants because of culturally bound differences in the assessed potency, reliability, and weight assigned to old-age stereotypes (e.g., the extent to which old age connotes energy depletion in the two cultures). Klatzky and Creswell (2014) sum up their approach by arguing that their model suggests that "priming should be promoted or discounted, according to whether factors present in the experimental context facilitate or impede access to mediators and heuristics or suggest that indirect sources of information are more or less reliable" (p. 56). The similarity with the situated-inference model is clear, and the ability of both models to accommodate the anchoring effects we have reviewed is readily apparent.

CONCLUSION

Putting aside the recent controversy about the replicability of some striking priming effects, there can be little doubt that behavior can be subtly and irrationally primed. We have focused on anchoring as a particularly well-documented illustration of this. However, the interpretation of such priming effects—and what they reveal about the mind and behavior—is altogether less clear. A common viewpoint is that priming arises from the automatic and unconscious activation of mental constructs, and that these constructs can have wide influences on behavior. In our view, a good portion of the current skepticism about priming is based on dissatisfaction with this framework. Disbelief about the priming effects themselves arises because, on alternative theoretical viewpoints, they appear implausible.

In the anchoring literature, researchers have marshaled evidence from studies of subliminal, incidental, and cross-modal anchoring, and from experiments on the extent to which individuals are or are not aware of and can or cannot control the influence of an anchor, to argue in support of this framework. An example is Morewedge and Kahneman's (2010) proposal that System 1, which carries out fast and automatic operations, is what drives many anchoring effects. We have argued here that this interpretation of anchoring is not strongly supported by the literature and is, indeed, in some respects contradicted by the evidence. For example, individuals can intentionally control the influence of anchors (Simmons et al., 2010) and have considerable insight into the extent to which anchors affect their estimates (e.g., Wilson et al., 1996). Anchors are typically very narrow in their influence across judgment dimensions, and from a Bayesian point of view, the evidence for incidental and cross-modal anchoring is at best inconclusive. We have evaluated the evidence in relation to three of the four standard criteria for automaticity (Bargh, 1994; Moors & De Houwer, 2006), namely absence of awareness of the prime, absence of awareness of the prime's effect on one's behavior, and uncontrollability of the prime's influence (the fourth criterion, persistence of the prime's influence even when cognitive resources are diminished, has received very little attention in anchoring studies). On each criterion, the evidence does not support the idea that anchoring can occur automatically. It is not necessary, in sum, to accept a dual-systems perspective in order to make sense of the varied phenomena associated with anchoring. Instead, the general principles underlying deliberative (System 2) thought are sufficient (Newell & Shanks, 2014; Shanks, 2007). On this alternative account, there are few (if any) truly automatic or unconscious processes, nor is activation a passive and obligatory phenomenon.

We acknowledge of course that anchoring is only one type of priming and that caution is advised in extrapolating our conclusions to other, perhaps very different, forms of priming. It is highly unlikely that there will turn out to be a single grand theory applicable to all forms of priming; indeed, the term *anchoring* itself refers to a range of phenomena that quite likely depend on distinct mental processes. But despite this, anchoring encompasses two key features that are central to other forms of priming: 1) it occurs without deliberate intent, and 2) it involves rich conceptual contents (e.g., magnitudes, semantic features) rather than narrow mental constructs.

Extraordinary claims require extraordinary evidence. We are not the first to point out that the incentive structures under which psychologists operate appear to discourage attempts at replicating published results (Asendorpf et al., 2013) and that insufficient effort has been devoted to replicating key results in experimental psychology (Makel, Plucker, & Hegarty, 2012; Simons, 2014). This is strikingly evident in the social cognition and anchoring fields. For example, it is very surprising that there have been no published attempts to replicate Critcher and Gilovich's (2008) demonstrations of incidental anchoring or Oppenheimer and colleagues' (2008) cross-modal anchoring effects. These (and other) findings are so important for our theoretical understanding of anchoring that they cry out for further exploration. After all, for many years it was almost universally accepted that accuracy motivation (induced by financial incentives) usually fails to diminish anchoring, and it was only because Simmons and colleagues (2010) undertook further replications of this phenomenon that they discovered that the influence of anchors can in fact be attenuated and that the earlier conclusion was premature. We urge researchers to place more emphasis on replication.

REFERENCES

Adaval, R., & Wyer, R. S. (2011). Conscious and nonconscious comparisons with price anchors: Effects on willingness to pay for related and unrelated products. *Journal of Marketing Research, 48*, 355-365.

Ariely, D., Loewenstein, G., & Prelec, D. (2003). "Coherent arbitrariness": Stable demand curves without stable preferences. *Quarterly Journal of Economics, 118*, 73-105.

Asendorpf, J. B., Conner, M., De Fruyt, F., De Houwer, J., Denissen, J. J. A., Fiedler, K., . . . Wicherts, J. M. (2013). Recommendations for increasing replicability in psychology. *European Journal of Personality, 27*, 108-119.

Bakker, M., & Wicherts, J. M. (2011). The (mis) reporting of statistical results in psychology journals. *Behavior Research Methods, 43*, 666-678.

Bargh, J. A. (1994). The four horsemen of automaticity: Awareness, intention, efficiency, and control in social cognition. In R. S. Wyer & T. K. Srull (Eds.), *Handbook of social cognition* (2nd ed., pp. 1-40). Hillsdale, NJ: Erlbaum.

Bargh, J. A. (2006). What have we been priming all these years? On the development, mechanisms, and ecology of nonconscious social behavior. *European Journal of Social Psychology, 36*, 147-168.

Bargh, J. A., Chen, M., & Burrows, L. (1996). Automaticity of social behavior: Direct effects of trait construct and stereotype activation on action. *Journal of Personality and Social Psychology, 71*, 230-244.

Bargh, J. A., & Huang, J. Y. (2009). The selfish goal. In G. B. Moskowitz & H. Grant (Eds.), *The psychology of goals* (pp. 127-150). New York: Guilford.

Bertamini, M., & Munafò, M. R. (2012). Bite-size science and its undesired side effects. *Perspectives on Psychological Science, 7*, 67-71.

Blankenship, K. L., Wegener, D. T., Petty, R. E., Detweiler-Bedell, B., & Macy, C. L. (2008). Elaboration and consequences of anchored estimates: An attitudinal perspective on numerical anchoring. *Journal of Experimental Social Psychology, 44*, 1465-1476.

Brewer, N. T., & Chapman, G. B. (2002). The fragile basic anchoring effect. *Journal of Behavioral Decision Making, 15*, 65-77.

Chapman, G. B., & Johnson, E. J. (1994). The limits of anchoring. *Journal of Behavioral Decision Making, 7*, 223-242.

Chapman, G. B., & Johnson, E. J. (2002). Incorporating the irrelevant: Anchors in judgments of belief and value. In T. Gilovich, D. Griffin, & D. Kahneman (Eds.), *The psychology of intuitive judgment: Heuristics and biases* (pp. 120-138). Cambridge, UK: Cambridge University Press.

Critcher, C. R., & Gilovich, T. (2008). Incidental environmental anchors. *Journal of Behavioral Decision Making, 21*, 241-251.

Dawson, M. E., & Reardon, P. (1973). Construct validity of recall and recognition postconditioning measures of awareness. *Journal of Experimental Psychology, 98*, 308-315.

Dijksterhuis, A., & van Knippenberg, A. (1998). The relation between perception and behavior, or how to win a game of Trivial Pursuit. *Journal of Personality and Social Psychology, 74*, 865-877.

Doyen, S., Klein, O., Pichon, C.-L., & Cleeremans, A. (2012). Behavioral priming: It's all in the mind, but whose mind? *PLOS ONE, 7*, e29081.

Englich, B., Mussweiler, T., & Strack, F. (2006). Playing dice with criminal sentences: The influence of irrelevant anchors on experts' judicial decision making. *Personality and Social Psychology Bulletin, 32*, 188-200.

Epley, N., & Gilovich, T. (2005). When effortful thinking influences judgmental anchoring: Differential effects of forewarning and incentives on self-generated and externally provided anchors. *Journal of Behavioral Decision Making, 18*, 199-212.

Epley, N., & Gilovich, T. (2006). The anchoring-and-adjustment heuristic: Why the adjustments are insufficient. *Psychological Science, 17*, 311-318.

Ericsson, K. A., & Simon, H. A. (1984). *Protocol analysis: Verbal reports as data.* Cambridge, MA: MIT Press.

Francis, G. (2012). Publication bias and the failure of replication in experimental psychology. *Psychonomic Bulletin & Review, 19*, 975-991.

Franks, J. J., Bilbrey, C. W., Lien, K. G., & McNamara, T. P. (2000). Transfer-appropriate processing (TAP) and repetition priming. *Memory & Cognition, 28*, 1140-1151.

Frederick, S. M., & Mochon, D. (2012). A scale distortion theory of anchoring. *Journal of Experimental Psychology: General, 141*, 124-133.

Gregory, R. L. (2005). The Medawar Lecture 2001 – Knowledge for vision: Vision for knowledge. *Philosophical Transactions of the Royal Society B, 360*, 1231-1251.

Greitemeyer, T., Kastenmüller, A., & Fischer, P. (2013). Romantic motives and risk-taking: An evolutionary approach. *Journal of Risk Research, 16*, 19-38.

Hogarth, R. M. (2014). Automatic processes, emotions, and the causal field. *Behavioral and Brain Sciences, 37*, 31-32.

Holender, D. (1986). Semantic activation without conscious identification in dichotic listening, parafoveal vision, and visual masking: A survey and appraisal. *Behavioral and Brain Sciences, 9*, 1-66.

Horner, A. J., & Henson, R. N. (2009). Bindings between stimuli and multiple response codes dominate long-lag repetition priming in speeded classification tasks. *Journal of Experimental Psychology: Learning, Memory, and Cognition, 35*, 757-779.

Kahneman, D. (2011). *Thinking, fast and slow.* New York: Farrar, Straus and Giroux.

Klatzky, R. L., & Creswell, J. D. (2014). An intersensory interaction account of priming effects—and their absence. *Perspectives on Psychological Science, 9*, 49-58.

Klein, O., Doyen, S., Leys, C., Magalhães de Saldanha da Gama, P. A., Miller, S., Questienne, L., & Cleeremans, A. (2012). Low hopes, high expectations: Expectancy effects and the replicability of behavioral experiments. *Perspectives on Psychological Science, 7*, 572-584.

Kruschke, J. K. (2013). Bayesian estimation supersedes the *t* test. *Journal of Experimental Psychology: General, 142*, 573-603.

Lachter, J., Forster, K. I., & Ruthruff, E. (2004). Forty-five years after Broadbent (1958): Still no identification without attention. *Psychological Review, 111*, 880-913.

Larrick, R. P. (2004). Debiasing. In D. J. Koehler & N. Harvey (Eds.), *Blackwell handbook of judgment and decision making* (pp. 316-337). Oxford, UK: Blackwell.

LeBoeuf, R. A., & Shafir, E. (2006). The long and short of it: Physical anchoring effects. *Journal of Behavioral Decision Making, 19*, 393-406.

Loersch, C., & Payne, B. K. (2011). The situated inference model: An integrative account of the effects of primes on perception, behavior, and motivation. *Perspectives on Psychological Science, 6*, 234-252.

Makel, M. C., Plucker, J. A., & Hegarty, B. (2012). Replications in psychology research: How often do they really occur? *Perspectives on Psychological Science, 7*, 537-542.

Matthews, W. J. (2011). What might judgment and decision making research be like if we took a Bayesian approach to hypothesis testing? *Judgment and Decision Making, 6*, 843-856.

McNamara, T. P. (1992). Priming and constraints it places on theories of memory and retrieval. *Psychological Review, 99*, 650-662.

Miller, J. (2000). Measurement error in subliminal perception experiments: Simulation analyses of two regression methods. *Journal of Experimental Psychology: Human Perception and Performance, 26*, 1461-1477.

Miller, J. K., Lloyd, M. E., & Westerman, D. L. (2008). When does modality matter? Perceptual versus conceptual fluency-based illusions in recognition memory. *Journal of Memory and Language, 58*, 1080-1094.

Moors, A., & De Houwer, J. (2006). Automaticity: A theoretical and conceptual analysis. *Psychological Bulletin, 132*, 297-326.

Morewedge, C. K., & Kahneman, D. (2010). Associative processes in intuitive judgment. *Trends in Cognitive Sciences, 14*, 435-440.

Mussweiler, T. (2001). The durability of anchoring effects. *European Journal of Social Psychology, 31*, 431-442.

Mussweiler, T., & Englich, B. (2005). Subliminal anchoring: Judgmental consequences and underlying mechanisms. *Organizational Behavior and Human Decision Processes, 98*, 133-143.

Mussweiler, T., & Strack, F. (1999). Comparing is believing: A selective accessibility model of judgmental anchoring. *European Review of Social Psychology, 10*, 135-167.

Mussweiler, T., & Strack, F. (2000). The use of category and exemplar knowledge in the solution of anchoring tasks. *Journal of Personality and Social Psychology, 78*, 1038-1052.

Mussweiler, T., Strack, F., & Pfeiffer, T. (2000). Overcoming the inevitable anchoring effect: Considering the opposite compensates for selective accessibility. *Personality and Social Psychology Bulletin, 26*, 1142-1150.

Newell, B. R., & Shanks, D. R. (2014). Unconscious influences on decision making: A critical review. *Behavioral and Brain Sciences, 37*, 1-61.

Northcraft, G. B., & Neale, M. A. (1987). Experts, amateurs, and real estate: An anchoring-and-adjustment perspective on property pricing decisions. *Organizational Behavior and Human Decision Processes, 39*, 84-97.

Oppenheimer, D. A., LeBoeuf, R. A., & Brewer, N. T. (2008). Anchors aweigh: A demonstration of cross-modality anchoring and magnitude priming. *Cognition, 106*, 13-26.

Pashler, H., Coburn, N., & Harris, C. R. (2012). Priming of social distance? Failure to replicate effects on social and food judgments. *PLOS ONE, 7*, e42510.

Pashler, H., & Harris, C. R. (2012). Is the replicability crisis overblown? Three arguments examined. *Perspectives on Psychological Science, 7*, 531-536.

Pratte, M. S., & Rouder, J. N. (2009). A task-difficulty artifact in subliminal priming. *Attention, Perception, & Psychophysics, 71*, 1276-1283.

Reitsma-van Rooijen, M., & Daamen, D. D. L. (2006). Subliminal anchoring: The effects of subliminally presented numbers on probability estimates. *Journal of Experimental Social Psychology, 42*(3), 380-387.

Roediger, H. L., & McDermott, K. B. (1993). Implicit memory in normal human subjects. In F. Boller & J. Grafman (Eds.), *Handbook of neuropsychology* (Vol. 8; pp. 63-131). Amsterdam: Elsevier.

Rouder, J. N., Morey, R. D., Speckman, P. L., & Pratte, M. S. (2007). Detecting chance: A solution to the null sensitivity problem in subliminal priming. *Psychonomic Bulletin & Review, 14*, 597-605.

Rouder, J. N., Speckman, P. L., Sun, D., Morey, R. D., & Iverson, G. (2009). Bayesian t tests for accepting and rejecting the null hypothesis. *Psychonomic Bulletin & Review, 16*, 225-237.

Schimmack, U. (2012). The ironic effect of significant results on the credibility of multiple-study articles. *Psychological Methods, 17*, 551-566.

Shanks, D. R. (2007). Associationism and cognition: Human contingency learning at 25. *Quarterly Journal of Experimental Psychology, 60*, 291-309.

Shanks, D. R., Newell, B. R., Lee, E. H., Balakrishnan, D., Ekelund, L., Cenac, Z., . . . Moore, C. (2013). Priming intelligent behavior: An elusive phenomenon. *PLOS ONE, 8*, e56515.

Simmons, J. P., LeBoeuf, R. A., & Nelson, L. D. (2010). The effect of accuracy motivation on anchoring and adjustment: Do people adjust from provided anchors? *Journal of Personality and Social Psychology, 99*, 917-932.

Simmons, J. P., Nelson, L. D., & Simonsohn, U. (2011). False-positive psychology: Undisclosed flexibility in data collection and analysis allows presenting anything as significant. *Psychological Science, 22*, 1359-1366.

Simons, D. J. (2014). The value of direct replication. *Perspectives on Psychological Science, 9*, 76-80.

Smith, A. R., Windschitl, P. D., & Bruchmann, K. (2013). Knowledge matters: Anchoring effects are moderated by knowledge level. *European Journal of Social Psychology, 43*, 97-108.

Strack, F., & Forster, J. (1995). Reporting recollective experiences: Direct access to memory systems? *Psychological Science, 6*, 352-358.

Strack, F., & Mussweiler, T. (1997). Explaining the enigmatic anchoring effect: Mechanisms of selective accessibility. *Journal of Personality and Social Psychology, 73*, 437-446.

Tenpenny, P. L. (1995). Abstractionist versus episodic theories of repetition priming and word identification. *Psychonomic Bulletin & Review, 2*, 339-363.

Tversky, A., & Kahneman, D. (1974). Judgment under uncertainty: Heuristics and biases. *Science, 185*, 1124-1131.

Wegener, D. T., Petty, R. E., Blankenship, K. L., & Detweiler-Bedell, B. (2010). Elaboration and numerical anchoring: Implications of attitude theories for consumer judgment and decision making. *Journal of Consumer Psychology, 20*, 5-16.

Williams, L. E., & Bargh, J. A. (2008). Keeping one's distance: The influence of spatial distance cues on affect and evaluation. *Psychological Science, 19*, 302-308.

Wilson, T. D., Houston, C. E., Etling, K. M., & Brekke, N. (1996). A new look at anchoring effects: Basic anchoring and its antecedents. *Journal of Experimental Psychology: General, 125*, 387-402.

UNDERSTANDING PRIME-TO-BEHAVIOR EFFECTS: INSIGHTS FROM THE ACTIVE-SELF ACCOUNT

S. Christian Wheeler
Stanford University

Kenneth G. DeMarree
University at Buffalo, SUNY

Richard E. Petty
Ohio State University

> In this paper, we provide a brief review of prime-to-behavior effects and discuss our theoretical model for such effects: the Active-Self Account. We also address recent discussions in the literature regarding the replicability of prime-to-behavior effects and outline features that can affect their existence and the likelihood of detecting such effects experimentally.

Behavioral priming refers to the phenomenon whereby exposure to a stimulus (e.g., a word or picture) or set of stimuli (e.g., sentences to unscramble) activates a concept, which in turn influences a subsequent behavioral response without awareness of the links among these elements. Put another way, priming can create a readiness to respond in particular ways without intention or awareness by the prime recipient. Researchers have known about priming effects for decades. Lashley (1951) first used the term "priming" to describe response preparedness in intentional serial behavioral sequences. Segal and Cofer (1960) were the first to demonstrate the sort of passive priming more typical of modern social psychological priming research, whereby simple exposure to a stimulus increases its use in subsequent contexts. Specifically, they showed that exposure to words in one task increased their usage in a subsequent free-association task. Primes can have effects beyond the activated construct itself, however. Constructs, when activated, can increase the accessibility of other constructs linked in memory. For example, people are quicker to identify whether a letter string is a word or not when they have previously been exposed to a semantically related word (e.g., Meyer and Sch-

---

Address correspondence to S. Christian Wheeler, 655 Knight Way, Stanford, CA 94305-7298; E-mail: christian.wheeler@stanford.edu.

vaneveldt, 1971). Constructs can be mentally linked in many different ways, such as through prior co-activation or even by sharing the same valence. For example, activated constructs can increase the speed with which people evaluate targets that are evaluated similarly, because exposure to an evaluative prime increases the accessibility of other similarly valenced targets (e.g., Fazio et al., 1986).

That primes can increase the accessibility of the constructs to which they refer as well as to other linked constructs in memory is beyond doubt. However, a more recent class of findings, prime-to-behavior effects, has generated more controversy. Prime-to-behavior effects refer to the phenomenon whereby primed constructs (e.g., the "elderly") affect observable behavior (e.g., walking speed). To the extent that one's active mental contents influence behavior, it should obviously be the case that primes, by affecting one's active mental contents, could also affect behavior. This effect is the focus of the present paper. Naturally, behavioral effects that are more causally distal from the prime should be more difficult to predict and obtain than more proximal effects, such as simple response facilitation. As one moves further downstream, the number of moderators and intervening processes can proliferate rapidly. A difficulty of prediction or obtaining an effect should not be confused with a lack of influence, however. In fact, behavioral priming effects can sometimes be larger than semantic priming effects, because they can activate downstream constructs (e.g., goals) that can have powerful and persistent effects on behavior. Because any one prime can activate a diversity of initial concepts, related concepts, and associated behaviors, any one study may not capture the predicted chain of events. Nonetheless, there are such a large number of reported prime-to-behavior effects in the literature from such a diverse array of scholars that their existence seems assured (see Dijksterhuis & Bargh, 2001; Loersch & Payne, 2011, 2014, this volume; Wheeler, DeMarree, & Petty, 2005, 2007, for reviews).

Our own work on priming has been focused on examining how and when primed constructs affect behavior (i.e., on what mechanisms are involved in prime-to-behavior effects and under what circumstances they operate). Early accounts of prime-to-behavior effects proposed relatively direct paths between construct activation and behavioral output. For example, the ideomotor account suggested that primed stereotypes automatically activate associated behavioral representations without any intervening processes. A similar but slightly more complex account, the auto-motive model (e.g., Bargh, Gollwitzer, Lee-Chai, Barndollar, & Trötschel, 2001), suggested that primes directly activate motivational representations, which in turn activate relevant behavioral routines to accomplish the goal.

Our own framework, the Active-Self Account (Wheeler et al., 2005; 2007), takes a different approach. This account builds on previous findings showing that primes can both selectively activate mental contents and be used to disambiguate perceptual targets (e.g., Higgins, Rholes, & Jones, 1977). According to the Active-Self Account, primes can increase the accessibility of primed and associated constructs, which in turn can shift the active self-concept. Put simply, primed constructs and their activated associates can be viewed as self-relevant, as applying to oneself or one's ongoing reactions, and these perceptions can in turn affect the behavior that subsequently occurs. Although the framework acknowledges that primes can also affect other constructs (e.g., one's interpretation of the environment or other people when those concepts are salient; Wheeler & Petty, 2001; Wheeler, DeMarree, & Petty, 2007), because the self is an available and ambiguous entity in many situations, it often absorbs the impact of the prime (see Loersch & Payne, 2011,

2014, this volume; Smeesters, Wheeler, & Kay, 2010; Wheeler & DeMarree, 2009, for further discussion). Below, we review the basic features of the Active-Self Account and some illustrative findings in support of those features. A full description of the model and review of the relevant literature is beyond the scope of this paper, but for other, more comprehensive reviews, see Wheeler and colleagues (2005; 2007) and Smeesters and colleagues (2010).

PRIMES CAN AFFECT THE ACTIVE SELF-CONCEPT

The Active-Self Account parallels prior theory about the self-concept in distinguishing between chronic and temporarily active self-concept contents (e.g., Markus & Kunda, 1986). The chronic self-concept refers to those characteristics of the self that reside in long-term memory, including self-knowledge, goals, beliefs, values, and the like (Markus & Wurf, 1987). It is called the chronic self-concept because it contains long-term content chronically available for activation. As noted above, not all content in memory is likely to be applied to judgment or action at any given moment. The content that is most accessible, all things being equal, is more likely to be applied. The active contents of the (perceived) self-concept are more likely to affect judgment and behavior than those contents that are not active. Because priming affects the accessibility of information, it should be capable of affecting which information is in the active self-concept, insofar as the active self-concept is malleable. Extensive research supports the notion that contextual factors can affect the active contents of the self-concept (DeSteno & Salovey, 1997; McConnell, 2011).

Considerable research also shows that very subtle influences such as primed concepts, even when subliminally activated, can affect one's active self-concept. Primed constructs such as meanness, helpfulness, and dishonesty affect one's self-views just as much as one's views of another target (Skowronski, Sedikides, Heider, Wood, & Scherer, 2010). Primes of thin or overweight people affect prime recipients' body image (Kawakami et al., 2012). And primes can affect not just one's perceived traits or characteristics, but also other prime-consistent content, such as feelings of luck (DeMarree, Wheeler, & Petty, 2005; Jiang, Cho, and Adaval, 2009), aggressiveness (DeMarree et al., 2005), or self-efficacy (Hansen & Wänke, 2009), as well as attitudes toward stereotype-relevant attitude-objects (Kawakami, Dovidio, & Dijksterhuis, 2003; Steele & Ambady, 2006). Interestingly, components of the active self-concept can be highly accessible, yet reside out of consciousness (e.g., in the case of implicit self-concept shifts). As a result, primes can potentially affect behavior via the active self-concept without awareness on the part of the prime recipient (see Wheeler et al., 2007, for more discussion).

Notably, primes can lead to both prime-congruent and prime-incongruent changes in the self-concept. For example, in accord with various theories of assimilation and contrast (e.g., Markman & McMullen, 2003; Mussweiler, 2003), exposure to a "smart" stereotype, such as the professor stereotype, increases the accessibility of "intelligent" in the active self-concept, whereas exposure to a more extreme "smart" exemplar, such as Einstein, increases the accessibility of "unintelligent" in the active self-concept (e.g., Dijksterhuis et al., 1998). Papers reporting both self-concept and behavioral shifts show congruent movement between the two (e.g., Dijksterhuis et al., 1998; Hundhammer & Mussweiler, 2012; Lebouf & Estes, 2004; Schubert & Häfner, 2003; Wheeler, DeMarree, & Petty, 2008; Wyer, Mazzoni, Perfect, Calvini, Neilens, 2010). That is, the prime's effect on the self-concept in one study parallels the prime's effect on behavior in other studies.

Several papers have tested self-concept and behavioral shifts within the same studies and found that primes' effects on behavior can be mediated by changes in the active self-concept. For example, young people primed with the elderly stereotype perceive themselves as more elderly stereotypic, walk more slowly, and exhibit poorer memory performance (Wyer, Neilens, Perfect, & Mazzoni, 2011). Further, self-perceptions of being like an elderly person mediated the behavioral effects. In a conceptually parallel finding, those primed with the cheerleader stereotype performed worse on an analytic test to the extent that the prime lowered self-views of intelligence (Galinsky, Wang, & Ku, 2008; for additional examples, see Hansen & Wänke, 2009; Jiang, et al., 2009; Pfeffer & Devoe, 2009). Although it is possible that behavioral shifts could occur in directions opposite to those of the active self-concept (e.g., when one successfully counteracts an undesired self-concept shift), the published effects to date have all shown active self-concept/behavior congruence, regardless of the consistency between the prime and the active self-concept shifts. These data are highly consistent with the Active-Self Account.

The reader may question how the self-concept could be involved in behavioral priming effects given that outgroup stereotypes have also been shown to affect behavior. Despite an outgroup stereotype being clearly inapplicable to a prime recipient in an objective sense (e.g., a young person is not elderly), much of the specific content of the stereotype can overlap with the self. For example, most European Americans have some degree of aggressive self-concept content, even though this content is a component of the African-American stereotype, and most young people are slow (elderly stereotype) on some occasions. As a result, outgroup stereotype primes can affect one's active self-concept by activating a biased subset of self-concept content (e.g., DeMarree et al., 2005; Wyer et al., 2011), what we call the biased activation account (Wheeler et al., 2007). Additionally, it is possible that non-self-relevant prime content could infiltrate the active self-concept. The boundaries between the self and non-self are nebulous. People are notoriously bad at identifying the sources of their own thoughts and feelings (e.g., Nisbett & Wilson, 1977), and they have limited access to their own inner states (Bem, 1967; Wilson, 2002). As a result, they could sometimes use primed constructs to disambiguate their current self-views, feelings, and attitudes, much like they use primed mental contents to disambiguate their reactions to others (e.g., Higgins et al, 1977; Srull & Wyer, 1979), what we call the expansion account (Wheeler et al., 2007). This need not be a conscious process of attribution, however. Rather, primed content could automatically be included in the construction of the active self-concept, as proposed by connectionist theories (e.g., Smith, 1996). For more on these two means of affecting the active self-concept, see discussion of the biased activation and expansion accounts in Wheeler and colleagues (2007).

MODERATORS OF PRIME-TO-BEHAVIOR EFFECTS

Many moderators of prime-to-behavior effects have been shown in the literature. A strength of the Active-Self Account is that it can make sense of these many moderators by relating those moderators to their effects on the active self-concept. A comprehensive review of these moderators is beyond the scope of this brief paper, but below, we review some of the more prominent moderation findings and show how they relate to the Active-Self Account.

Determining the Extent of Assimilation. Many prime-to-behavior effects reported in the literature are assimilation effects. That is, the prime leads behavior to be more similar to that implied by the primed content. A number of moderators determine the *extent* of assimilation that occurs. According to the active-self account, one way to understand these moderators of extent is to understand how those moderators relate to the extent of active self-concept change. Specifically, features that affect the extent to which primes can shift the active self-concept should likewise affect the magnitude of prime-to-behavior effects. Indeed, as noted earlier, a number of studies have shown that the degree of self-concept change mediates the impact of a prime on behavior change. In addition to these mediational studies, a number of other findings in the literature support the active-self account.

First, those with prime-relevant self-concept inconsistencies show larger priming effects on behavior. For example, people who believe they have both African-American stereotype-consistent (e.g., lazy) and stereotype-inconsistent (e.g., industrious) attributes subsequently express more stereotype-consistent attitudes (e.g., supporting affirmative action) following an African-American stereotype prime (DeMarree, Morrison, Wheeler, & Petty, 2011). Similarly, those made self-uncertain also show larger priming effects on the self-concept (Morrison, Johnson, & Wheeler, 2012). Presumably, ambiguities in the self-concept render it more subject to construction and, hence, make the prime more influential in guiding behavior.

Second, individual differences in the way primed content is processed can also moderate the extent of prime-to-behavior effects. Private self-consciousness can either increase or decrease prime-to-behavior effects, depending on which facet of self-consciousness (self-reflectiveness or internal state awareness) is dominant in that context (see Dijksterhuis & van Knippenberg, 2000; Hull, Slone, Meteyer, & Matthews, 2002). Specifically, self-reflectiveness, which is associated with self-relevant processing directed towards obtaining self-understanding, magnifies prime-to-behavior effects (Wheeler, Morrison, DeMarree, & Petty, 2008). This is because processing primed content in self-relevant ways increases prime-to-behavior effects (e.g., Hull et al., 2002; Wheeler, Jarvis, & Petty, 2001). Internal state awareness, which by contrast is associated with greater awareness of one's internal states and resistance of the self-concept to change, reduces prime-to-behavior effects (Wheeler et al., 2008).

Low self-monitors show larger prime-induced shifts in the active self-concept and behavior than do high self-monitors (DeMarree, Wheeler, & Petty, 2005). Low and high self-monitors do not appear to differ in their access to their actual internal states, but low self-monitors are more *responsive* to information believed to be diagnostic of them (e.g., Fiske & von Hendy, 1992). Hence, subtle primes are more likely to shift the active self-concepts of low self-monitors because they are perceived as self-relevant. Additionally, because low self-monitors act consistently with their internal states and use them to guide behavior, these shifts in the active self-concept are more likely to be reflected in resulting behavior.

Last, actively relating primed content to the self can increase priming effects on the active self-concept and behavior. For example, taking the perspective of an elderly person, as opposed to remaining objective, makes participants walk more slowly and act more conservatively, consistent with the elderly stereotype (Ku, Wang, & Galinsky, 2010). Writing about an African American from the first-person perspective (vs. third-person perspective) makes one perform more poorly on a math test (Wheeler, Jarvis, & Petty, 2001).

In summary, structural features and processing orientations that make the active self-concept susceptible to change increase the magnitude of prime-to-behavior effects. Additionally, those most likely to act consistently with their active self-concepts exhibit the largest prime-to-behavior effects. These findings point to the key role of the active self-concept in determining the effects of primes on behavior.

Determining Assimilation versus Contrast. Initially, most of the prime-to-behavior effects published in the literature were assimilation effects. Now, however, a large number of contrast effects, whereby primes lead to more prime-*inconsistent* behavior, have been shown. Contrast effects are difficult for many models of prime-to-behavior effects to explain, and those that do predict contrast effects do not generally handle the wide variety of known contrast effects very well.

According to the active-self account, primed constructs can cause contrast in behavior due to the activation of contrasting content in the self-concept. For example, as noted above, exposure to a "smart" stereotype, such as the professor stereotype, increases the accessibility of "intelligent" in the active self-concept, whereas exposure to a more extreme "smart" exemplar, such as Einstein, increases the accessibility of "unintelligent" in the active self-concept (e.g., Dijksterhuis et al., 1998). The latter effect occurs because "Einstein" is more concrete and/or discrepant from the self than "professor" (Mussweiler, 2003). Features of the prime that make it likely to be viewed as a discrepant comparison standard increase the likelihood of contrast (Sherif, Taub, & Hovland, 1958). Similarly, a processing orientation that promotes looking for dissimilarities (Mussweiler, 2003) or evaluating oneself against a comparison standard (Markman & McMullen, 2003) increase the likelihood of contrast in self-perceptions.

These well-established social comparison phenomena are borne out in prime-to-behavior effects as well, supporting the role of the active self-concept in such phenomena. For example, salience of one's self-identity (Schubert & Häfner, 2003) or one's group-identity (Spears, Gordijn, Dijksterhuis, & Stapel, 2004) can foster viewing oneself as distinct from outgroup primes and hence lead to contrast in behavior. Identifying strongly with the ingroup leads to the same effects (Hall & Crisp, 2008). Similarly, disliking (Cesario, Plaks, & Higgins, 2006) and feeling distant from outgroups (Ledgerwood & Chaiken, 2007) promote contrast from outgroup primes. Independence (Bry, Follenfant, & Meyer, 2008) and dissimilarity (Haddock, Macrae, & Fleck, 2002) mindsets, both of which emphasize differences from others, do the same. These findings are remarkably consistent in showing that features that emphasize oneself as distinct, distant, or different from prime content facilitate contrast in the active self-concept and in behavior. Without understanding how the moderating variables affect the direction of active self-concept change, one would be ill equipped to predict most of these effects.

OTHER MECHANISMS FOR PRIME-TO-BEHAVIOR EFFECTS

The active-self account is a perception-based account in that primes are proposed to bias the prime recipient's ongoing conception or construal of him- or herself in the moment. As we and others have written elsewhere (e.g., Loersch & Payne, 2011, 2014, this volume; Smeesters et al., 2010; Wheeler & DeMarree, 2009; Wheeler & Petty, 2001), other types of perceptions, such as construals of the situation or of others, can sometimes be biased by primes, particularly when they are ambiguous to the perceiver and are the focus of the perceiver's attention. Shifts in perceptions of these other targets should follow the same basic principles as shifts in the perceptions of the self, and they could occur through both the biased activation and expansion model mechanisms described above. For example, a prime could bias the specific subset of chronically available information about a situation or another person that is currently accessible. Similarly, the representation of a situation or another person could be expanded to include content activated by the prime. Nonetheless, given the chronic availability of self-related content and the importance of self-related thoughts in directing behavior, regardless of the situation, we believe that the active-self account can hold explanatory power in a wide variety of contexts.

REPLICABILITY OF PRIMING EFFECTS

Recently, the replicability of prime-to-behavior effects has come under question (e.g., Shanks et al., 2013), though priming effects are not alone in receiving such scrutiny (see e.g., openscienceframework.org; psychfiledrawer.org), and concerns even extend to presumably more established areas, such as medical research (Ioannidis, 2005). Why are priming effects sometimes difficult to reproduce? Like many other effects in social psychology and other fields, there are a number of potential reasons. First, as discussed above with respect to prime-to behavior effects, there are many moderators that have been established. With so many moderators, it is now clear that behavioral priming effects are most likely to occur under specific conditions or among specific people, and this was not always clear from the initial research. That is, any initial study reporting an effect might have contained certain "background" conditions for the preponderance of the subjects (e.g., a focus on the self), whereas replication efforts might not, making them less likely to obtain the effect.

Although well-known papers have found main effects of primes on relevant outcomes (Bargh, Chen, & Burrows, 1996; Dijksterhuis & van Knippenberg, 1998), ignoring the studies that find moderation patterns (or just remembering the conditions under which significant effects emerged) might lead people to overestimate the generalizability of prime-to-behavior effects across all people and settings. Notably, many of the moderation studies do not find significant overall effects of the primes, instead finding effects only among some subset of the sample or under certain conditions. Ignoring potential moderating factors will make it more difficult to detect effects.

Further, many factors can intervene to limit prime-to-behavior effects. For example, even those who would otherwise be affected by a prime may not be so if their current motivations or concerns do not align with the primed concepts (e.g., Loersch, Durso, & Petty, 2013; Macrae & Johnston, 1998; Strahan, Spencer, & Zanna, 2002). Additionally, if people lack confidence in their thoughts (such as if they are feeling low in power or are depressed), primes will fail to affect behavior even when they do affect the prime-recipient's thoughts (e.g., DeMarree et al., 2012; see Briñol & Petty, 2009, for a review). Of course, not all moderators are necessarily relevant to all studies, but researchers should do their best to identify the individual difference variables that are most relevant as well as the situational factors most likely to maximize the intended effects, and include these in their research.

In addition, it is important to pay attention to what the various moderators tell us about the conditions under which priming effects are likely to occur. Most notably, factors that influence people's explanations for the activated content are particularly important. As we have noted, one key reason that a prime can influence a person's judgment is because a behaviorally relevant perceptual target (such as the self) is mistakenly seen as the source of a primed concept (e.g., Wheeler et al., 2007; Wheeler & DeMarree, 2009; see also Loersch & Payne, 2011, 2014, this volume). Classic research on attribution as well as contemporary work in social cognition more generally (Higgins, 1996) has identified ambiguity, applicability, and salience as key factors that drive such attributions.

So, if factors such as self-ambiguity or self-focused attention are present, activated concepts may be used to disambiguate self-perceptions, resulting in self-concept assimilation (DeMarree et al., 2011; Wheeler, DeMarree et al., 2008; Wheeler, Morrison et al., 2008). These changed self-perceptions will then influence behavior to the extent that the self is relevant for and used to guide action. If, instead, there are salient and/or ambiguous social or situational targets available or salient in one's mind, activated concepts may be used to disambiguate these targets (e.g., DeMarree & Loersch, 2009; Kay, Wheeler, Bargh, & Ross, 2004; Loersch et al., 2013). However, if these targets are not relevant for behavior, no behavioral changes are expected (DeMarree & Loersch, 2009). Hence, primes may or may not affect behavior depending on the prime recipient's focus, the availability and ambiguity of a relevant perceptual target, and the relevance of that target for behavior.

This highlights several key implications for the replication of priming effects. Most critically, researchers should not assume that a given prime can only have one particular type of effect (Bargh et al., 2001; DeMarree & Loersch, 2009; Schwarz, 2004). Activating the concept of *competitive*, for example, could influence people's self-perceptions, their perceptions of another person, their perceptions of the situation, their goals, and so forth (Wheeler et al., 2007; Wheeler & DeMarree, 2009). Any number of features of the experimental setting or study materials could influence participants' explanations of the activated content. For example, if the experimenter remains visible to participants and behaves in a sufficiently ambiguous manner, he or she could be viewed as the source of the accessible competitive content. If the dependent measure in such a study were to involve the competitiveness of negotiation offers between two participants, the prime would be less likely to have a behavioral effect, as it would have been used to form an impression of the experimenter whose competitiveness may have been seen as irrelevant to participants' behavior. That is, a null effect on the intended dependent measure is not necessarily a sign that the prime did not affect participants' judgments or behavior in any way.

Interestingly, in a complex social world, one implication is that a diversity of potential effects of an activated concept can emerge. Several factors (e.g., a person's focus of attention, the availability of ambiguous self-conceptions, social targets, or situational factors) can determine the target to which this activated concept is attributed, and the relevance of that target for action will determine whether the effects are entirely cognitive (e.g., seeing a passerby as more intelligent) or if they have implications for one's own behavior (e.g., deciding not to compete with a debate partner who is seen as more intelligent).

With this in mind, it becomes critical to carefully manage the experimental situation. Indeed, the social psychology laboratory is desirable as a context in which a researcher can gain control over many irrelevant features of the situation and maximize the chances that the independent variable will have the intended effect. Researchers should take care to make sure that the intended judgment target is salient to people. This can be done, in part, by limiting their interactions with other people (unless the other people are the intended target) during the study (Wyer et al., 2011). Just as researchers typically select contexts and participants that will maximize demonstration of an effect if it exists, a careful experimenter will also choose dependent measures that are likely to be influenced by the prime *given the experimental context*. For example, if the lab setup is such that participants will always be able to see the experimenter, researchers could consider using primed constructs and dependent measures that are relevant to people's perceptions of the experimenter.

In addition to the above reasons, which are derived from our theoretical perspective on prime-to-behavior effects, there are a number of very general methodological considerations that researchers should keep in mind when attempting to replicate *any* research finding. Ideally, all study materials should be pretested to determine their suitability for the target population and situation. Each participant pool, experimental context, mode of study delivery, and so forth can have different characteristics which might make study materials more or less likely to work in a given setting. Our presumption here is that most experimental social psychology research is driven by showing the relationship among conceptual variables (e.g., primes of various sorts can influence behavior of various sorts) as well as mediators and moderators of those relationships. Such research is not generally aimed at testing hypotheses about how large such effects are. Stated differently, independent and dependent variables are deliberately chosen to maximize the chances of showing an effect and are not chosen to represent the pool of exemplars that could or do represent these variables in the real world.

Thus, on the independent variable side of the study, the prime induction should be pretested to determine whether it leads to an increase in accessibility of the intended construct (e.g., using a lexical decision task following the prime induction) and that the induction is not too blatant. If a prime is too blatant and people identify its true source and attempt to correct for it (Wegener & Petty, 1997), priming effects can be eliminated or even reversed (Loersch & Payne, 2012; Mussweiler & Neumann, 2000; Strack, Schwarz, Bless, Kubler, & Wänke, 1993). In addition, sample differences, such as in people's motivation to think carefully (in general or about the experiment), could lead participants to be more likely to identify and correct for a potential biasing agent such as a prime (Petty, DeMarree, Briñol, Horcajo, & Strathman, 2008). Finally, variation in the racial, ethnic, age, or gender composition of a given university or national sample could cause the same prime induction to produce differing degrees of concept activation or even to the activation of different content (e.g., if different participant populations have different prime associations; Wheeler & Berger, 2007).

On the dependent variable side of the study, it is of central importance to make sure that the dependent variable is likely to be sensitive to any prime-induced effects. The dispersion of participants' responses to the dependent variable should be examined. If participants' responses are very uniform or are subject to ceiling or floor effects, then the dependent variable is less likely to be affected by a prime. For example, if a researcher at a junior college attempts to replicate an intelligence priming effect initially observed at an Ivy League institution, using the original dependent measure might not be appropriate, as floor effects might likely occur. Instead, researchers should endeavor to create a dependent variable that has similar properties *in the population* to the original study materials (e.g., if participants in the initial study answered 60% of trivia questions correctly with a standard deviation of 15%, researchers should attempt to develop a measure with a similar distribution).

Of course, characteristics of the population are important to consider, but even seemingly irrelevant characteristics of the setting might also matter. It is important to consider that just as primes or other independent variables can have many outcomes other than the intended one, so too are dependent variables influenced by many factors other than the intended one. For example, the length of a hallway or the average time or distance between classes at a particular university could affect the speed at which students walk down the hallway after an experiment. Thus, even if two samples have the same average walking speed and variance, it could be that in one sample 70% of the walking speed is determined by the short time and long distance between classes but in another sample these factors account for only 50% of the variance, leaving more to be affected by a prime. Although it is likely impossible to determine all of the relevant factors that might influence the presence or magnitude of a priming effect in a given context, careful construction of an experimental setting, accompanied by open-minded consideration of possible influences should a failure to replicate emerge, could help not only explain a successful or unsuccessful study, but also lend additional insight into the nature of prime-to-behavior effects.

Together, these considerations suggest that replications of priming studies might at best hope to replicate the direction of an effect (or effects) observed in an original study, but not the effect size. In fact, because of the considerations above, effect sizes are likely to be considerably smaller even in so-called "exact" replications. This is because even a replication study using the same independent variable (IV) (e.g., unscrambling sentences about the elderly) and the same dependent variable (DV) (e.g., walking speed) as an original study, though using the exact same materials, cannot be exact in its other features (the participants, the time, the background features of the experimental context, the meaning of the IV in the participants' minds, other possibly unique influences on the DV, etc.). These uncontrolled extraneous factors that likely enhanced the effect size in an original study, if not present in the replication study, will lead to a smaller effect, thus requiring a larger sample to produce a significant result. Researchers finding non-significant results in the same direction as the original result could test whether the addition of their studies in a meta-analysis enhances or diminishes the likelihood that an initial effect was reliable.

Because the purpose of much social psychological research is theory testing rather than application, priming researchers should be encouraged if their direction of effects replicates in new populations and settings. It should not be too surprising (or discouraging) if effect sizes do not generalize (Petty & Cacioppo, 1996). This is not to say that prime-to-behavior effects have no practical utility. Rather, it means that when one wishes to use primes to influence behavior for a particular group in a particular domain, the same kind of pretesting that occurred for the original study should begin anew to determine how the independent and dependent variables need to be modified for the particular purpose of interest. Ultimately, however, as a basic science, social psychologists are often interested in *how* and *why* various factors influence people's judgments and behavior. Priming is one tool that psychologists can use to investigate these questions, and the exploration of these questions should not be limited to a specific experimental paradigm. Researchers may want to find procedures that work in their experimental context, and then use those procedures to further probe the nature of human thought and behavior.

CONCLUSION

At first glance, prime-to-behavior effects may seem incredible. How could something as simple as exposure to mere words affect one's overt behavior? Much of our work in this domain has been aimed at taking something that appears magical and revealing that it actually has a rather mundane mechanism. That primes can affect one's mental processes is beyond question at this point. That one's mental processes can drive behavior seems similarly so. Through understanding these linkages more fully, one can better isolate when and how primes will affect behavior and see that sometimes ordinary processes can have surprising consequences.

REFERENCES

Bargh, J. A., Chen, M., & Burrows, L. (1996). Automaticity of social behavior: Direct effects of trait construct and stereotype activation on action. *Journal of Personality and Social Psychology, 71*, 230-240. doi:10.1037/0022-3514.71.2.230

Bargh, J. A., Gollwitzer, P. M., Lee-Chai, A., Barndollar, K., & Trötschel, R. (2001). The automated will: Nonconscious activation and pursuit of behavioral goals. *Journal of Personality and Social Psychology, 81*, 1014-1027. doi:10.1037/0022-3514.81.6.1014

Bem, D. J. (1967). Self-Perception: An alternative interpretation of cognitive dissonance phenomena. *Psychological Review, 74*(3), 183-200. doi:10.1037/h0024835

Briñol, P., & Petty, R. E. (2009). Persuasion: Insights from the self-validation hypothesis. In M. P. Zanna (Ed.), *Advances in experimental social psychology* (Vol. 41, pp. 69-118). New York: Elsevier.

Bry, C., Follenfant, A., & Meyer, T. (2008). Blonde like me: When self-construals moderate stereotype priming effects on intellectual performance. *Journal of Experimental Social Psychology, 44*(3), 751-757. doi:10.1016/j.jesp.2007.06.005

Cesario, J., Plaks, J. E., & Higgins, E. T. (2006). Automatic social behavior as motivated preparation to interact. *Journal of Personality and Social Psychology, 90*(6), 893-910. doi:10.1037/0022-3514.90.6.893

DeMarree, K. G., & Loersch, C. (2009). Who am I and who are you? Priming and the influence of self versus other focused attention. *Journal of Experimental Social Psychology, 45*, 440-443. doi:10.1016/j.jesp.2008.10.009

DeMarree, K. G., Loersch, C., Briñol, P., Petty, R. E., Payne, B. K., & Rucker, D. D. (2012). From primed construct to motivated behavior: Validity perceptions in automatic goal pursuit. *Personality and Social Psychology Bulletin, 38*, 1659-1670. doi: 10.1177/0146167212458328

DeMarree, K. G., Morrison, K. R., Wheeler, S. C., & Petty, R. E. (2011). Self-ambivalence and resistance to subtle self-change attempts. *Personality and Social Psychology Bulletin, 37*, 674-686. doi:10.1177/0146167211400097

DeMarree, K. G., Wheeler, S. C., & Petty, R. E. (2005). Priming a new identity: Self-monitoring moderates the effects of nonself primes on self-judgments and behavior. *Journal of Personality and Social Psychology, 89*, 657-671. doi:10.1037/0022-3514.89.5.657

DeSteno, D., & Salovey, P. (1997). Structural dynamism in the concept of self: A flexible model for a malleable concept. *Review of General Psychology, 1*, 389-409. doi: 10.1037/1089-2680.1.4.389

Dijksterhuis, A., & Bargh, J. A. (2001). The perception-behavior expressway: Automatic effects of social perception on social behavior. In M. P. Zanna (Ed.), *Advances in experimental social psychology* (Vol. 33, pp. 1-40). San Diego, CA: Academic Press. doi:10.1016/S0065-2601(01)80003-4

Dijksterhuis, A., & Van Knippenberg, A. (2000). Behavioral indecision: Effects of self-focus on automatic behavior. *Social Cognition, 18*(1), 55-74. doi:10.1521/soco.2000.18.1.55

Dijksterhuis, A., & van Knippenberg, A. (1998). The relation between perception and behavior, or how to win a game of Trivial Pursuit. *Journal of Personality and Social Psychology, 74*, 865-877. doi:10.1037/0022-3514.74.4.865

Dijksterhuis, A., Spears, R., Postmes, T., Stapel, D., Koomen, W., Knippenberg, A. V., & Scheepers, D. (1998). Seeing one thing and doing another: Contrast effects in automatic behavior. *Journal of Personality and Social Psychology, 75*(4), 862-871. doi:10.1037/0022-3514.75.4.862

Fazio, R. H., Sanbonmatsu, D. M., Powell, M. C., & Kardes, F. R. (1986). On the automatic activation of attitudes. *Journal of Personality and Social Psychology, 50*, 229-238. doi:10.1037/0022-3514.50.2.229

Fiske, S. T., & von Hendy, H. M. (1992). Personality feedback and situational norms can control stereotyping processes. *Journal of Personality and Social Psychology, 62*(4), 577-596.

Galinsky, A. D., Wang, C. S., & Ku, G. (2008). Perspective-takers behave more stereotypically. *Journal of Personality and Social Psychology, 95*(2), 404–419. doi:10.1037/0022-3514.95.2.404

Haddock, G., Macrae, C. N., & Fleck, S. (2002). Syrian science and smart supermodels: On the when and how of perception-behavior effects. *Social Cognition, 20*(6), 461-479. doi:10.1521/soco.20.6.461.22976

Hall, N. R., & Crisp, R. J. (2008). Assimilation and contrast to group primes: The moderating role of ingroup identification. *Journal of Experimental Social Psychology, 44*(2), 344-353. doi:10.1016/j.jesp.2007.07.007

Hansen, J., & Wänke, M. (2009). Think of capable others and you can make it! Self-efficacy mediates the effect of stereotype activation on behavior. *Social Cognition, 27*, 76-88. doi: 10.1521/soco.2009.27.1.76

Higgins, E. T. (1996). Knowledge activation: Accessibility, applicability, and salience. In E. T. Higgins & A. W. Kruglanski (Eds.), *Social psychology: Handbook of basic principles* (pp. 133-168). New York: Guilford.

Higgins, T. E., Rholes, W. S., & Jones, C. R. (1977). Category accessibility and impression formation. *Journal of Experimental Social Psychology, 13*(2), 141-154.

Hull, J. G., Slone, L. B., Meteyer, K. B., & Matthews, A. R. (2002). The nonconsciousness of self-consciousness. *Journal of Personality and Social Psychology, 83*(2), 406-424. doi:10.1037/0022-3514.83.2.406

Hundhammer, T., & Mussweiler, T. (2012). How sex puts you in gendered shoes: Sexuality-priming leads to gender-based self-perception and behavior. *Journal of Personality and Social Psychology, 103*(1), 176-193. doi:10.1037/a0028121

Ioannidis, J. P. A. (2005). Why most published research findings are false. *PLoS Med, 2*, e124. doi: 10.1371/journal.pmed.002012

Jiang, Y., Cho, A., & Adaval, R. (2009). The unique consequences of feeling lucky: Implications for consumer behavior. *Journal of Consumer Psychology, 19*(2), 171-184. doi:10.1016/j.jcps.2009.02.010

Kawakami, K., Dovidio, J. F., & Dijksterhuis, A. (2003). Effect of social category priming on personal attitudes. *Psychological Science, 14*(4), 315-319.

Kawakami, K., Phills, C. E., Greenwald, A. G., Simard, D., Pontiero, J., Brnjas, A., et al. (2012). In perfect harmony: Synchronizing the self to activated social categories. *Journal of Personality and Social Psychology, 102*(3), 562–575. doi:10.1037/a0025970

Kay, A. C., Wheeler, S. C., Bargh, J. A., & Ross, L. (2004). Material priming: The influence of mundane physical objects on situational construal and competitive behavioral choice. *Organizational Behavior and Human Decision Processes, 95*, 83-96. doi:10.1016/j.obhdp.2004.06.003

Kay, A. C., Wheeler, S. C., & Smeesters, D. (2008). The situated person: Effects of construct accessibility on situation construals and interpersonal perception. *Journal of Experimental Social Psychology, 44*, 275-291. doi:10.1016/j.jesp.2007.05.005

Ku, G., Wang, C. S., & Galinsky, A. D. (2010). Perception through a perspective-taking lens: Differential effects on judgment and behavior. *Journal of Experimental Social Psychology, 46*, 792-798. doi: 10.1016/j.jesp.2010.04.001

Lashley, K. S. (1951). The problem of serial order in behavior. In L. A. Jeffress (Ed.), *Cerebral mechanisms in behavior: The Hixon symposium* (pp. 112-136). New York: Wiley.

LeBoeuf, R. A., & Estes, Z. (2004). "Fortunately, I'm no Einstein": Comparison relevance as a determinant of behavioral assimilation and contrast. *Social Cognition, 22*(6), 607-636. doi:10.1521/soco.22.6.607.54817

Ledgerwood, A., & Chaiken, S. (2007). Priming us and them: Automatic assimilation and contrast in group attitudes. *Journal of Personality and Social Psychology, 93*(6), 940-956. doi:10.1037/0022-3514.93.6.940

Loersch, C., Durso, G. R. O., & Petty, R. E. (2013). Vicissitudes of desire: A matching mechanism for subliminal persuasion. *Social Psychological and Personality Science, 4*, 624-631.

Loersch, C., & Payne, B. K. (2011). The situated inference model: An integrative account of the effects of primes on perception, behavior, and motivation *Perspectives on Psychological Science, 6*, 234-252. doi:10.1177/1745691611406921

Loersch, C., & Payne, B. K. (2012). On mental contamination: The role of (mis)attribution in behavior priming. *Social Cognition, 30*, 241-252.

Loersch, C., & Payne, B. K. (2014). Situated inferences and the what, who, and where of priming. This volume.

Macrae, C. N., & Johnston, L. (1998). Help, I need somebody: Automatic action and inaction. *Social Cognition, 16*, 400-417.

Markman, K. D., & McMullen, M. N. (2003). A reflection and evaluation model of comparative thinking. *Personality and Social Psychology Review, 7*(3), 244-267. doi:10.1207/S15327957PSPR0703_04

Markus, H., & Kunda, Z. (1986). Stability and malleability of the self-concept. *Journal of Personality and Social Psychology, 51*(4), 858-866. doi:10.1037/0022-3514.51.4.858

Markus, H. R., & Wurf, E. (1987). The dynamic self-concept: A social psychological perspective. *Annual Review of Psychology, 38*, 299-337. doi: 10.1146/annurev.ps.38.020187.001503

McConnell, A. R. (2011). The Multiple Self-Aspects Framework: Self-concept representation and its implications. *Personality and Social Psychology Review, 15*, 3–27. doi:10.1177/10888.

Meyer, D. E., & Schvaneveldt, R. W. (1971). Facilitation in recognizing pairs of words: Evidence of a dependence between retrieval operations. *Journal of Experimental Psychology, 90*(2), 227-234. doi:10.1037/h0031564

Morrison, K. R., Johnson, C. S., & Wheeler, S. C. (2012). Not all selves feel the same certainty: Assimilation to primes among individualists and collectivists. *Social Psychological and Personality Science, 3*(1), 118-126. doi:10.1177/1948550611411310

Mussweiler, T. (2003). Comparison processes in social judgment: Mechanisms and consequences. *Psychological Review,*

110(3), 472-489. doi:10.1037/0033-295X.110.3.472

Mussweiler, T., & Neumann, R. (2000). Sources of mental contamination: Comparing the effects of self-generated versus externally provided primes. *Journal of Experimental Social Psychology, 36*, 194-206. doi:10.1006/jesp.1999.1415

Nisbett, R. E., & Wilson, T. D. (1977). Telling more than we can know: Verbal reports on mental processes. *Psychological Review, 84*(3), 231-259. doi:10.1037/0033-295X.84.3.231

Petty, R. E., & Cacioppo, J. T. (1996). Addressing disturbing and disturbed consumer behavior: Is it necessary to change the way we conduct behavioral science? *Journal of Marketing Research, 33*, 1-8.

Petty, R. E., DeMarree, K. G., Briñol, P., Horcajo, J., & Strathman, A. J. (2008). Need for cognition can magnify or attenuate priming effects in social judgment. *Personality and Social Psychology Bulletin, 34*, 900-912. doi:10.1177/0146167208316692

Pfeffer, J., & DeVoe, S. E. (2009). Economic evaluation: The effect of money and economics on attitudes about volunteering. *Journal of Economic Psychology, 30*(3), 500-508. doi:10.1016/j.joep.2008.08.006

Schubert, T. W., & Häfner, M. (2003). Contrast from social stereotypes in automatic behavior. *Journal of Experimental Social Psychology, 39*(6), 577-584. doi:10.1016/S0022-1031(03)00034-9

Schwarz, N. (2004). Metacognitive experiences in consumer judgment and decision making. *Journal of Consumer Psychology, 14*, 332-348.

Segal, S. J., & Cofer, C. N. (1960). The effect of recency and recall on word association. *American Psychologist, 15*, 451.

Shanks, D. R., Newell, B. R., Lee, E. H., Balakrishnan, D., Ekelund, L., Cenac, Z., et al. (J. Daunizeau, Ed.). (2013). Priming intelligent behavior: An elusive phenomenon. *PLOS ONE, 8*(4), e56515. doi:10.1371/journal.pone.0056515.s001

Sherif, M., Taub, D., & Hovland, C. I. (1958). Assimilation and contrast effects of anchoring stimuli on judgments. *Journal of Experimental Psychology, 55*(2), 150-155. doi:10.1037/h0048784

Skowronski, J. J., Sedikides, C., Heider, J. D., Wood, S. E., & Scherer, C. R. (2010). On the road to self-perception: Interpretation of self-behaviors can be altered by priming. *Journal of Personality, 78*(1), 361-391. doi:10.1111/j.1467-6494.2009.00619.x

Smeesters, D., Wheeler, S. C., & Kay, A. C. (2010). Indirect prime-to-behavior effects. In M. Zanna (Ed.), *Advances in experimental social psychology* (Vol. 42, pp. 259-317). New York: Elsevier. doi:10.1016/S0065-2601(10)42005-5

Smith, E. R. (1996). What do connectionism and social psychology offer each other? *Journal of Personality and Social Psychology, 70*(5), 893-912. doi:10.1037/0022-3514.70.5.893

Spears, R., Gordijn, E., Dijksterhuis, A., & Stapel, D. A. (2004). Reaction in action: Intergroup contrast in automatic behavior. *Personality and Social Psychology Bulletin, 30*(5), 605-616. doi:10.1177/0146167203262087

Srull, T. K., & Wyer, R. S. (1979). The role of category accessibility in the interpretation of information about persons: Some determinants and implications. *Journal of Personality and Social Psychology, 37*(10), 1660-1672. doi:10.1037/0022-3514.37.10.1660

Steele, J. R., & Ambady, N. (2006). "Math is Hard!" The effect of gender priming on women's attitudes. *Journal of Experimental Social Psychology, 42*(4), 428-436. doi:10.1016/j.jesp.2005.06.003

Strack, F., Schwarz, N., Bless, H., Kubler, A., & Wänke, M. (1993). Awareness of the influence as a determinant of assimilation versus contrast. *European Journal of Social Psychology, 23*, 53-62.

Strahan, E. J., Spencer, S. J., & Zanna, M. P. (2002). Subliminal priming and persuasion: Striking while the iron is hot. *Journal of Experimental Social Psychology, 38*, 556-568. doi: 10.1016/S0022-1031(02)00502-4

Wegener, D. T., & Petty, R. E. (1997). The flexible correction model: The role of naive theories of bias in bias correction. In M. P. Zanna (Ed.), *Advances in experimental social psychology* (Vol., 29, pp. 141-208). San Diego, CA: Academic Press.

Wheeler, S. C., & Berger, J. (2007). When the same prime leads to different effects. *Journal of Consumer Research, 34*, 357-368.

Wheeler, S. C., & DeMarree, K. G. (2009). Multiple mechanisms of prime-to-behavior effects. *Social and Personality Psychology Compass*, *3*(4), 566-581. doi:10.1111/j.1751-9004.2009.00187.x

Wheeler, S. C., & Petty, R. E. (2001). The effects of stereotype activation on behavior: A review of possible mechanisms. *Psychological Bulletin*, *127*(6), 797-826. doi:10.1037/0033-2909.127.6.797

Wheeler, S. C., DeMarree, K. G., & Petty, R. E. (2005). The roles of the self in priming-to-behavior effects. In A. Tesser, J. V. Wood, & D. A. Stapel (Eds.), *On building, defending, and regulating the self: A psychological perspective* (pp. 245-271). New York: Psychology Press.

Wheeler, S. C., DeMarree, K. G., & Petty, R. E. (2007). Understanding the role of the self in prime-to-behavior effects: The active-self account. *Personality and Social Psychology Review*, *11*(3), 234-261. doi:10.1177/1088868307302223

Wheeler, S. C., DeMarree, K. G., & Petty, R. E. (2008). A match made in the laboratory: Persuasion and matches to primed traits and stereotypes. *Journal of Experimental Social Psychology*, *44*, 1035-1047. doi:10.1016/j.jesp.2008.03.007

Wheeler, S. C., Jarvis, W. B. G., & Petty, R. E. (2001). Think unto others: The self-destructive impact of negative racial stereotypes. *Journal of Experimental Social Psychology*, *37*(2), 173-180. doi:10.1006/jesp.2000.1448

Wheeler, S. C., Morrison, K. R., DeMarree, K. G., & Petty, R. E. (2008). Does self-consciousness increase or decrease priming effects? It depends. *Journal of Experimental Social Psychology*, *44*, 882-889. doi:10.1016/j.jesp.2007.09.002

Wilson, T. D. (2002). *Strangers to ourselves*. Cambridge, MA: Harvard University Press.

Wyer, N. A., Mazzoni, G., Perfect, T. J., Calvini, G., & Neilens, H. L. (2010). When not thinking leads to being and doing. *Social Psychological and Personality Science*, *1*(2), 152-159.

Wyer, N. A., Neilens, H., Perfect, T. J., & Mazzoni, G. (2011). Automatic and ironic behavior are both mediated by changes in the self-concept. *Journal of Experimental Social Psychology*, *47*, 1300-1303. doi:10.1016/j.jesp.2011.05.008

Wyer, N. A., Perfect, T. J., Neilens, H., Mazzoni, G., & Roper, J. (2011). With or without you: Determinants of postsuppression behavior. *Social Psychological and Personality Science*, *2*, 272-276. doi:10.1177/1948550610389081

REPLICABILITY AND MODELS OF PRIMING: WHAT A RESOURCE COMPUTATION FRAMEWORK CAN TELL US ABOUT EXPECTATIONS OF REPLICABILITY

Joseph Cesario
Michigan State University

Kai J. Jonas
University of Amsterdam

In this chapter, we argue that whether or not a replication attempt is informative is dependent on the accuracy of one's underlying model to explain the effect, as it is the explanatory model that enumerates the contingencies necessary for producing the effect. If the model is incorrect, then a researcher may unknowingly change variables that the model says are irrelevant but which are really essential, rendering the replication results ambiguous. The expectation that effects of priming on social behavior should be widely invariant makes sense only under the assumptions of strict direct expression and spreading activation models, yet it has been shown that these models cannot adequately explain findings from the priming literature. We describe one model of priming that predicts variability across experimental contexts and populations: *the resource computation model*. We highlight variables that have been uncovered under the assumptions of this model that cannot be accounted for by direct expression models and which can explain replication failures. The model is also consistent with evolutionary understandings of the mind, in which information from multiple sources beyond just stimulus information is incorporated into behavioral decisions. To the degree that anything other than a strict, direct expression, spreading activation model is correct, the expectation that priming of social behaviors should be widely invariant is unreasonable.

The material is based on work supported by the National Science Foundation under award No. BCS-1230281 to the first author.

Address correspondence to Joseph Cesario, Psychology Building, 316 Physics Road - Room 255, East Lansing, MI 48824; E-mail: cesario@msu.edu or to Kai J. Jonas, Sociale Psychologie & Cognitive Science Center, Universiteit van Amsterdam, Weesperplein 4, 1018 XA Amsterdam; E-mail: k.j.jonas@uva.nl.

A researcher publishes an intriguing priming effect showing that subliminal exposure to faces of black males increases participants' aggressiveness in response to provocation (Bargh, Chen, & Burrows, 1996). A second researcher decides to attempt a replication of this effect by repeating the original experiment. What are the appropriate expectations for the replicability of such effects of priming, and how does the model used to explain such effects influence these expectations?

In this chapter, we argue that the expectation that the effects of priming should be widely invariant (and, thus, easily replicable) is reasonable only if one holds a direct expression, non-motivational model of such effects.[1] Researchers holding such expectations tend to operate under spreading activation models found in cognitive psychology (e.g., Collins & Loftus, 1975). These models accurately describe some types of effects of priming (such as facilitated processing of semantically—related words; Meyer & Schvaneveldt, 1971; Neely, 1977), and indeed these models were proposed in early work as a way to explain priming of more complex social and goal-directed behaviors (e.g., Bargh et al., 1996). However, more recent research (for a summary see Jonas, 2013) has demonstrated that spreading activation models alone cannot account for priming of social behaviors in all instances. Such models assume a single perceiver who encounters a social category stimulus in an environment devoid of other actors or objects, and with no desires or goals with respect to the target other—in short, a social, physical, and motivational landscape that offers little contextual richness in which behavior is entirely a function of stimulus features.

More recent models, in contrast, outline a large set of contingencies that would serve to reduce, eliminate, or reverse priming effects if not met. Such contingencies include whether the person likes or dislikes the primed category (Cesario, Plaks, & Higgins, 2006); whether a person has interdependent versus independent self-construal (Bry, Follenfant, & Meyer, 2008); whether a primed goal is associated with ingroup versus outgroup members (Loersch, Aarts, Payne, & Jefferis, 2008); or whether the prime is self- or other-generated (Mussweiler & Neumann, 2000). We describe one such model that outlines a set of contingencies, the resource computation model, and summarize recent evidence in support of it (see Loersch & Payne, 2011, 2014, this volume, for another such model). We conclude that the expectation that effects of priming should be consistent across a wide range of experimental contexts and populations is misguided, inconsistent with understandings of the evolved design of the mind, and should be reconsidered in light of more complete and accurate models of priming.

EXPECTATIONS OF REPLICABILITY

Every effect of priming has some set of contingencies that must be met in order for the effect to occur; that is, all priming is conditional (see also Bargh, 1989). One's theory or model for explaining a given effect of priming is fundamental precisely because it directs the researcher to those variables that are the key con-

---

1. Priming refers to a wide range of effects of the presentation of a stimulus, including everything from semantic priming (e.g., Neely, 1977; Posner & Snyder, 1975) to goal priming (e.g., Shantz & Latham, 2009). In this chapter, we refer exclusively to the effects of presenting social category members on automatic cognitive and behavioral responses. Such research is often referred to as social priming, goal priming, or automatic social behavior. Whether any of the arguments advanced herein apply to any other type of priming is unknown at this time.

tingencies necessary to produce the effect. Different theories will enumerate a different set of necessary contingencies (see also Asendorpf et al., 2013). Therefore, if a researcher is operating under an inaccurate model, he or she may be failing to take into account key variables. Indeed, the researcher may inadvertently change contingencies which are necessary to produce the effect but which are viewed as merely arbitrary or incidental.

To illustrate with the opening example, how might one's model for explaining the effects of priming *black male* influence which contingencies are seen as necessary and thus influence one's expectations of replicability? In the earliest work on priming social behaviors, such effects of priming were explained with *direct expression* models, which were essentially spreading activation models plus an unspecified link from cognition to behavior. Bargh and colleagues (Bargh & Chartrand, 1999; Bargh et al., 1996; Dijksterhuis & Bargh, 2001) explained their effects with the *perception-behavior link*, which enumerated the following three steps: 1) perception of the prime event caused activation of a corresponding mental representation; 2) activation of that representation spread to associated, stored information; and 3) information with increased activation was more likely to be executed when given the appropriate circumstance, due simply to its increased activation. Steps 1 and 2 are the traditional spreading activation model; step 3 is the vague link that "explains" why information with increased activation is more likely to be executed. For example, perception of subliminal pictures of young black males activates the mental representation of this category, activation spreads to associated information such as "aggressive," and the mere increase in activation of "aggressive" then makes it more likely that the person will behave in an aggressive way when provoked.

Suppose that such direct expression, spreading activation models are correct. Just like any other model, this model outlines a set of features that are necessary to produce the effect, and *as long as these contingencies are met*, it is reasonable to expect that the effect should be replicated. In the presence of repeated failures to produce the effect when meeting such contingencies, we rightly conclude that the original demonstration of the effect was likely Type I error.

What are the contingencies outlined by this and similar spreading activation models? The required contingencies are very straightforward and fairly easy to realize in any replication attempt. They include only: 1) the prime event itself (e.g., that people perceive subliminal pictures of young black males); 2) associations between the representation activated by the prime and the relevant stored information to be executed (e.g., that people associate black males with aggression); and 3) the appropriate circumstance to allow expression of the behavior (e.g., that people are provoked by an experimenter in a situation that allows for an aggressive response to be executed). Early research operating under such a model found that these contingencies did indeed influence the effects of priming, as when Dijksterhuis and colleagues found that the strength of association between the category *elderly* and the trait *forgetful* mediated the degree of memory impairment after priming of the category *elderly* (Dijksterhuis, Aarts, Bargh, & van Knippenberg, 2000).

It is easy to see why researchers operating under this kind of spreading activation model would expect priming effects to be widely replicable and why failed replication attempts would lead to the conclusion that the original demonstrations were Type I error. If one wants to replicate this effect, the required contingencies *as outlined by the model* are easy to achieve. For the first contingency, the prime event can be replicated exactly (as long as researchers are willing to share stimuli), and we know that changes to the prime stimuli or prime duration would change the expected effect (Higgins, 1996). For the second contingency, one can (and should) measure the association between the primed category and the measured trait through lexical decision tasks, output order, or other indirect measures, to ensure that participants do in fact have strong associations between, for example, black males and aggressiveness. Finally, it is a fairly straightforward matter to reproduce the appropriate circumstance by provoking the participant in the same manner as in the original demonstration.[2]

However, suppose spreading activation models are not the correct type of model to explain such effects of priming. In this case, the variables listed above might be necessary but not sufficient to produce the effect, as additional contingencies might also be needed. If this is the case, then a researcher seeking to replicate the effect may unintentionally change or lose necessary contingencies that he or she views as incidental or unimportant, thereby undermining or even reversing the priming effect. This may lead the researcher to erroneously conclude that the original effect was Type I error. Rather than that inference, the correct conclusion might simply have been that the researcher was operating under the wrong model, one that failed to identify the necessary contingencies to obtain the effect.

RESOURCE COMPUTATION MODEL OF AUTOMATICITY

Recently, we have proposed that automatic social behaviors following priming be understood as the output of a computational process that assesses what a person can and cannot accomplish in response to others (Cesario & Jonas, 2013). This computation includes an assessment of one's social, bodily, and structural resources, information that serves as input into decision processes concerning different courses of action. Social resources define what behaviors are possible and likely to be successful given the support of reliable others present. Bodily resources define what behaviors are possible and likely given one's current bodily states, including body position and physiology. Structural resources define what behaviors are possible and likely given the physical structure of the environment, including the presence or absence of action-relevant objects (Faber & Jonas, 2013). The computation involves integrating these features to lead to selection of one behavioral output over another (e.g., fight vs. flight, shoot or don't shoot, and so on).[3]

The model begins by proposing that perception of others (including perception from priming category members) initiates self-regulatory systems to prepare the body for effective interactions with the target other (Cesario, Plaks, & Higgins,

---

2. Even assuming a simple model, differences across broad segments of the population exist which may serve to undermine any one of the three required contingencies. The assumption that black males would prime aggressive behavior may not hold in societies in which the black stereotype is less clear, as in the Netherlands, for example, where one most likely would be able to replicate the effect with Arab faces (De Dreu et al., 2011).

3. We use the term computation as an indicator that such influences can and should be cognitively modeled. We (Cesario & Pleskac, in preparation) have recently begun a line of research modeling shoot/no shoot decisions in a first-person shooter task using a two-stage dynamic signal detection model, which models response times and error rates (see Pleskac & Busemeyer, 2010).

2006; Jonas & Sassenberg, 2006). In order for a person to effectively interact with others, decision calculations for such interactions must incorporate information about available resources for preparing and executing different behavioral response options. Only if such information is used as input into the decision-making process can behavior be regulated in an effective way. For example, human and nonhuman animal decisions about aggressive responses in contest situations follow game-theoretic logic and incorporate information about the presence of coalitional members (i.e., social resources). This is because such information changes the likelihood of successful aggressive actions and changes the costs that may be incurred by such behaviors (as costs can be distributed among group members if others are present; see, e.g., Benson-Amram et al., 2011; Fessler & Holbrook, 2013; McComb, Packer, & Pusey, 1994; Wilson, Britton, & Franks, 2002).

Importantly, this model of automatic behavior following priming is consistent with evolutionary accounts of the mind. The mind is not just similar to a computer, it is a computer in the sense that it is a computational organ: it takes informational inputs and regulates the body according to a set of evolved psychological adaptations (see Tooby & Cosmides, 2005). If the mind is to regulate the body with even the most remote bit of success, it must take into account information beyond just the information about the target other. In other words, stored knowledge about a social category member cannot be the sole determinant of behavioral output. Direct expression models of automatic behavior essentially argue that priming can be understood entirely as a function of activated stereotype content. In the case of behavior following priming of black males, this would mean that the brain had evolved to respond with aggression whenever aggression was perceived, regardless of one's coalition, whether one was lying prone or standing tall, or had objects for defense available. This cannot be the case, and such a model is inconsistent with what is known about nonhuman animal behavior (see Gawronski & Cesario, 2013).

Rather than behavior following priming being determined exclusively by the direct expression of primed stored content, a host of variables relevant to effective behavioral regulation combine to determine automatic responses to social category primes. Returning to the original point about replicability, a range of variables can be predicted to influence replication attempts *a priori*.

In what follows, we describe some recent experiments in support of the resource computation model, highlighting along the way how the model pointed to variables that should be important in producing certain effects of priming *given the model* but would have been regarded as irrelevant under other models (particularly non-motivational spreading activation models).

INITIAL FINDINGS SUPPORTING A SELF-REGULATORY ACCOUNT

In one of the first demonstrations that spreading activation models could not account for social behavior following priming, we modeled several experiments after the original Bargh and colleagues' (1996) findings, but with twists that pitted a direct expression, spreading activation account (as proposed by Bargh et al.) against a self-regulatory account (Cesario et al., 2006). First, we considered the study in which participants are subliminally primed with pictures of black males and are then provoked into an aggressive response. Instead of priming the black male category, however, we primed the category of *gay male* (vs. *straight male* or no prime). According to direct spreading activation accounts, priming *gay male* should result in decreased hostility, as the stereotype of gay males contains, almost universally, the stereotype of femininity or passivity. On the other hand, if a self-regulatory response is being prepared, we would expect that priming a negatively evaluated outgroup male, such as *gay male* (all participants were heterosexual), should result in more negative and aggressive responses. Indeed, priming *gay male* resulted in greater aggressiveness following provocation than either priming *straight male* or a no-prime control condition. These results do not readily follow from a model that considers spreading activation of activated stereotype content to exclusively drive priming effects.

Next, we again took an earlier, classic finding and modified it to produce a study that was able to test contrasting predictions from self-regulatory versus spreading activation accounts (Cesario et al., 2006, Study 2). Here, we took Bargh and colleagues' (1996) study showing that priming of the elderly stereotype (vs. a no-prime control condition) resulted in people walking more slowly and asked whether such responses should vary by participants' attitudes toward the elderly. According to direct spreading activation accounts, as long as the stored content *slow* is associated with the category *elderly*, then priming this category should result in slow walking speed, regardless of one's liking or disliking of the elderly. From a self-regulatory perspective, on the other hand, attitude toward the target group is a variable of central importance, given that effective behavior is defined very differently for liked and disliked others. To the extent that participants had positive attitudes toward the elderly, we predicted and found that they walked more slowly following priming, as one slows down to maintain contact with a liked, slow other. On the other hand, to the extent that participants had negative attitudes toward the elderly, we predicted and found that they *walked more quikkly following elderly priming*, presumably as a way to distance themselves from the disliked, slow other. Importantly, the degree to which participants associated the elderly with slow walking did not vary as a function of whether they held positive or negative attitudes toward them.

This study is particularly instructive for questions about replicability, given that a clear moderator was identified (attitudes toward the elderly) that could eliminate or even reverse the priming effect in a given sample, depending on the sample-wide level of this variable. Considering the widespread attention afforded to a failure to replicate the original Bargh and colleagues' (1996) finding (Doyen, Klein, Pichon, & Cleeremans, 2012), the assessment of such a moderator, among others, could help illuminate why failures can occur. But under the assumptions of a direct, spreading activation model, the only conditions for the effect to be obtained would be: 1) participants are primed with the category; 2) participants associate the elderly with slow walking; and 3) participants are given an opportunity to walk. If these conditions are met, then the replication attempt should be successful—or else one concludes that the original demonstration was Type I error, as many critics were quick to do. But for the replication attempt to be informative, the relevant contingencies *must* be in place, and these contingencies are defined by the explanatory model to which one adheres. It is becoming increasingly clear that spreading activation models cannot account for priming social behaviors, and therefore the expectations of replicability *derived from such models* are also becoming increasingly untenable.

EVIDENCE SUPPORTING STRUCTURAL RESOURCES

While the above two studies provided support for a general self-regulatory account (as opposed to a direct expression, spreading activation model), in another series of studies we tested the specific resource contingencies outlined above (social, bodily, and structural).[4] We first studied the possibility that structural resources would change automatic cognitive responses following priming if the structure of the physical environment changed which behaviors could be executed in response to a social category prime (Cesario et al., 2010). Specifically, we asked whether the physical environment of a person when primed with an aggressive target would influence the nature of the response to the prime. Basing our predictions on nonhuman animal models of defensive threat behavior, we predicted that whether participants were in a physical environment that allowed versus restricted fleeing behavior would influence the behavior prepared in response to the prime of *young black male*. If young black males are seen by white undergraduates as threatening outgroup members, then a defensive response should be prepared during priming. However, if this response takes into account which behaviors can actually be executed given the physical environment, then those participants in an environment allowing for flight behavior should show escape-related preparation, whereas those in an environment preventing flight behavior should show fight-related preparation.

To test these predictions, in one of the studies presented we primed participants with pictures of either young black males or young white males and tested the automatic activation of fight- versus escape-related action semantics. We then assessed the degree to which participants associated black males with danger (using a variant of Fazio's sequential priming task; Fazio, Jackson, Dunton, & Williams, 1995), reasoning that participants would prepare a defensive threat response only to the degree that they associated black males with danger. Crucially, the entire experiment took place while participants were seated either in an enclosed, restrictive space (a sound-resistant booth) or in an open field. In other words, the current structural resources either allowed for escape-related behavior to be executed in response to the prime or not. Consistent with predictions, we found that the relative activation of fight- versus escape-related words differed as a function of whether participants were in the booth or the field *and* the degree to which participants associated blacks with danger. When participants were in the booth, the more they associated black males with danger, the greater the activation of fight-related words. In the open field, however, the more participants associated black males with danger, the more they showed increased activation of escape-related words.

In addition to the primary finding that the structural environment influences automatic responses to primes, a further moderator was obtained in that the effect was contingent on the degree of association between black males and danger. The latter would be predicted from a direct expression account, while the former could not. If a researcher is operating under such a model, it would appear entirely

---

4. We do not discuss here our research on bodily resources, given that the research on this resource is the least developed of the three types of resources (see Cesario & McDonald, 2013, for research on how bodily resources, such as physical posture, can be understood as an input into the calculation of what one can accomplish).

reasonable to change this feature of the experimental context without any loss to the expectation of replicability. Indeed, what is more likely is that this feature of the experimental setup would not even register as an important variable precisely because the model says that it should not matter in obtaining the effect.[5]

A similar contingency, one not explained by spreading activation models, is the absence or presence of response-relevant objects in the current environment. If we consider again the black priming–aggression effect, responses could also be driven by other objects present (or absent) that one might use in relation to the primed category. While a bike may facilitate a flight response, a baseball bat may facilitate a defensive aggression response. Further, and building on the relevance of context introduced before, it would be difficult for spreading activation models to account for the effects of present objects on varying responses to social category primes. While one's representation of a social category undoubtedly contains links with objects used regularly and stably by the category, objects used in relation to the category are variable across contexts and are dependent on one's current motivation toward the category, resisting simple associative links. For example, one might associate bats with black males due to a connection with athleticism (black males are good athletes and routinely use bats for this purpose), and one might associate wheelchairs with the elderly due to a connection with frailty (the elderly typically use wheelchairs for transport due to frailty of old age). Spreading activation models might well predict activation of bats or wheelchairs when priming black males or the elderly, respectively. But it would be quite a different matter for spreading activation models to predict that bicycles should be activated by black males to the extent that one associates black males with danger and bicycles being a good means to flee, or to predict that wheelchairs should only be activated in response to the elderly if one has the goal to transport the elderly, but not the goal to rehabilitate them. Moreover, the relevance of the object is only given through the situation; in a different situation, the same object could be rendered useless.

Initial evidence for such an object co-determined response comes from research by Faber and Jonas (2013). Within an eye-tracking paradigm, these authors showed that a social category prime in a matching context led to more attention for response-relevant means. For example, in a sequential priming paradigm, attention for cheering devices was higher only after priming athlete and a stadium context, compared to a shop context or for irrelevant objects. These data show that social categories in matching contexts also increase attention to response-relevant objects.

EVIDENCE SUPPORTING SOCIAL RESOURCES

In a recent line of research, we have begun to investigate the way in which the presence of ingroup members changes automatic responses following priming of social categories. Ingroups are important insofar as the presence of reliable coali-

---

5. This study also illustrates further complications with replication attempts and the difficulty of trying to reproduce exactly the situation of a prior experiment. For instance, we took great care to ensure that participants would not encounter other students during their participation in the experiment, the reason being that seeing other university students might constitute a social resource, and the presence of coalitions is known to influence the likelihood of escape versus fight behavior (e.g., see Benson-Amram et al., 2011). The next section on social resources details this logic in more depth.

tion members changes the range of responses available to a person. If behavior in response to social category primes is to be effective, it must take into account the presence of others—ingroups both increase the likelihood that certain actions can be successfully executed and distribute costs of risky actions across group members.

There is evidence from a wide range of social species showing that the presence of others is taken into the calculus of which of several behavioral responses to execute, especially when it comes to defensive threat regulation. One illustrative example involving wild hyenas is provided by Benson-Amram and colleagues (2011). These researchers played the sounds of stranger (i.e., outgroup) hyenas to wild hyenas through a concealed speaker and assessed whether a target hyena hearing the sounds would flee or approach. These researchers found that a strong predictor of this behavioral choice was numerical advantage: the ratio of the number of ingroup hyenas present to the number of outgroup hyena voices. The greater this ratio, the more likely hyenas were to approach the unknown outgroup voices. This influence of one's coalition (in this case, familiar ingroup hyenas) is consistent with a game theoretic perspective on animal conflict (Maynard Smith, 1979; Maynard Smith & Price, 1973), and it appears that hyenas were computing the relative strength of the ingroup and outgroup coalitions in making decisions about different courses of action.

Returning to the case of priming social categories, then, the presence of one's coalition should affect the automatic responses to the social category, as the presence of the ingroup as a resource can change the potential costs incurred by risky actions and make certain behaviors more likely to be effective and successful.

We have so far studied responses to two different social categories and the ways in which being surrounded by other group members can influence the action tendencies automatically elicited in response to the primes (Cesario & Jonas, 2013). Across studies, our methodology has been similar: participants complete a task measuring automatic reactions to primes, but do so in the experimental room either alone or with a group of other ingroup members (with their shared ingroup identity made salient).

In a first study, we looked at how automatic responses to *police* primes changed depending on participants' currently available social resources. Specifically, we assessed reaction times in a lexical decision task to words related to *rioting* in response to police (or control) primes, while participants completed the task either alone or surrounded by an ingroup. Rioting is a behavioral response that can only be done with others; you cannot riot alone. We predicted and found that *police* primes led to increased accessibility of *riot*-related words only when participants were surrounded by others, not when they were alone. In other words, automatic cognitive processes took into account the social situation of the individual.

In a second set of studies (including two direct replications), we tested several predictions that follow from a resource computation account using a different kind of automatic reaction, that of whites' automatic evaluation of young black males. Physically formidable outgroup males would have been a recurrent evolutionary threat, and the mind likely evolved computational programs to assess coalitional numerosity (see, e.g., Kurzban, Tooby, & Cosmides, 2001; Navarrete, McDonald, Molina, & Sidanius, 2010). Therefore, physically formidable black males would, for whites, constitute an outgroup threat. Here, we tested the idea that (physically formidable) black males would no longer be automatically negatively evaluated when participants were surrounded by their racial ingroup, reflecting the fact that ingroup members change what strategic responses are deemed necessary in response to threat.

If the presence of one's coalition changes the computation of action possibility, then two predictions would follow. First, a physically formidable outgroup male requires vigilance and should be negatively evaluated when a person is alone (and therefore less able to incur the costs of aggression and less able to inflict costs on others; see also Cesario & Navarrete, 2014). Second, such vigilance and negativity should be attenuated when one is surrounded by one's coalition because one now has the resources to manage the threat. If automatic reactions from priming were indeed sensitive to the presence of social resources, then we should detect these changes in typical indirect measures of attitudes.

To test these predictions, participants completed two implicit association tests (IAT), either alone or surrounded by their ingroup. They completed both a stereotype IAT, which assesses the association between blacks and physicality (compared to whites and mentality), and an evaluative IAT, which assesses the association between blacks and negativity (compared to whites and positivity; see Amodio & Devine, 2006). We then examined the correlation between scores on each of these two measures, comparing this relationship between those participants who completed both measures alone and those who completed both measures surrounded by the ingroup. If the presence of others changes which responses a person computes as possible and effective in response to a potential threat, then the correlation between these two measures should depend on whether participants were alone or in the presence of the ingroup. Specifically, we found that when participants were alone, a positive correlation between responses on these two measures was obtained: the more black males were stereotyped as physical, the more they were negatively evaluated. However, we found that when participants were surrounded by their ingroups, this correlation was attenuated: A physically formidable outgroup male no longer carried the same negative evaluation.

Returning to the theme of the expectations for replicability, the resource computation model *predicts a priori* that the presence of others should matter for priming effects because automatic responses from priming are strategic and reflect functional preparation for interaction, at the cognitive level. In contrast, a direct expression or spreading activation model *predicts* that whether a participant is alone or surrounded by others should not matter in the least for priming effects, as priming effects are triggered merely by the presence of the appropriate stimulus (and not what actions are possible given the presence of others). Therefore, whether a researcher is a proponent of one model or the other directly influences expectations of replicability because each model describes for the researcher those variables that can be changed (or not changed) during a replication attempt.

CONCLUSION

What are the appropriate expectations for the replicability of the effects of priming? In this chapter, we have argued that one's model for explaining such effects directly and wholly informs such expectations, because the explanatory model enumerates the contingencies necessary for producing the effect in question. If direct expression, spreading activation models are correct in explaining these effects, then a certain set of contingencies are needed. These contingencies, which include the presence of the stimulus, association between the stimulus and the response in question, and the opportunity to execute the response, would naturally lead to the expectation of widespread invariance, given that such contingencies are very easy to implement in an experimental replication. In the presence of repeated unsuccessful replications of an effect of priming, one would rightly conclude that the original effect was likely Type I error.

To the extent that a spreading activation model is insufficient to explain the effects of priming, however, then one's expectations of invariance are unreasonable and unfounded. This is because the contingencies in place, which are believed to be necessary and sufficient for producing the effect, are in fact insufficient. Recent research has shown that spreading activation models cannot fully account for the effects of priming, and several more complex models have arisen in recent years, all of which enumerate a long list of additional contingencies necessary to produce such effects. We described one such model in the current chapter, the resource computation model. If correct, it suggests that a range of additional contingencies—beyond just those proposed by spreading activation models—must be in place in order to obtain effects of priming. This model is consistent with evolutionary understandings of the mind, in which information from multiple sources beyond just stimulus information is incorporated into behavioral decisions. The model directly undermines the expectation that effects of priming should be widely replicable across varying experimental contexts and populations.

We conclude on a final caveat. It is important to note that the argument outlined in this chapter should *not* be used as an excuse for poor research practices on the part of priming researchers, who might be publishing false findings due to a combination of researcher degrees of freedom, questionable research practices, and file drawer activity (see, e.g., Pashler, & Wagenmakers, 2012; Simmons, Nelson, & Simonsohn, 2011). While it may be tempting to explain away every failure in terms of unknown moderators, to do so would be to undermine the self-correcting nature of science. Moreover, priming researchers themselves have been insufficiently concerned with data reporting and collection practices and have contributed to the current state of confusion regarding the reliability of priming results. In other writings, we chart out a path for both priming researchers and critics to advance in a constructive way, and we provide recommendations for priming researchers to increase the quality of our research (see Cesario, 2014).

REFERENCES

Amodio, D. M., & Devine, P. G. (2006). Stereotyping and evaluation in implicit race bias: Evidence for independent constructs and unique effects on behavior. *Journal of Personality and Social Psychology, 91*, 652-661.

Asendorpf, J. B., Conner, M., de Fruyt, F., de Houwer, J., Denissen, J. J. A., Fiedler, K. (2013). Recommendations for increasing replicability in psychology. *European Journal of Personality, 27*, 108-119. doi:10.1002/per.1919

Bargh, J. A. (1989). Conditional automaticity: Varieties of automatic influence in social perception and cognition. In J. S. Uleman & J. A. Bargh (Eds.), *Unintended thoughts* (pp. 3-51). New York: Guilford.

Bargh, J. A., & Chartrand, T. L. (1999). The unbearable automaticity of being. *American Psychologist, 54*, 462-479.

Bargh, J. A., Chen, M., & Burrows, L. (1996). Automaticity of social behavior: Direct effects of trait construct and stereotype activation on action. *Journal of Personality and Social Psychology, 71*, 230-244. doi:10.1037/0022-3514.71.2.230

Benson-Amram, S., Heinen, V. K., Dryer, S. L., & Holekamp, K. E. (2011). Numerical assessment and individual call discrimination by wild spotted hyaenas, Crocuta crocuta. *Animal Behaviour, 82*, 743-752.

Bry, C., Follenfant, A., & Meyer, T. (2008). Blonde like me: When self-construals moderate stereotype priming effects on intellectual performance. *Journal of Experimental Social Psychology, 44*, 751-757. doi:10.1016/j.jesp.2007.06.005

Cesario, J. (2014). Priming, replication, and the hardest science. *Perspectives on Psychological Science, 9*(1), 40-48.

Cesario, J., & Jonas, K. J. (2013). *The role of ingroups in action preparation: A resource computation framework for automatic responses*. Manuscript in preparation.

Cesario, J., & McDonald, M. M. (2013). Bodies in context: Power poses as a computation of action possibility. *Social Cognition, 31*, 260-274.

Cesario, J., & Navarrete, C. D. (2014). Perceptual bias in threat distance: The critical roles of in-group support and target evaluations in defensive threat regulation. *Social Psychological and Personality Science, 5*(1), 12-17.

Cesario, J., Plaks, J. E., Hagiwara, N., Navarrete, C. D., & Higgins, E. T. (2010). The ecology of automaticity: How situational contingencies shape action semantics and social behavior. *Psychological Science, 21*, 1311-1317. doi:10.1177/0956797610378685

Cesario, J., Plaks, J. E., & Higgins, E. T. (2006). Automatic social behavior as motivated preparation to interact. *Journal of Personality and Social Psychology, 90*, 893-910. doi:10.1037/0022-3514.90.6.893

Cesario, J., & Pleskac, T. J. (in preparation). *Computational modeling of racial bias in the First-Person Shooter Task*.

Collins, A. M., & Loftus, E. F. (1975). A spreading-activation theory of semantic priming. *Psychological Review, 82*, 407-428.

De Dreu, C. K. W., Greer, L. L., Van Kleef, G. A., Shalvi, S., & Handgraaf, M. J. J. (2011). Oxytocin promotes human ethnocentrism. *Proceedings of the National Academy of Sciences, 108*, 1262-1266. doi:www.pnas.org/cgi/doi/10.1073/pnas.1015316108

Doyen, S., Klein, O., Pichon, C.-L., & Cleeremans, A. (2012). Behavioral priming: It's all in the mind, but whose mind? *PLOS ONE, 7*, e29081. doi:10.1371/journal.pone.0029081

Dijksterhuis, A., Aarts, H., Bargh, J. A., & van Knippenberg, A. (2000). On the relation between associative strength and automatic behavior. *Journal of Experimental Social Psychology, 36*, 531-544. doi:10.1006/jesp.2000.1427

Dijksterhuis, A., & Bargh, J. A. (2001). The perception-behavior expressway: Automatic effects of social perception on social behavior. *Advances in Experimental Social Psychology, 33*, 1-40.

Faber, T. W., & Jonas, K. J. (2013). Perception in a social context: Attention for response-functional means. *Social Cognition, 31*, 301-314.

Fazio, R. H., Jackson, J. R., Dunton, B. C., & Williams, C. J. (1995). Variability in automatic activation as an unobtrusive measure of racial attitudes: A bona fide pipeline? *Journal of Personality and Social Psychology, 69*, 1013-1027.

Fessler, D. M. T., & Holbrook, C. (2013). Friends shrink foes: The presence of comrades decreases the envisioned physical formidability of an opponent. *Psychological Science, 24*, 797-802. doi:10.1177/0956797612461508

Gawronski, B., & Cesario, J. (2013). Of mice and men: What animal research can tell us about context effects on automatic responses in humans. *Personality and Social Psychology Review, 17*, 187-215. doi:10.1177/1088868313480096

Higgins, E. T. (1996). Knowledge activation: Accessibility, applicability, and salience. In E. T. Higgins & A. W. Kruglanski (Eds.), *Social psychology: Handbook of basic principles* (pp. 133-168). New York: Guilford.

Jonas, K. J. (2013). Automatic behavior – Its social embedding and individual consequences. *Social and Personality Psychology Compass, 7/9*, 689-700.

Jonas, K. J., & Sassenberg, K. (2006). Knowing how to react: Automatic response priming from social categories. *Journal of Personality and Social Psychology, 90*, 709-721.

Kurzban, R., Tooby, J., & Cosmides, L. (2001). Can race be erased? Coalitional computation and social categorization. *Proceedings of the National Academy of Sciences, 98*, 15387-15392.

Loersch, C., Aarts, H., Payne, B. K., & Jefferis, V. E. (2008). The influence of social groups on goal contagion. *Journal of Experimental Social Psychology, 44*, 1555-1558. doi:10.1016/j.jesp.2008.07.009

Loersch, C., & Payne, B. K. (2011). The situated inference model: An integrative account of the effects of primes on perception, behavior, and motivation. *Perspectives on Psychological Science, 6*, 234-252.

Loersch, C., & Payne, B. K. (2014). Situated inferences and the what, who, and where of priming. This volume.

Maynard Smith, J. (1979). Game theory and the evolution of behavior. *Proceedings of the Royal Society B, 205*, 475-488.

Maynard Smith, J., & Price, G. R. (1973). The logic of animal conflict. *Nature, 246*, 15-18.

McComb, K., Packer, C., & Pusey, A. (1994). Roaring and numerical assessment in contests between groups of female lions, Panthera leo. *Animal Behaviour, 47*, 379-387.

Meyer, D. E., & Schvaneveldt, R. W. (1971). Facilitation in recognizing pairs of words: Evidence of a dependence between retrieval operations. *Journal of Experimental Psychology, 90*, 227-234.

Mussweiler, T., & Neumann, R. (2000). Sources of mental contamination: Comparing the effects of self-generated versus externally provided primes. *Journal of Experimental Social Psychology, 36*, 194-206. doi:10.1006/jesp.1999.1415

Navarrete, C. D., McDonald, M. M., Molina, L. E., & Sidanius, J. (2010). Prejudice at the nexus of race and gender: An outgroup male target hypothesis. *Journal of Personality and Social Psychology, 98*, 933-945.

Neely, J. H. (1977). Semantic priming and retrieval from lexical memory: Roles of inhibitionless spreading activation and limited-capacity attention. *Journal of Experimental Psychology: General, 106*, 226-254.

Pashler, H., & Wagenmakers, E. J. (2012). Editors' introduction to the special section on replicability in psychological science: A crisis of confidence? *Perspectives on Psychological Science, 7*, 528-530. doi:10.1177/1745691612465253

Pleskac, T. J., & Busemeyer, J. R. (2010). Two-stage dynamic signal detection: A theory of choice, decision time, and confidence. *Psychological Review, 117*, 864-901. doi:10.1037/a0019737

Posner, M. I., & Snyder, C. R. R. (1975). Attention and cognitive control. In R. L. Solso (Ed.), *Information processing and cognition: The Loyola symposium* (pp. 55-85). Hillsdale, NJ: Erlbaum.

Shantz, A., & Latham, G. P. (2009). An exploratory field experiment of the effect of subconscious and conscious goals on employee performance. *Organizational Behavior and Human Decision Processes, 109*, 9-17. doi:10.1016/j.obhdp.2009.01.001

Simmons, J. P., Nelson, L. D., & Simonsohn, U. (2011). False-positive psychology: Undisclosed flexibility in data collection and analysis allows presenting anything as significant. *Psychological Science, 22*, 1359-1366. doi:10.1177/0956797611417632

Tooby, J., & Cosmides, L. (2005). Conceptual foundations of evolutionary psychology. In D. M. Buss (Ed.), *Handbook of evolutionary psychology* (pp. 5-67). Hoboken, NJ: Wiley.

Wilson, M. L., Britton, N. F., & Franks, N. R. (2002). Chimpanzees and the mathematics of battle. *Proceedings of the Royal Society B, 269*, 1107-1112.

SITUATED INFERENCES AND THE WHAT, WHO, AND WHERE OF PRIMING

Chris Loersch
University of Colorado

B. Keith Payne
University of North Carolina at Chapel Hill

> We describe the situated inference model and discuss how it may contribute to better understanding priming effects and their absence. The model suggests that priming effects result when primes make certain ideas more likely to come to mind and those ideas are misattributed to one's own thoughts, interpreted in light of situational affordances. This perspective organizes a range of moderators identified in previous priming studies. We also describe new research that has tested the model's predictions. Finally, we consider the implications of the model for debates about the nature and replicability of priming effects on higher order cognition and behavior.

Sometimes simple ideas combine to create something surprising. The effects of incidental stimuli (primes) on higher order thought and behavior are surely surprising, and this has contributed to both enthusiasm and skepticism about priming effects. We have argued that the appearance and disappearance of priming effects can be understood based on the combination of three simple premises.

The first is that primes tend to increase the accessibility of related information, making certain thoughts and feelings more likely to come to mind. The second is that people tend to assume that their thoughts and feelings are about whatever they are attending to at the moment (even when the thoughts were actually caused by something else; see Higgins, 1998). And the third is that people tend to use accessible thoughts and feelings to guide responses to the situations in which they find themselves. From this perspective, priming is expected only when all three of these processes coincide. Stated simply, priming effects result when primes make certain ideas more likely to come to mind and those ideas are misattributed to one's own thoughts, interpreted in light of situational affordances. To know how a

---

Address correspondence to Chris Loersch, University of Colorado, Department of Psychology and Neuroscience, E328–B Muenzinger Hall, Boulder, CO 80309-0345; E-mail: chris.loersch@Colorado.edu.

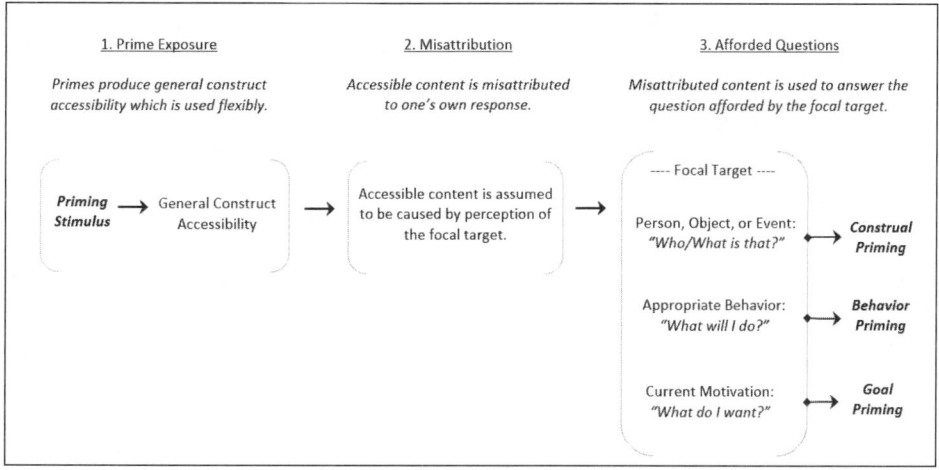

FIGURE 1. The Situated Inference Model

prime will affect behavior, we need to know *what* thoughts are activated, *who* these thoughts are attributed to, and *where* (e.g., in what context) people can apply them.

Some important consequences fall naturally out of these basic ideas. They help explain, for example, why a single prime might have a variety of different effects, such as altering judgments in one study, motives in another, and behaviors in yet another. They also help explain why priming effects may sometimes be found but other times may be elusive. In this paper, we summarize the situated inference model (Loersch & Payne, 2011) in which we have formalized these ideas. We highlight recent empirical findings predicted by the theory, and consider the implications for recent debates about the replicability and context-specificity of priming effects.

THE SITUATED INFERENCE MODEL

CORE MECHANISMS

Accessibility. According to the situated inference model, priming effects emerge through a basic three-step process (see Figure 1). This begins (Step 1) with a prime increasing the accessibility of related information. Accessibility is generally understood to mean the likelihood that a given piece of information will be retrieved from memory (Tulving & Pearlstone, 1966) and used in subsequent processing (Higgins, 1996). Many kinds of information can be made accessible, including (for example) mental content that is semantically (Neely, 1991), experientially (Bearce & Rovee-Collier, 2006; Conway, 1990), or affectively (Fazio, Sanbonmatsu, Powell, & Kardes, 1986; Payne, Cheng, Govorun, & Stewart, 2005) related to the primed stimulus. These basic accessibility effects do not necessarily rely on the conscious act of perception (de Groot, 1983; Fowler, Wolford, Slade & Tassinary, 1981; Marcel, 1983) and can be produced by subliminally presented stimuli (Jacoby, Lindsay, & Toth, 1992). As such, both conscious and nonconscious processing of a priming stimulus can produce the initial change in construct accessibility from which higher order social priming effects emerge.

Misattribution. The increase in accessibility resulting from priming has often been viewed as having an immediate effect on responses. For example, accounts of goal (Bargh, 1990; Chartrand & Bargh, 1996) and behavior priming (Dijksterhuis & Bargh, 2001) often assume a direct effect of primes on behavior, unmediated by further thought processes. We suggest, in contrast, that this simple change in accessibility does not produce a direct effect on judgment or behavior. Instead, primes affect responses when this accessible content is mistakenly attributed to one's own internal thoughts and feelings about whatever is in the focus of attention (Step 2). People will tend to act in ways consistent with the implications of those thoughts and feelings, but what are the implications? It depends on the demands and opportunities afforded by the situation.

Afforded Questions. The meaning of primed information for the person depends on the particular question(s) afforded by the situation (Step 3). Notably, different situations afford different questions, and this can cause the same accessible content to produce very different effects. For example, although being asked to think about another person and their personality traits affords the question, "What type of person are they," being asked to think about yourself will instead afford the question, "What type of person am I?" To the extent that prime-related content is misattributed to the focal target, these two situations will produce two distinct priming effects, differentially producing changes in other versus self-perception (e.g., a more aggressive personality in one's friend vs. the self; DeMarree & Loersch, 2009).

Although this example demonstrates how the situated inference model accounts for the variable effects of primes on perception and judgment (i.e., construal priming), this same process can be used to understand behavior and goal priming as well. This is because some situations naturally afford questions about how to behave, or what one wants. When this occurs, accessible content that becomes misattributed to one's response to these questions will affect the behavioral (or motivational) inferences that are drawn. Again, this can cause the same accessible content to produce very different downstream consequences. If, for example, one mistakenly assumes that hostility-related thoughts are accessible because of their desire to aggress, then a behavioral priming effect may emerge (e.g., more intense punishing behavior; Carver, Ganellen, Froming, & Chambers, 1983; see also Bargh, Gollwitzer, Lee-Chai, Barndollar, & Trotschel, 2001). In this way, the situated inference model naturally provides an answer to the "many effects of one prime problem" that Bargh (2006) identified as a central second-generation issue for the field. A single prime produces a myriad of downstream effects because its misattributed accessibility can have very different inferential implications across situations.

This process need not be conscious or deliberate. Instead, just as with attributional processes in other domains (e.g., spontaneous trait inferences; Newman & Uleman, 1990), these processes have been shown to occur outside of conscious awareness (Jones, Fazio, & Olson, 2009; Loersch, Durso, & Petty, 2013; Loersch & Payne, 2012). Indeed, we view the basic process of using accessible information to infer the answer to environmentally afforded questions as a constant and obligatory aspect of the decision-making system, one that simply cannot operate at a solely conscious level. Because the environment continuously affords different questions as one seeks to understand the situation and determine how best to interact with the people and objects present, consciously attending to every decision would be untenable. Even without conscious involvement, however, the inference process we propose allows the mind to naturally integrate one's past learning history with the constraints of the current situation to guide behavior in a contextually appropriate matter. It is only because of the challenges of accurate source monitoring that this process introduces errors and produces priming effects.

THE FLEXIBLE USE OF ACCESSIBLE INFORMATION

Because the situated inference model proposes that accessible content simply serves as a source of information in the decision-making process (see also Jefferis & Fazio, 2008), various metacognitive factors (Briñol & DeMarree, 2012) and mindset manipulations (Fujita & Trope, 2014, this volume) can exert important influences on the process. For example, any variable that affects the perceived validity of prime-related content will modulate its impact on judgment and behavior. When the accessible information is seen as highly valid (e.g., because it is associated with trust, confidence, ease, fluency, etc.), it will be especially likely to produce a priming effect. If the same content is instead associated with feelings of invalidity, then it will not produce an assimilative effect and may even lead to contrast effects if the metacognitive cues are strong enough to produce a correction motive (Wegener & Petty, 1995). Mindset manipulations can have similar effects because they also alter the way accessible information is used. For example, mindsets can cause people to habitually compare accessible content to a salient standard, a process that can cause the same prime to produce very different effects depending on whether people focus their comparison on similarities or differences (Crusius & Mussweiler, 2012; Mussweiler & Damisch, 2008).

MODERATORS OF PRIMING EFFECTS

Since the original demonstrations of the basic priming effects, many of the publications in this area have documented the operation of various moderators. Although this isn't well explained by models that emphasize direct, automatic effects, the situated inference model's proposed process naturally captures many of the key moderators that have been identified. In the following section, we discuss some of the important moderators and highlight how they are accounted for by our perspective. Because the model suggests that construal, behavior, and goal priming all occur through the same basic process, the following discussion will not be concerned with the exact type of outcome which is moderated. Readers interested in such a breakdown are encouraged to refer to our initial presentation of the model (Loersch & Payne, 2011, pp. 240-247). Following this review of past research, we briefly summarize new research that has directly tested moderating variables as specifically predicted by the situated inference model.

KNOWN MODERATORS AFFECTING MISATTRIBUTION

Aspects of the Priming Event. Because prime-related accessibility will only produce a priming effect when misattributed to an alternative source, the model predicts that any variable affecting the likelihood of misattribution will be an important moderator. Evidence for this hypothesis can be seen throughout the literature, as many of the identified moderators directly relate to the confusability of prime-related content with the target of judgment. For example, primes that are especially distinctive are unlikely to be misattributed to alternative targets because the information they make accessible isn't vague or general enough to be confused with other sources. Because of this, highly distinctive primes can only exert an influence on the decision-making process by serving as a comparison standard that highlights how different the target of judgment is from the accessible construct (Moskowitz & Skurnik, 1999; Mussweiler, 2003). These stimuli, such as animals with extreme features (e.g., using sharks to prime fierceness) or a specific person with known traits (e.g., using Albert Einstein to prime intelligence), often produce contrast effects rather than prime-consistent responses (see Dijksterhuis et al., 1998; Herr, Sherman, & Fazio, 1983).

Information made accessible by a prime is also difficult to misattribute when the priming manipulation is particularly blatant or salient. Under these conditions, the true source of the accessibility is obvious, and assimilative priming effects are prevented. This is why it is especially important that participants in a priming experiment do not perceive a direct connection between a priming manipulation and the dependent measure (Bargh & Chartrand, 2000). When misattribution is prevented in this manner, the most likely way for the prime to exert an effect is if individuals feel that it will bias their judgment and engage in effortful, motivated correction (Martin, 1986; Wegener & Petty, 1995). It is for this reason that blatant (Martin, Seta, & Crelia, 1990; Newman & Uleman, 1990, Petty, DeMarree, Briñol, Horcajo, & Strathman, 2008) or well-remembered priming manipulations (Lombardi, Higgins, & Bargh, 1987) generally produce contrast effects on judgment or behavior. It is important to note, however, that blatant priming will not inevitably induce these correction efforts. In particular, if people mistakenly believe the prime-related content is self-generated, this information may still be confused with that person's response to the current situation. In these cases, misattribution can still occur and the primes produce assimilation effects (Moskowitz & Roman, 1992; Mussweiler & Neumann, 2000).

Aspects of the Target. The likelihood of misattribution can depend upon factors that are related to the target of judgment as well. When the target of attention is highly distinctive, only a very limited subset of information is relevant, thereby decreasing the number of dimensions on which it is susceptible to priming effects (Higgins, Rholes, & Jones, 1977). In contrast, highly ambiguous targets (e.g., novel or nonsense animals like "jabos" or "lemphors," Herr et al., 1983) are especially likely to show priming effects because they are non-distinct and their characteristics can be plausibly confused with many different types of accessible content.

Another target-related moderator that uniquely applies to goal and behavior priming is the self-concept. The role of the self-concept in these priming effects (Wheeler, DeMarree, & Petty, 2007, 2014, this volume) makes manipulations that target self-perceptions especially effective at producing behavioral changes (DeMarree & Loersch, 2009). It is perhaps for this reason why priming inductions that require participants to self-generate the behavioral content from memory (e.g., by recalling their past behaviors or imagining their actions while role-playing as a stereotyped target; DeMarree et al., 2012; Galinsky, Wang, & Ku, 2008; Wheeler &

Petty, 2001) have been successful at producing such effects. Because the primes are self-generated, they are easily confused with personal motives and thoughts about how to behave, and are unlikely to instantiate correction motives.

Situational Factors. Finally, there are a number of situational factors that can affect the likelihood of misattribution. By reducing the ability to accurately check the source of accessible information, cognitive load manipulations such as increased time pressure (Payne, Lambert, & Jacoby, 2002) and multiple-task requirements (van Boven & Robinson, 2012) increase the impact of primes. Conversely, other factors prevent misattribution by motivating people to pay special attention to the source of accessible content. When one is suspicious that they may have been exposed to subliminal primes, for example, they are less likely to misattribute prime-related content to their own thoughts about how to behave (Verwijmeren, Karremans, Bernritter, Stroebe, & Wigboldus, 2013). In the realm of behavior and goal priming, high levels of self-consciousness (induced, for example, by the presence of a mirror) can also prevent primes from impacting behavior (Dijksterhuis & van Knippenberg, 2000). Because high self-consciousness is associated with increased salience of personal goals and standards (Carver & Scheier, 1978), fewer constructs are able to be misattributed to the active self-concept.

KNOWN MODERATORS AFFECTING THE USE OF ACCESSIBLE INFORMATION

Target of Focus. Although the above misattribution-related moderators are most important for determining if a prime will produce *any* effect, moderators that affect the type of question afforded by the environment are critical for determining exactly *what* that effect is. Because different targets of focus often afford unique questions, manipulations of this variable frequently cause the same prime to produce very different effects (Jefferis & Fazio, 2008). In one study (DeMarree & Loersch, 2009), participants were subliminally primed with social stereotypes related to either hostility (African Americans) or passivity (Buddhist monks). They then spent a few minutes thinking about either their own lifestyle and personality or those of their best friend. These targets afford different questions ("Who am I?" vs. "Who are they?"), thereby causing a single prime to differentially affect self versus other perceptions of trait aggression.

This same basic processes can also be used to explain the moderating role of personal need in the subliminal persuasion literature (Strahan, Spencer, & Zanna, 2002; Veltkamp, Aarts, & Custers, 2008). Because having a strong need (e.g., being very thirsty) causes people to search the environment for ways to achieve the goal, it too can be used as a manipulation of attentional focus. This can make primes that relate to the need (and therefore provide an answer to the basic question afforded by it) particularly effective (Karremans, Stroebe, & Claus, 2006).

Metacognitive Cues. Because prime-related content is used as information for answering afforded questions, any variable that changes the way people use this information will influence the final priming effect. Although not always framed as an influence of metacognitive cues, such effects have been obtained by several labs. For example, positive affect is seen as a cue that one should use mental content, whereas negative affect is seen as a cue that current thoughts should not be trusted (Briñol, Petty, & Barden, 2007; Schwarz & Clore, 1988). Accordingly, assimilative priming effects are seen when the primed content is associated with feelings of positivity and reversed when associated with feelings of negativity (Aarts, Custers, & Holland, 2007; Cesario, Plaks, & Higgins, 2006; Custers & Aarts, 2005; Fishbach & Labroo, 2007).

Because they also alter how accessible content is used, mindset manipulations can have similar moderating effects. For example, participants can be trained to habitually compare accessible content with a salient standard, looking for ways in which the two constructs are similar or different, depending on the mindset that is activated. While similarity mindsets cause judgment and behavior to assimilate to the prime, comparison mindsets cause contrast effects (Crusius & Mussweiler, 2012; Mussweiler & Damisch, 2008). Other mindsets (Fujita & Trope, 2014, this volume) can also affect priming by generally causing people to approach decision making in either an open or cautious manner, trust or distrust their current thoughts, or differentially focus on answering concrete versus abstract questions afforded by the environment.

NEW EMPIRICAL SUPPORT FOR THE MODEL

Core Processes. Although the situated inference model was developed only recently, a number of studies have been conducted to directly test its hypotheses. One of the most central predictions is that primes shape responses mainly when accessible information is misattributed to one's own internal reaction. Loersch and Payne (2012) tested this idea by priming subjects with subliminally presented and masked words related to either profit or equity, before participants played an economic game which contrasted those two motives. During the priming task, participants were instructed to stare at the computer monitor while clearing their minds of all thoughts. Half of the participants were (correctly) told that the flashes they saw during the priming task could make some thoughts more likely to come to mind. This instruction encouraged participants to attribute their thoughts to an external source. The other half were told that the flashed stimuli would make it harder to generate thoughts. This instruction encouraged an internal attribution for thoughts because whatever information came to mind did so in spite of external interference. As expected, participants' decisions in the economic game were influenced by the primes only when internal attributions were encouraged. A second study replicated these effects by priming "fast" versus "slow." Again, primes influenced the speed of subsequent responses only when participants were encouraged to attribute primed thoughts to their own minds. Responses in the external attribution conditions tended toward contrast effects.

A second critical prediction of the model is that primes should affect responses by providing a meaningful answer to the questions afforded by the situation. Loersch, Durso, and Petty (2013) tested this hypothesis by subliminally priming participants with words related to the concept "clean" or "dirty." They then presented participants with a set of cleaning products to be evaluated, and manipulated the question afforded by framing the attitude question in two ways. One group was asked, "Considering your potential need for this product, how desirable is it?" In this condition, participants primed with dirty liked the cleaning products more than those primed with clean. The other group was asked, "Considering this product's physical state, how desirable is it?" In this condition, participants primed with clean liked the products more than those primed with dirty. These results highlight the role of afforded questions in producing priming effects, and suggest that the downstream consequences of priming critically depend on what participants do with the accessible information.

A third important prediction of the model is that the consequences of priming depend on metacognitive inferences about whatever thoughts or feelings come to mind. In some recent work, we tested a variety of manipulations which have been shown in previous research to influence whether participants consider their momentary thoughts to be valid or invalid (DeMarree et al., 2012). For example, participants in a position of power assume that their thoughts are more valid than the powerless. Participants also assume that thoughts that come easily to mind are more valid than thoughts that come with difficulty. Across several kinds of manipulations (power, subjective ease, and confidence), assimilative priming effects were only seen when participants were induced to experience a sense of thought validity after priming. Consistent with the predictions of the situated inference model, the same primes instead produced contrast when associated with feelings of invalidity.

The model makes similar predictions about general mindsets related to information validity. In one recent study, participants were instructed to "go with their gut" when making a social judgment during the experiment. They then read information about a target individual while being subliminally primed with either positive or negative masked images. Those individuals who were given the mindset to make decisions based on their intuitive gut feelings were more affected by the subliminal primes than participants given instructions to simply read the information (Loersch, McCaslin, & Petty, 2011; see also Croizet & Fiske, 2000; De Houwer & Smith, 2012, for similar findings with affective primes).

Sequential Priming. Typically, behavioral priming is discussed separately from sequential priming. In sequential priming, within-subjects procedures are frequently used as implicit measures to assess individual differences in attitudes or other associations. In a typical study, primes (e.g., black and white faces) are presented for a short duration immediately before a target (e.g., a valenced word or a Chinese ideograph, see Fazio et al., 1986; Payne et al., 2005). Although participants are instructed to respond only to the target (e.g., by categorizing it as positive or negative), the typical finding is that the primes influence behavior by making individuals more likely to judge the target in a prime-congruent manner. Some implicit measures (e.g., the affect misattribution procedure or AMP; Payne et al., 2005) may produce their effects through the same basic process proposed by the situated inference model. That is, the downstream consequences of the information made accessible by the primes is expected to influence subsequent decisions and actions when mistakenly assumed to reflect one's thoughts and feelings about the subsequent target. This misattributed content should then be used in a contextually sensitive manner to answer whatever question is afforded by the current situation.

Evidence for these predictions was recently obtained by Gawronski and Ye (2014). Within the context of the AMP, it was shown that a prime can make a variety of information accessible (including both affective and semantic content) and that the precise influence of that activated content depends on the current question afforded by the situation. For example, when participants were asked to judge the animacy of Chinese ideographs in the AMP (i.e., "Does this object represent an animate or inanimate object?"), the animacy information made accessible by a prime (e.g., kitten, maggot, pleasure, garbage, etc.) was misattributed to the ideograph target. When the same primes and targets were presented but participants were instead asked to judge the ideograph's valence (i.e., "Does this object represent a positive or negative object?"), the prime's evaluative content instead affected judgments.

Implicit–Explicit Correlations. Across a great deal of research, there have been relatively low correlations between these implicit measures and corresponding explicit measures designed to measure the same construct (e.g., attitudes toward African Americans; see Cameron, Brown-Iannuzzi, & Payne, 2012). Critically, because it makes predictions about the process by which prime-related accessibility impacts judgment and behavior, the situated inference model can be used to help understand the conditions under which implicit measures will predict explicit judgments.

For example, in one study, we measured individual differences in affective responses to same-sex couples using a sequential priming task (i.e., the AMP). Next, we asked one group to consider reasons that the feelings experienced during the priming task were intentional. Another group was asked to consider reasons that their feelings might be unintentional. Finally, we measured explicit homophobia. The basic affective reactions measured by the priming task were more likely to be endorsed as explicit homophobia (resulting in higher implicit-explicit correlations) when participants were randomly assigned to consider their feelings as intentional (Cooley, Payne, & Phillips, 2014). Consistent with the situated inference model, metacognitive inferences regarding intention determined whether primed content was used to answer the question afforded by the homophobia questionnaire.

CONTEXT-SPECIFICITY AND REPRODUCIBILITY

A great deal of attention has been given to recent failures to replicate some classic priming effects (e.g., Doyen, Klein, Pichon, & Cleeremans, 2012; Shanks et al., 2013). Although there has been substantial debate over the meaning of these results, we suspect that much of the controversy has to do with predicting only simple, direct effects of a prime. While this impression is consistent with some well-known theories and early results, it is largely inconsistent with the sizeable literature on priming moderators that has developed over the years.

A strength of the situated inference model is that it provides a framework that naturally accounts for many moderators. Indeed, when one considers the situated nature of priming, it is no surprise primes affect judgment and behavior differently in different labs and in samples from different populations. Humans are not automatons. As one can see simply by observing daily life, our species is incredibly adept at modifying behavior to meet the needs of the current situation. By reconciling the automatic nature of priming effects with the social reality that our behavior is highly contextualized, the situated inference model helps emphasize this fact.

Interestingly, our perspective suggests that priming both is and is not a ubiquitous phenomenon. On one hand, the model outlines a basic decision-making process that is continually active. Information in the environment makes related mental content accessible and that information can potentially be used to guide judgment and behavior. This process is "priming" in the narrow sense that a stimulus has made related information more accessible. The counterintuitive priming effects that have been the focus of debate occur through the same process, except that they are accompanied by a source monitoring error in which people mistake the true source of accessible information. In this sense, priming must be a less frequent occurrence because these are a subset of all times that information becomes accessible. Although every billboard, traffic sign, and overheard conversation we pass during a walk down the street may indeed prime us, this information will only have surprising effects on behavior if misattributed to one's internal thoughts and then used to answer some question afforded within a subsequent situation.

The same reasoning applies when considering how easily priming effects should emerge in exact replication attempts. Our model suggests that three presumably independent processes must co-occur. The primes must make the same mental content accessible for a new subset of participants, these individuals must then mistakenly attribute this information to their own thoughts about whatever dependent measure is targeted, and they need to view these thoughts as important and relevant to the particular question afforded by that dependent measure. Many factors can easily disrupt one or more of these processes, thereby making even exact replications more challenging than might be expected. Different subject populations might possess different stereotype content or have relatively weaker associations between the primes and the critical concept that needs to be activated. Because of this, replication studies testing a sample of participants that differs from the original sample are less likely to be successful simply because the associations and cultural contexts may differ. For example, Shanks and colleagues (2013) sampled participants from ages 18–79, recruited from both universities and general communities in England, Sweden, Greece, and Australia.

Similarly, the presence of any alternative target to which the accessible content can be misattributed can easily "dilute" the priming effect by causing some subset of participants to misattribute prime-related accessibility to an unanticipated source. Finally, the suspicion that one is being manipulated can make participants distrustful, leading them to question their current thoughts. Such a process could easily prevent a priming effect (Loersch & Payne, 2012; Verwijmeren et al., 2013) even in an otherwise perfect replication. Moving forward, priming studies should measure and report subjects' perceptions and suspicions, preferably in ways that could be compared across samples to evaluate this possibility.

The reasoning outlined above suggests that priming should not be expected to be a robust and ubiquitous phenomenon. Instead, it will inevitably be contextualized. This does not mean that priming is not real or that it is not important, but simply that it will occur in a context-specific manner. By emphasizing this fact, the situated inference model helps make sense not only of existing studies, but also some failures to replicate past research. For example, although frequently categorized as a "failure to replicate," Doyen and colleagues (2012) actually provides positive evidence for behavioral priming. In contrast to past research (Bargh, Chen, & Burrows, 1996), there was no direct effect of priming on behavior, but the primed constructs did interact with the affordances created by experimenter expectancies. Thus, just as we have argued, the effects of the primes depended on the current situation and its behavioral affordances (see also Klein et al., 2012).

One criticism of past priming studies is that they sometimes showed large effect sizes and yet did not always replicate in later studies. Some authors have suggested that this indicates publication bias, in which large effects were selectively published. That is possible, but the context-specificity of priming suggests that unmeasured moderators could also explain these discrepancies. As we reviewed above, a variety of moderators can cause priming effects to be eliminated and in some cases to reverse. It is entirely possible that a priming effect in a sample with a particular set of assumptions, traits, and so forth could be large, and in another sample, with another set of assumptions, traits, and so forth, the effect could be absent. It would not be surprising that a hundred American undergraduates might respond differently to a prime than a hundred German community members. This is not a question specific to priming research. It is a basic issue of sampling and generalizability that is an issue in many areas of research. Of course, large representative samples would be an ideal solution, but resource constraints necessarily limit that possibility for many studies. If priming is highly context-specific, then much more attention should be paid in future studies (both original tests and replications) to carefully describing and controlling the social context.

CONCLUSIONS

The situated inference model sheds light on several controversies in the priming literature. It helps explain why a single prime can produce many different downstream consequences. It also clarifies how various situational factors will make priming effects appear and disappear. Although earlier models of priming suggested that stimuli could exert direct control over judgment and behavior, the contextual nature of priming effects is not well captured by these accounts. The large literature documenting various priming moderators suggests that priming does not follow this simple, direct, unchanging route. In contrast, the situated inference model acknowledges the basic, contextualized nature of behavior. In doing so, it highlights the power of the situation for shaping how primes have their effects, and how they do not.

REFERENCES

Aarts, H., Custers, R., & Holland, R. W. (2007). The nonconscious cessation of goal pursuit: when goals and negative affect are coactivated. *Journal of Personality and Social Psychology, 92,* 165-178.

Bargh, J. A. (1990). Auto-motives: Preconscious determinants of thought and behavior. In E. T. Higgins & R. M. Sorrentino (Eds.), *Handbook of motivation and cognition: Foundations of social behavior* (Vol. 2; pp. 93-130). New York: Guilford.

Bargh, J. A. (2006). Agenda 2006: What have we been priming all these years? On the development, mechanisms, and ecology of nonconscious social behavior. *European Journal of Social Psychology, 36,* 147-168.

Bargh, J. A., & Chartrand, T. (2000). Studying the mind in the middle: A practical guide to priming and automaticity research. In H. Reis & C. Judd (Eds.), *Handbook of research methods in social psychology* (pp. 253-285). New York: Cambridge University Press.

Bargh, J. A., Chen, M., & Burrows, L. (1996). Automaticity of social behavior: Direct effects of trait construct and stereotype activation on action. *Journal of Personality and Social Psychology, 71*, 230-244.

Bargh, J., Gollwitzer, P. M., Lee-Chai, A., Barndollar, K., & Trotschel, R. (2001). The automated will: Nonconscious activation and pursuit of behavioral goals. *Journal of Personality and Social Psychology, 81*, 1014-1027.

Bearce, K. H., & Rovee-Collier, C. (2006). Repeated priming increases memory accessibility in infants. *Journal of Experimental Child Psychology, 93*, 357-376.

Briñol, P., & DeMarree, K. G. (2012). *Social metacognition.* New York: Psychology Press.

Briñol, P., Petty, R. E., & Barden, J. (2007). Happiness versus sadness as a determinant of thought confidence in persuasion: A self-validation analysis. *Journal of Personality and Social Psychology, 93*, 711-727.

Cameron, C. D., Brown-Iannuzzi, J., & Payne, B. K. (2012). Sequential priming measures of implicit social cognition: A meta-analysis of associations with behaviors and explicit attitudes. *Personality and Social Psychology Review, 16*, 330-350.

Carver, C. S., Ganellen, R. J., Froming, W. J., & Chambers, W. (1983). Modeling: An analysis in terms of category accessibility. *Journal of Experimental Social Psychology, 19*, 403-421.

Carver, C. S., & Scheier, M. F. (1978). Self-focusing effects of dispositional self-consciousness, mirror presence, and audience presence. *Journal of Personality and Social Psychology, 36*(3), 324-332. doi:10.1037/0022-3514.36.3.324

Cesario, J., Plaks, J. E., & Higgins, E. T. (2006). Automatic social behavior as motivated preparation to interact. *Journal of Personality and Social Psychology, 90*, 893-910.

Chartrand, T. L., & Bargh, A. (1996). Automatic activation of impression formation and memorization goals: Nonconscious goal priming reproduces effects of explicit task instructions. *Journal of Personality and Social Psychology, 71*, 464-478.

Conway, M. A. (1990). Associations between autobiographical memories and concepts. *Journal of Experimental Psychology: Learning, Memory, and Cognition, 16*, 799-812.

Cooley, E., Payne, B. K., & Phillips, K. J. (2014). Implicit bias and the illusion of conscious ill will. *Social Psychological and Personality Science, 5*(4), 500-507.

Croizet, J.-C., & Fiske, S. T. (2000). Moderation of priming by goals: Feeling entitled to judge increases judged usability of evaluative primes. *Journal of Experimental Social Psychology, 36*(2), 155-181. doi:10.1006/jesp.1999.1397

Crusius, J., & Mussweiler, T. (2012). To achieve or not to achieve? Comparative mindsets elicit assimilation and contrast in goal priming. *European Journal of Social Psychology, 42*, 780-788. doi:10.1002/ejsp.873

Custers, R., & Aarts, H. (2005). Positive affect as implicit motivator: On the nonconscious operation of behavioral goals. *Journal of Personality and Social Psychology, 89*, 129-142.

de Groot, A. M. (1983). The range of automatic spreading activation in word priming. *Journal of Verbal Learning & Verbal Behavior, 22*, 417-436.

De Houwer, J., & Smith, C. (2012). Go with your gut! Effects of affect misattribution procedures become stronger when participants are encouraged to rely on their gut feelings. *Social Psychology, 44*(5), 299-302.

DeMarree, K. G., & Loersch, C. (2009). Who am I and who are you? Priming and the influence of self versus other focused attention. *Journal of Experimental Social Psychology, 45*, 440-443. doi:10.1016/j.jesp.2008.10.009

DeMarree, K. G., Loersch, C., Briñol, P., Petty, R. E., Payne, B. K., & Rucker, D. D. (2012). From primed construct to motivated behavior: Validation processes in goal pursuit. *Personality & Social Psychology Bulletin, 38*, 1659-1670.

Dijksterhuis, A., & Bargh, J. A. (2001). The perception-behavior expressway: Automatic effects of social perception on social behavior. In M. P. Zanna (Ed.), *Advances in experimental social psychology* (Vol. 33; pp. 1-40). San Diego: Academic Press.

Dijksterhuis, A., Spears, R., Postmes, T., Stapel, D., Koomen, W., Knippenberg, A. v., et al. (1998). Seeing one thing and doing another: Contrast effects in automatic behavior. *Journal of Personality and Social Psychology, 75*, 862-871.

Dijksterhuis, A., & van Knippenberg, A. (2000). Behavioral indecision: Effects of self-focus on automatic behavior. *Social Cognition, 18*(1), 55-74. doi:10.1521/soco.2000.18.1.55

Doyen, S., Klein, O., Pichon, C. L., & Cleeremans, A. (2012). Behavioral priming: It's all in the mind, but whose mind? *PLOS ONE, 7*, e29081. doi:10.1371/journal.pone.0029081

Fazio, R. H., Sanbonmatsu, D. M., Powell, M. C., & Kardes, F. R. (1986). On the automatic activation of attitudes. *Journal of Personality and Social Psychology, 50*, 229-238.

Fishbach, A., & Labroo, A. (2007). Be better or be merry: How mood affects self-control. *Journal of Personality and Social Psychology, 93*, 158-173.

Fowler, C. A., Wolford, G., Slade, R., & Tassinary, L. (1981). Lexical access with and without awareness. *Journal of Experimental Psychology: General, 110*, 341-362.

Fujita, K., & Trope, Y. (2014). Structured vs. unstructured regulation: On procedural mindsets and the mechanisms of priming effects. This volume.

Galinsky, A. D., Wang, C. S., & Ku, G. (2008). Perspective-takers behave more stereotypically. *Journal of Personality and Social Psychology, 95*, 404-419.

Gawronski, B., & Ye, Y. (2014). What drives priming effects in the affect misattribution procedure? *Personality and Social Psychology Bulletin, 40*, 3-15.

Herr, P. M., Sherman, S. J., & Fazio, R. H. (1983). On the consequences of priming: Assimilation and contrast effects. *Journal of Experimental Social Psychology, 19*, 323-340.

Higgins, E. T. (1996). Knowledge activation: Accessibility, applicability, and salience. In E. T. Higgins & A. W. Kruglanski (Eds.), *Social psychology: Handbook of basic principles* (pp. 133-168). New York: Guilford.

Higgins, E. T. (1998). The aboutness principle: A pervasive influence on human inference. *Social Cognition, 16*, 173-198.

Higgins, E. T., Rholes, W. S., & Jones, C. R. (1977). Category accessibility and impression formation. *Journal of Experimental Social Psychology, 13*(2), 141-154.

Jacoby, L. L., Lindsay, D. S., & Toth, J. P. (1992). Unconscious influences revealed: Attention, awareness, and control. *American Psychologist, 47*, 802-809.

Jefferis, V. E., & Fazio, R. H. (2008). Accessibility as input: The use of construct accessibility as information to guide behavior. *Journal of Experimental Social Psychology, 44*, 1144-1150.

Jones, C. R., Fazio, R. H., & Olson, M. A. (2009). Implicit misattribution as a mechanism underlying evaluative conditioning. *Journal of Personality and Social Psychology, 96*, 933–948. doi:10.1037/a0014747

Karremans, J. C., Stroebe, W., & Claus, J. (2006). Beyond Vicary's fantasies: The impact of subliminal priming and brand choice. *Journal of Experimental Social Psychology, 42*, 792-798.

Klein, O., Doyen, S., Leys, C., Gama, P. A. M. de S. da, Miller, S., Questienne, L., & Cleeremans, A. (2012). Low hopes, high expectations expectancy effects and the replicability of behavioral experiments. *Perspectives on Psychological Science, 7*, 572-584. doi:10.1177/1745691612463704

Loersch, C., Durso, G. R. O., & Petty, R. E. (2013). Vicissitudes of desire: A matching mechanism for subliminal persuasion. *Social Psychological and Personality Science, 4*(5), 624-631. doi:10.1177/1948550612471975

Loersch, C., McCaslin, M. J., & Petty, R. E. (2011). Exploring the impact of social judgeability concerns on the interplay of associative and deliberative attitude processes. *Journal of Experimental Social Psychology, 47*, 1029-1032. doi:10.1016/j.jesp.2011.03.024

Loersch, C., & Payne, B. K. (2011). The Situated Inference Model: An integrative account of the effects of primes on perception, behavior, and motivation. *Perspectives on Psychological Science, 6*, 234-252. doi:10.1177/1745691611406921

Loersch, C., & Payne, B. K. (2012). On mental contamination: The role of (mis) attribution in behavior priming. *Social Cognition, 30*, 241-252. doi:10.1521/soco.2012.30.2.241

Lombardi, W. J., Higgins, E. T., & Bargh, J. A. (1987). The role of consciousness in priming effects on categorization: Assimilation versus contrast as a function of awareness of the priming task. *Personality and Social Psychology Bulletin, 13*, 411-429.

Marcel, A. J. (1983). Conscious and unconscious perception: Experiments on visual masking and word recognition. *Cognitive Psychology, 15*, 197-237.

Martin, L. L. (1986). Set/reset: Use and disuse of concepts in impression formation. *Journal of Personality and Social Psychology, 51*, 493-504.

Martin, L. L., Seta, J. J., & Crelia, R. A. (1990). Assimilation and contrast as a function of people's willingness and ability to expend effort in forming an impression. *Journal of Personality and Social Psychology, 59*, 27-37.

Moskowitz, G. B., & Roman, J. (1992). Spontaneous trait inferences as self-generated primes: Implications for conscious social judgment. *Journal of Personality and Social Psychology, 62*, 728-738.

Moskowitz, G. B., & Skurnik, W. (1999). Contrast effects as determined by the type of prime: Trait versus exemplar primes initiate processing strategies that differ in how accessible constructs are used. *Journal of Personality and Social Psychology, 76*, 911-927.

Mussweiler, T. (2003). Comparison processes in social judgment: Mechanisms and consequences. *Psychological Review, 110*, 472-489.

Mussweiler, T., & Damisch, L. (2008). Going back to Donald: How comparisons shape judgmental priming effects. *Journal of Personality and Social Psychology, 95*(6), 1295-1315. doi:10.1037/a0013261

Mussweiler, T., & Neumann, R. (2000). Sources of mental contamination: Comparing the effects of self-generated versus externally provided primes. *Journal of Experimental Social Psychology, 36*, 194-206.

Neely, J. H. (1991). Semantic priming effects in visual word recognition: A selective review of current findings and theories. In D. Besner & G. W. Humphreys (Eds.), *Basic processes in reading: Visual word recognition* (pp. 264-336). Hillsdale, NJ: Erlbaum.

Newman, L. S., & Uleman, S. (1990). Assimilation and contrast effects in spontaneous trait inference. *Personality and Social Psychology Bulletin, 16*, 224-240.

Payne, B. K., Cheng, C. M., Govorun, O., & Stewart, B. D. (2005). An inkblot for attitudes: Affect misattribution as implicit measurement. *Journal of Personality and Social Psychology, 89*(3), 277-293. doi:10.1037/0022-3514.89.3.277

Payne, B. K., Lambert, A. J., & Jacoby, L. L. (2002). Best laid plans: Effects of goals on accessibility bias and cognitive control in race-based misperceptions of weapons. *Journal of Experimental Social Psychology, 38*(4), 384-396.

Petty, R. E., DeMarree, K. G., Briñol, P., Horcajo, J., & Strathman, A. J. (2008). Need for cognition can magnify or attenuate priming effects in social judgment. *Personality and Social Psychology Bulletin, 34*, 900-912.

Shanks, D. R., Newell, B. R., Lee, E. H., Balakrishnan, D., Ekelund, L., Cenac, Z., Kawadia, F., & Moore, C. (2013). Priming intelligent behavior: An elusive phenomenon. *PLOS ONE, 8*, e56515. doi:10.1371/journal.pone.0056515

Schwarz, N., & Clore, G. L. (1988). How do I feel about it? Informative functions of affective states. In K. Fiedler & J. Forgas (Eds.), *Affect, cognition, and social behavior* (pp. 44-62). Toronto: Hogrefe International.

Strahan, E. J., Spencer, S. J., & Zanna, M. P. (2002). Subliminal priming and persuasion: Striking while the iron is hot. *Journal of Experimental Social Psychology, 38*, 556-568.

Tulving, E., & Pearlstone, Z. (1966). Availability versus accessibility of information in memory for words. *Journal of Verbal Learning and Verbal Behavior, 5*, 381-391.

van Boven, L., & Robinson, M. D. (2012). Boys don't cry: Cognitive load and priming increase stereotypic sex differences in emotion memory. *Journal of Experimental Social Psychology, 48*, 303-309. doi:10.1016/j.jesp.2011.09.005

Veltkamp, M., Aarts, H., & Custers, R. (2008). On the emergence of deprivation-reducing behaviors: Subliminal priming of behavior representations turns deprivation into motivation. *Journal of Experimental Social Psychology, 44*, 866-873.

Verwijmeren, T., Karremans, J. C., Bernritter, S. F., Stroebe, W., & Wigboldus, D. H. J. (2013). Warning: You are being primed! The effect of a warning on the impact of subliminal ads. *Journal of Experimental Social Psychology, 49*(6), 1124-1129.

Wegener, D. T., & Petty, E. (1995). Flexible correction processes in social judgment: The role of naive theories in corrections for perceived bias. *Journal of Personality and Social Psychology, 68*, 36-51.

Wheeler, S. C., DeMarree, K. G., & Petty, R. E. (2007). Understanding the role of the self in prime-to-behavior effects: The active self account. *Personality and Social Psychology Review, 11*, 234-261.

Wheeler, S. C., DeMarree, K. G., & Petty, R. E. (2014). Understanding prime-to-behavior effects: Insights from the active-self account. This volume.

Wheeler, S. C., & Petty, R. E. (2001). The effects of stereotype activation on behavior: A review of possible mechanisms. *Psychological Bulletin, 127*, 797-826.

PRIMING: CONSTRAINT SATISFACTION AND INTERACTIVE COMPETITION

Tobias Schröder and Paul Thagard
University of Waterloo

> Priming influences holistic representations of social situations and subsequent actions through interactive competition among relevant concepts such as the prime, the self, a partner, or other features of the environment. The constraints among these representations stem from culturally shared affective meanings of concepts acquired in socialization. Our theory is implemented in a localist connectionist model, which in simulations reproduced major experimental results on priming. The neural plausibility of our proposal comes from semantic pointers, a neural mechanism that integrates symbolic concepts with underlying emotional and sensorimotor processes. The compositional nature of semantic pointers also explains the interaction of priming with more deliberate and intentional forms of social cognition.

There is overwhelming evidence for the power of representations that are made cognitively accessible to influence seemingly unrelated social perceptions, decisions, and actions—a phenomenon often referred to as social priming (Molden, 2014, this volume). However, the precise mechanisms that cause this influence have remained poorly understood. The question of what kinds of primes cause what kinds of consequences in what kinds of situations has puzzled many (e.g., see Bargh, 2006). We recently proposed that understanding social priming as parallel constraint satisfaction gives rise to a comprehensive theoretical explanation of the phenomenon, which allows precise predictions about the likely effects of priming procedures in many different situations (Schröder & Thagard, 2013). Our proposal was targeted at instances of behavioral priming, where an action is the dependent variable (e.g., Bargh, Chen, & Burrows, 1996), but we think it is also applicable to other cases, for example in impression formation (see Loersch & Payne, 2011; 2014, this volume, for a review of different domains of social priming).

Tobias Schröder was awarded a research fellowship by the Deutsche Forschungsgemeinschaft (German Research Foundation; # SCHR 1282/1-1) to support this work. Paul Thagard's work is supported by the Natural Sciences and Engineering Research Council of Canada. Address correspondence to Paul Thagard at pthagard@connect.uwaterloo.ca.

In neural networks, parallel constraint satisfaction is a competitive mechanism in which the activation of a representation results from the combination of excitation between compatible elements and inhibition between incompatible elements (McClelland & Rumelhart, 1981). We showed that this mechanism explains many cases of behavioral priming if we assume that the constraints among elements of a representation stem from culturally shared affective meanings of relevant social concepts. Affective meanings are the emotional components of concepts, typically measured along the cross-culturally universal dimensions of affective experience, evaluation-valence, potency-control, and activity-arousal (Osgood, May, & Miron, 1975). We also demonstrated the neural plausibility of our explanation of priming with a neurocomputational model based on Eliasmith's (2013) new semantic pointer architecture for human cognition, which overcomes the dichotomy between symbolic and connectionist accounts of the mind. Semantic pointers are distributed patterns of neural activity that have symbol-like properties through their capacity to recursively bind deeper representations in multiple modalities. The capacity of semantic pointers to expand into their underlying somatosensory and motor representations explains the observation that the activation of symbolic concepts through priming may eventually lead to associated physical actions as in priming-to-behavior experiments (Schröder & Thagard, 2013).

Here, we will review our theory of priming as constraint satisfaction, but also extend it in significant ways that reflect recent advances. We describe a plausible mechanism for how brains may compute competition among multiple distributed representations, further supporting our previous claims about the neural plausibility of our theory of priming. We use our new neural theory of intentional action (Schröder, Stewart, & Thagard, in press) to show that our constraint-satisfaction account also gives explanations of the interplay between automatic, priming-based cognition and more deliberate, effortful thinking. This advanced version of our theory makes extensive use of the richer capabilities of semantic pointers, which in contrast to classic constraint-satisfaction explanations of the mind respect the compositional, relational, and partially embodied nature of conceptual representations.

PRIMING AS PARALLEL CONSTRAINT SATISFACTION

While evidence for priming is abundant, prior theoretical explanations have been diverse and sometimes competing, focusing on the cognitive accessibility of specific aspects of a situation like stereotypes, traits, goals and motivations, or self-concepts (e.g., Bargh et al., 1996; Loersch & Payne, 2011; Wheeler & DeMarree, 2009). We have proposed that these perspectives can be unified by considering priming as a form of parallel constraint satisfaction, where the constraints stem from affective meanings of the concepts that are used to represent the situation (Schröder & Thagard, 2013).

PARALLEL CONSTRAINT SATISFACTION

The human mind can be viewed as a network of positive and negative constraints among elements such as stereotypes, traits, roles, emotions, or actions. For example, a positive constraint exists between the stereotype of a stigmatized group and a negative action such as displaying hostility, because these representations are compatible with each other. However, a negative constraint exists between displaying hostility toward a member of a stigmatized group and a view of oneself as friendly and tolerant, because these representations are mutually exclusive (Rogers, Schröder, & Scholl, 2013). Parallel constraint satisfaction is the mechanism by which a decision or course of action arises from amalgamating all the different elements into a holistic, coherent *Gestalt*. Psychologists have shown repeatedly that people have a tendency to avoid the tensions resulting from perceived incompatibilities.

While early versions of such psychological consistency theories were restricted to very few elements (e.g., Heider, 1946; Osgood & Tannenbaum, 1955), connectionist constraint-satisfaction networks provide richer capabilities to model the dynamic interactions of multiple cognitions in parallel (Read & Simon, 2012; Simon & Holyoak, 2002; Thagard, 2000). In these networks, the elements of representations are modeled as nodes and the positive (negative) constraints as excitatory (inhibitory) connections between nodes. All the nodes have a degree of activation, which either adds to or inhibits the activation of the connected nodes. Typically, such a network settles in a stable pattern of some activated and some inhibited elements after a small number of iterative exchanges of activation between its nodes. This behavior models the how the activation of a construct in any given situation is a result of interactive competition among all the representations evoked by that situation. The emergent pattern of activated and inhibited concepts in a stabilized constraint network is then interpretable as the *Gestalt*-like, coherent interpretation of the specific situation. Parallel constraint satisfaction is a general psychological mechanism that explains many cognitive and social phenomena such as person perception, stereotyping, legal inference, and political ideologies (e.g., Homer-Dixon et al., 2013; Kunda & Thagard, 1996; Read & Simon, 2012; Thagard, 2000; 2003).

We have argued that parallel constraint satisfaction also explains behavioral priming, and possibly priming in general (Schröder & Thagard, 2013). It has been shown that the effectiveness of priming procedures can depend on many factors including peoples' self-concepts, relationship goals, and features of the environment (e.g., Cesario, Plaks, Hagiwara, Navarrete, & Higgins, 2010; Fitzsimons & Bargh, 2003; Wheeler, DeMarree, & Petty, 2007). In other words, priming is subject to many constraints. Whereas previous theoretical explanations have focused on some of these particular constraints, we see them as operating together in parallel.

AFFECTIVE MEANINGS

Bargh (2006) suggested that the sources of constraints on priming effects are the conceptual structures that organize people's minds. More specifically, we have proposed that affective meanings of social concepts (Osgood et al., 1975) are crucial, as they are largely shared by members of one culture and therefore provide a computationally efficient mechanism for automatically aligning people's social perceptions and actions with cultural meaning structures (Heise, 2007; 2010; Schröder, Netzel, Schermuly, & Scholl, 2013). We thus suggest a multi-level explanation of priming, where parallel constraint satisfaction operates at the individual level while the maintenance of affective meanings is a social mechanism.

There is abundant evidence for the organization of affective meaning along three universal dimensions of emotional experience (Fontaine, Scherer, Roesch, & Ellsworth, 2007; Osgood et al., 1975). Evaluation-valence (E) relates to the goodness versus badness of things, potency-control (P) to judgments of strength versus weakness, and activity-arousal (A) to excitement versus quietness. These dimensions can be considered as aspects of cognitive appraisal in the generation of emotion (Rogers, Schröder, & von Scheve, 2014; Scherer, Dan, & Flykt, 2006). They also have large semantic overlap with warmth (E) and competence (P and to some extent A), considered by many as the universal dimensions of social cognition (Fiske, Cuddy, & Glick, 2007; Kervyn, Fiske, & Yzerbyt, 2013; Rogers et al., 2013).

Culturally shared conceptual structures, which guide social cognition in general and priming in particular, can be viewed as relatively stable distributions of social concepts over the resulting affective EPA space. Empirically, culture-specific EPA vectors of concepts are determined with the semantic differential, a technique where samples of cultural informants provide ratings of the concepts along bipolar adjective scales relating to the three dimensions (Heise, 2010; Osgood, Suci, & Tannenbaum, 1957). Typically, there is high within-culture agreement and overtime stability about the relative positioning of stereotypes, identities, actions, and other representations in affective space (Ambrasat von Scheve, Schauenburg, Conrad, & Schröder, 2014; Heise, 2010). Affective-meaning differences across cultures are meaningfully related to known properties of these cultures, such as individualism-collectivism, power distance, or masculinity (Schröder, Rogers, Ike, Mell, & Scholl, 2013; cf. Hofstede, 2001).

Given the universality of the evaluation-potency-activity space of affective meaning, its overlap with core dimensions of social cognition, and the clear evidence for the stable cultural consensus about social representations in the affective space, we think that affective meanings provide a parsimonious operationalization of the complex conceptual structures that govern behavioral priming effects (cf. Bargh, 2006). In the seminal studies that led to the development of the semantic differential, Osgood and colleagues (1957) found that roughly half of the semantic relations between symbolic concepts can be explained by evaluation, potency, and activity, while many more and much more context-specific dimensions of meaning are required to explain the other half. In the context of social priming, this means that affective meanings will not be the only sources of constraints that explain all cases of priming in all circumstances; however, evaluation-potency-activity configurations of primes, situations, and behaviors will be a good approximation of the semantic relations underlying priming effects in many cases. With the simulation model described in the next section, we have shown that this is true in important instances of behavioral priming.

A LOCALIST CONNECTIONIST MODEL OF BEHAVIORAL PRIMING

We have implemented our view of priming as constraint satisfaction, where the constraints are given by culturally shared affective meanings, in a connectionist network model depicted in Figure 1. The model is a modification of the earlier IMP model of impression formation by Kunda and Thagard (1996). We have used

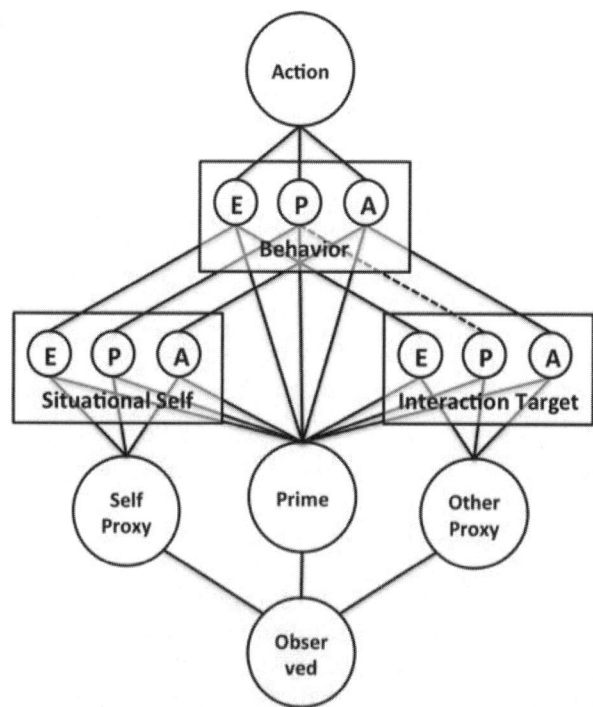

FIGURE 1. Parallel-constraint-satisfaction model of priming effects. Adapted from "The affective meanings of automatic social behaviors: Three mechanisms that explain priming." By T. Schröder and P. Thagard, 2013, *Psychological Review*, p. 262. Copyright 2012 by the American Psychological Association.

it to simulate important instances of behavioral priming experiments (Schröder & Thagard, 2013). These successful simulations support our claim that our theory provides a plausible explanation of a wide range of phenomena.

The "observed" node in the bottom row of Figure 1 activates the primed concept as well as symbolic representations of self and the target person of the interaction. In simulations of behavioral priming experiments, the generic nodes are replaced with more specific concepts, for example *rude* versus *polite* for the prime node in our simulation of Bargh and colleagues' (1996) first classic demonstration of behavioral priming. In this experiment, participants primed with rudeness were more likely to interrupt the experimenter during a conversation than participants primed with politeness. In our model, the *prime*, *self*, and *other* input concepts excite (or inhibit) activation of evaluation-valence (E), potency-control (P), and activity-arousal (A) patterns of self, target, and ultimately behavior, representing the affective meanings of the concepts. The degree of excitation or inhibition (i.e., the connection weights in the model) is determined by empirical EPA measures of the concepts from previous studies (e.g., Heise, 2010; Schröder et al., 2013). The top node is a symbolic action representation (i.e., the dependent variable in prime-to-behavior experiments) and will be either activated or inhibited once the network has reached a stable state after running the iterative constraint-satisfaction algorithm. Then, we can compare the degree of activation of the action node across different conceptual inputs, which correspond to experimental conditions, with the behavior patterns observed in the simulated experiments.

In the case of Bargh and colleagues' (1996) priming of rudeness versus politeness, the simulation works as follows. From Francis and Heise's (2006) repository of affective meanings, which is based on EPA ratings of 1,500 concepts by Indiana University students (for details, see Heise, 2010), we take the values for "rude" (E = -2.69, P = -0.74, A = 0.60) and "polite" (E = 2.86, P = 1.68, A = 0.41) to scale the connection weights between the prime node and the self, behavior, target EPA nodes displayed in Figure 1. Similarly, for the connections between the self node and EPA nodes, we used ratings of "myself as I really am" (E = 1.97, P = 0.75, A = 1.04; from Schröder et al., 2013). For the target node, we used Francis and Heise's (2006) ratings of "student" (E = 1.93, P = 0.92, A = 1.20) and for the behavior node those of "interrupt" (E = -1.51, P = -0.12, A = 1.15), which was the dependent variable in the Bargh and colleagues' (1996) experiment.

We ran the simulation 1,000 times for each experimental condition, to simulate different individual participants of the experiment with slightly varying self-sentiments, affective representations of rudeness or politeness, and perceptions of target persons. In each run of the simulation, we determined the exact scaling factor for the excitatory and inhibitory connections in the network (see Figure 1) by drawing from a Gaussian distribution centered at the above-mentioned empirical EPA profiles. Constraint satisfaction is computed by updating the activation values of all the nodes according to the summed input they receive from all the other nodes. The update is repeated iteratively until a stable network configuration is reached, where no longer any node changes its activation (for a technical details, see the appendix of Schröder & Thagard, 2013). In the simulation of Bargh's experiment, we thus obtained 1,000 different stable network states for each the rudeness and the politeness condition. In each case, the activation parameter of the behavior node, representing the action of interrupting the experimenter (Bargh et al., 1996), had a characteristic value. A higher value of the behavior node in a simulation corresponds to a higher likelihood of a participant of the original experiment to interrupt the experimenter.

Consistent with the data reported by Bargh and colleagues (1996), we found that the average activation of the behavior "interrupt" was significantly higher in the simulations that took rudeness as priming input compared to politeness. If we interpret any positive activation value as the execution of the action and any negative activation value as refraining from the action, our simulations suggest that more than 90% of the participants primed with rudeness would interrupt the experimenter, while less than 5% of those primed with politeness would do so (Schröder & Thagard, 2013, Figure 4). This result exaggerates the effect size of the original findings, but clearly reproduces their data patterns. We may thus conclude that our theory of priming as constraint satisfaction, implemented in the simulation model depicted in Figure 1, explains the results of Bargh and colleagues' (1996) first, now-classic demonstration of behavioral priming.

Following the same procedure, we showed that our model reproduces the results of additional well-known priming experiments. As explained in detail for Bargh's rudeness priming, in each case we simulated the different experimental conditions by scaling the excitatory and inhibitory connections of the model in Figure 1 with empirically based affective meanings of concepts appropriate to the specific context. By showing that the same model, where only the specific input varies, reproduces the data patterns of a variety of important experiments, we were able to show that our theory of priming as constraint satisfaction integrates diverse and sometimes competing explanations, such as direct trait and stereotype activation (Bargh et al., 1996), motivations to interact (Cesario, Plaks, & Higgins, 2006), relationship goals (Fitzsimons & Bargh, 2003), and self-concept activation (Smeesters, Yzerbyt, Corneille, & Warlop, 2009).

THE NEURAL COMPUTATION OF PRIMING

Localist neural networks such as the one displayed in Figure 1 have important limitations. For example, they lack the ability to represent syntactical and structural information such as the difference between *John loves Mary* and *Mary loves John*. Also, their components and parameters do not map onto properties of biologically realistic neurons. Both shortcomings can be overcome with the new semantic pointer architecture of Eliasmith (2013), which provides a biologically plausible theory of human cognition. To demonstrate the neural plausibility of our account of priming, we provided a neurocomputational model of the proposed mechanisms based on Eliasmith's approach (Schröder & Thagard, 2013). After a brief summary of the semantic pointer approach to priming, we extend our theory by describing a new and more sophisticated neural implementation of a competition mechanism (Thagard & Stewart, 2013).

SEMANTIC POINTERS

Semantic pointers are patterns of neural firing activity whose structure is a consequence of information compression operations implemented in neural connections (Eliasmith, 2013). The term "pointer" comes from computer science where it refers to a kind of data structure that gets its value from a machine address to which it points. Semantic pointers can be decomposed into the underlying representational structures, thereby enabling the cognitive system to control flows of information across different modalities. In line with Barsalou's (1999) claim that symbols are higher-level representations of perceptual components based on sensorimotor experience, Eliasmith distinguishes between shallow (abstract, symbolic) and deep (perceptual, experiential) meanings. The decompression of shallow into deep meanings is crucial for understanding behavioral priming, since it specifies how high-level symbolic representations set off the low-level motor representations that ultimately govern physical actions (Schröder & Thagard, 2013).

The semantic pointer approach combines so-called vector symbolic architectures of human cognition (in particular Plate, 2003) with the neural engineering framework (NEF) developed by Eliasmith and Anderson (2003). Vector symbolic architectures describe semantic and syntactical relations of concepts in terms of vector operations (for review, see Stewart & Eliasmith, 2012). The NEF provides mathematical tools to encode representations of vectors in patterns of firing in neural populations, and mathematical transformations of vectors in the connection weights between populations of firing neurons (Eliasmith & Anderson, 2003). The key idea is that neurons have fixed preferred direction vectors, signifying that the likelihood of a neuron to spike is contingent on the similarity of a represented vector to an optimal vector, which elicits the strongest reaction of the neuron (Georgopoulos, Schwartz, & Kettner, 1986). Different neurons in the same population can have different preferred direction vectors. This results in a unique pattern of neural activity for a specific vector. In the same neural population, similar vectors will elicit similar firing patterns.

Space limitations prevent detailed discussion of the technical details of the semantic pointer architecture here (see Eliasmith, 2013; Eliasmith et al. 2012; Eliasmith & Anderson, 2003). We consider it a milestone in providing a synthesis, not just a hybrid, of symbolic and neural network approaches to understanding the mind. Spaun (for Semantic Pointer Architecture Unified Network), a functional simulation model of the human brain consisting of 2.5 million artificial neurons, is capable of carrying out basic cognitive tasks such as perception, classification, memory retrieval, and motor control (Eliasmith et al., 2012).

A NEUROCOMPUTATIONAL MODEL OF BEHAVIORAL PRIMING

We have used the semantic pointer idea to demonstrate the neural plausibility of our proposed theory of priming, complementing our explanations at the psychological and cultural levels by one at the brain level. The model, which is depicted in Figure 2, is similar to the localist model in that it employs the same psychological constraints on automatic social behaviors (i.e., conceptual representations of the prime, the self, and a target person) and the same empirical evaluation-potency-activity (EPA) vectors of social concepts as operationalization of culturally shared conceptual structures. The main difference is that concepts are no longer represented as single nodes, but rather as distributed patterns of activity in populations of biologically plausible artificial neurons, loosely tied to the known anatomy of social cognition and action control (e.g., Cunningham & Zelazo, 2007; Tsakiris & Haggard, 2010). Of course, the anatomical structure of our model is highly simplified. In reality, affective processing not only occurs in the amygdala as indicated in Figure 2, but in widely distributed neural networks that include many additional brain areas (Lindquist, Wager, Kober, Bliss-Moreau, & Barrett, 2012; Thagard & Schröder, in press). Whether computational mechanisms operate in localized or distributed neural populations is an empirical matter; for detailed discussions, see Schröder & Thagard (2013).

As shown in Figure 2, the primed concept, the self, and a target person are represented as patterns of activity in artificial neural populations tied to sensory and prefrontal areas of the brain, respectively. These patterns are summed up in a neural group, for which the anterior cingulate cortex (ACC) is a plausible brain structure, and then passed on to another group, possibly representing the supplemental motor area, where they initiate a physical action.

We used this model to simulate the classic behavioral priming experiment by Bargh and colleagues (1996), where participants primed with rudeness were more likely to interrupt an interpreter than participants primed with politeness (Schröder & Thagard, 2013). The simulation works as follows. We took empirically based evaluation-potency-activity (EPA) vectors for the primes ("rude" versus "polite"), the self ("myself as I really am"), a target person ("student"), and the behavior that was the dependent variable in the experiment ("interrupt") from published repositories of affective meaning, as described above for the localist constraint-network model. We then used the mathematical procedures from the Neural Engineering Framework (Eliasmith & Anderson, 2003) to create unique

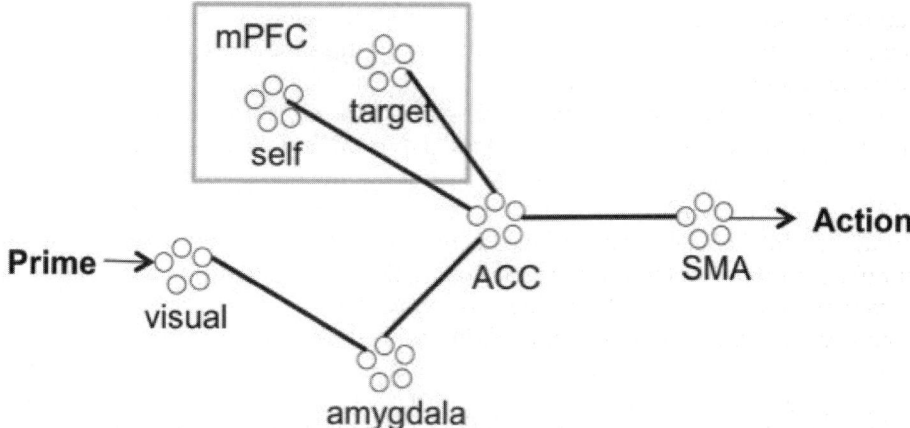

FIGURE 2. Neurocomputational model of behavioral priming. mPFC = medial prefrontal cortex. ACC = anterior cingulate cortex. SMA = supplemental motor area. Adapted from "The affective meanings of automatic social behaviors: Three mechanisms that explain priming." By T. Schröder and P. Thagard, 2013, Psychological Review, p. 270. Copyright 2012 by the American Psychological Association.

patterns of simulated neural spiking activity for each of the EPA vectors. In the rudeness (politeness) condition of the experiment, we thus had a spike pattern in the *visual* neural population from Figure 2 that represented the affective meaning of "rude" ("polite"). In both conditions, we implemented the same spike patterns for "myself as I really am" and "student" in the *self* and *target* populations of the mPFC displayed in Figure 2. The ACC population aggregated the incoming activity from all three representations and passed the combined pattern of activity on to the SMA population. We then compared the resulting activity in SMA to the activity pattern given through encoding the EPA vector for "interrupt" with the Neural Engineering Framework. The result of the simulation was that the similarity of the activity in SMA with the pattern for "interrupt" was high (low), when the pattern for "rude" ("polite") was active in *visual* (for details, see Schröder & Thagard, 2013). This simulation served to substantiate our claim that our proposed theory of priming as resulting from satisfying constraints given by affective meanings of concepts is compatible with current theorizing about computational mechanisms in the brain. However, one of the limitations of this model is that summing up patterns in ACC is not a very sophisticated constraint-satisfaction mechanism.

A NEURAL MECHANISM FOR COMPETITION AMONG SEMANTIC POINTERS

A more elaborate neural theory of priming needs a competition mechanism akin to what occurs in localist connectionist models as the result of excitatory and inhibitory links between units that represent whole concepts. In order to explain phenomena concerning consciousness and attention, Thagard and Stewart (2013) describe how competition can occur among semantic pointers that are distributed across thousands or millions of neurons. According to the semantic pointer competition theory of consciousness, consciousness is a neural process resulting from three mechanisms: representation by firing patterns in neural populations, binding of representations into more complex representations called semantic pointers, and competition among semantic pointers to capture the most important aspects of an organism's current state.

Two semantic pointers do not require separate neural populations, but can just be different patterns of firing in the same neural population resulting from connections among the neurons. These patterns are produced by binding inputs from other neural populations that carry sensory, motor, emotional, or verbal information. Terry Stewart figured out how to implement competition among semantic pointers by means of recurrent connections among the neurons in a neural population that captures more than one semantic pointer. These recurrent connections ensure, for example, that input of information about small animals will produce competition between the semantic pointers for dissimilar concepts like *cat* versus *dog*. This competition affects not only the classification of the animals as cats or dogs, but also the extent to which the winning concept contributes to attention and consciousness (Thagard & Stewart, 2013). In the context of priming, such a competition mechanism helps explain how priming can have many different psychological consequences, depending on the specific context (Bargh, 2006; Loersch & Payne, 2011). On a methodological level, the simulation result that constraint satisfaction can be achieved by populations of spiking neurons justifies the continued use of the much simpler localist models for explanations of social cognition despite their obvious limitations in biological plausibility.

PRIMING AND INTENTIONAL BEHAVIOR

We believe that constraint satisfaction not only explains automatic social perceptions and actions following priming, but also the interactions of these automatic processes with more intentional forms of decision making and planning (e.g., Fishbein & Ajzen, 2010). Social psychologists have proposed various dual process models, which differ in their details but share the general view that social cognition and action result from the dynamic interplay of relatively automatic, fast, and implicit kinds of information processing with relatively deliberate, flexible, and explicit kinds (for review, see Deutsch & Strack, 2006). We have proposed a new theory of intentions as semantic pointers that provides a computational implementation of dual process models and overlaps with the neurocomputational priming model discussed above (Schröder, Stewart, & Thagard, in press). The model, whose neural components are depicted in Figure 3, capitalizes on the capacities of the semantic pointer approach to model the compositional structure of concepts as well as rule-based reasoning within distributed networks.

In this theory, intentions are semantic pointers that result from binding representations of situations, emotional evaluation, actions, and sometimes the self. Intentions may cause actions, when the semantic pointer decompresses into the underlying motor components (i.e., the deep meanings), much as in behavioral priming discussed above. Intentions fail to cause actions when information flowing through the direct perception-action pathway (sensory brain areas, amygdala, ACC, and SMA in Figure 3) competes with an intention. For example, under high cognitive load, people's eating behavior is guided more by their implicit attitudes

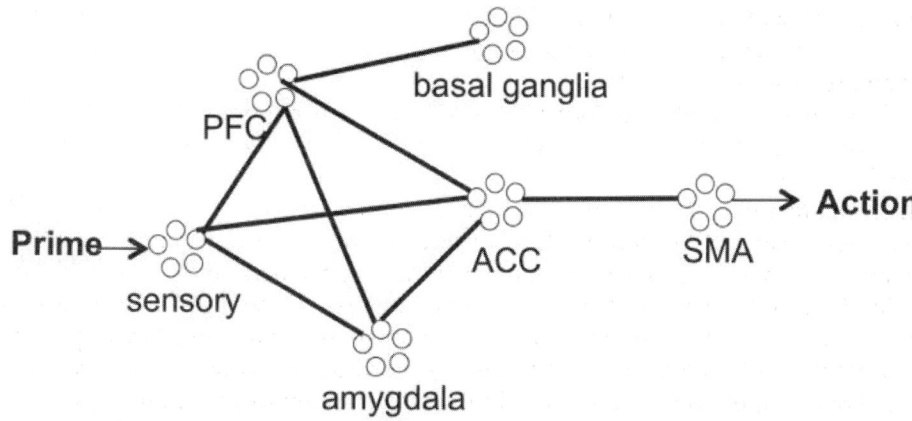

FIGURE 3. Components of a neurocomputational model of intentional action, with an added priming input. PFC = medial prefrontal cortex. ACC = anterior cingulate cortex. SMA = supplemental motor area. Adapted from Figure 3 in Schröder, Stewart, and Thagard (in press), © 2013 Cognitive Science Society, Inc.

toward food than by their deliberate choices (Friese, Hofmann, & Wänke, 2008). However, if enough cognitive resources are available, people are often able to override their impulses and even engage in long-term planning (Fishbein & Ajzen, 2010). This is one of the reasons why priming does not always have straightforward linear effects. Not only do primes compete with other conceptual representations such as the self or a target person, but also with richer semantic pointers like intentions that result from recursive processes in the brain.

Figure 3 shows how our intention model largely overlaps with the priming model discussed above and depicted in Figure 2. The main differences are the addition of a cortico-limbic feedback loop, following Cunningham and Zelazo (2007), which allows intentional processes to override the automatic initial reactions following priming, and the inclusion of the basal ganglia for deliberate, rule-based decision making (following Stewart, Bekolay, & Eliasmith, 2012). Other differences between the components of the models are minor. The *visual* population in Figure 2 corresponds to the broader *sensory* area in Figure 3. The *medial* PFC in Figure 2 is a structure for representing self-other relations, while the intention model in Figure 3 uses the broader PFC for performing more general computations.

Taken together, these models provide a comprehensive account of the full range of social cognition, from priming-based automatic inference and action to deliberate reasoning and decision making, all using constraint satisfaction. For example, a particular person who is primed with rudeness, as in the Bargh and colleagues' (1996) experiment, might have just started working in a department store and received corporate training about being polite to customers. For this person, Bargh's experimental setting might cause the impulsive tendency to interrupt the experimenter through the sensory-amygdala-ACC pathway in Figure 3, but also trigger a conscious deliberation about the appropriateness of interrupting someone in the PFC-basal ganglia decision-making networks, which might override the initial tendency via the PFC-amygdala-ACC feedback loop.

RELATED WORK

We think that our constraint-satisfaction theory of priming integrates many previous attempts to explain the phenomenon of social priming (for detailed discussion, see Schröder & Thagard, 2013). The semantic pointer mechanism specifies the nature of the semantic link between symbolic perceptions such as traits or stereotypes and physical behaviors (Bargh et al., 1996). Measurements of culturally shared affective meanings of large numbers of social objects with the semantic differential technique, which we used as inputs for our simulations, substantiate and mathematically model the notion of complex conceptual structures, which guide social priming (Bargh, 2006).

Interpersonal motivations and goals specific to certain kinds of relationships, hypothesized to underlie priming by some authors (e.g., Cesario et al., 2006; Eitam & Higgins, 2010; Fitzsimons & Bargh, 2003), are not directly encoded in our models, but dynamically emerge from the computation of constraint satisfaction because of the relational configuration of affective meanings of the self and the target persons of the interaction. We do not think that there is a strong dichotomy between the cognitive activation of concepts and motivation. All concepts evoke affective meanings (Heise, 2007; Osgood et al., 1975). The motivation to enact a certain interpersonal behavior can be parsimoniously modeled by a constraint-satisfaction mechanism that picks an emotionally coherent behavior, without requiring goals or motivations as special classes of concept. This result was not only shown by some of our simulations with the priming model depicted in Figure 1 (e.g., see the simulation of an experiment by Fitzsimons & Bargh, 2003, in Schröder & Thagard, 2013), but also by the large body of work on affect control theory (e.g., Heise, 2007; 2010; Rogers et al., 2013; Schröder, Netzel et al., 2013). Affect control theory states that the maintenance of affective meanings is the primary motivation that underlies social interaction, causing individuals to automatically align their behavior with the social order.

We think that our approach might help elucidate the distinction between cognitive accessibility and activation, as theorized by Eitam and Higgins (2010). On their relevance-of-a-representation (ROAR) account, an "accessible" representation needs a signal of relevance in order to become "active" and thus able to influence further cognitive processes. On our account, whether a concept that is made accessible through priming influences subsequent actions, and is thus "active" in the Eitam and Higgins' sense, is a matter of computing constraint satisfaction in the neural network. The affective meaning of the prime could be understood precisely as a "signal of relevance." The constraint-satisfaction algorithm will reject primes (i.e., deactivate them) whose affective meanings are incompatible with the overall network structure (see Figure 1). "Incompatibility of affective meanings" might translate to a lack of relevance in the sense of the ROAR model.

Our theory is also compatible with the self-activation theory of priming (e.g., Wheeler et al., 2007), whose proponents have repeatedly demonstrated that people's susceptibility to priming depends on the semantic interactions between primed concepts and people's self knowledge. We think that this prime*self interaction is simply an instance of constraint satisfaction, and our model, which incorporates a representation of the self, provides a computational specification of the self-activation account.

According to Loersch & Payne (2011), priming effects result from misattributing the content of a prime to the objects of the environment that are currently in the focus of the primed person's attention. Our proposal that primes influence the representation of a situation through constraint satisfaction is quite similar to the misattribution idea, although our approach implies a more holistic, amalgamated representation of the situation. In some ways, Loersch and Payne's model is broader than ours, as we focused on behavioral priming and neglected other priming phenomena, such as in-person perception and impression formation. However, we believe that this shortcoming can be overcome easily as the conceptual ingredients to our theory—constraint satisfaction and affective meanings—have been widely applied to modeling impression formation (e.g., Kunda & Thagard, 1996; Heise, 2007; 2010; Schröder, 2011). It is thus likely possible to apply the model of Figure 1 to social priming experiments, where the dependent variable is not a behavior, but some kind of social perception.

CONCLUSION

We have described social priming as a process of constraint satisfaction that can be performed by neural networks through interactive activation and competition. We have proposed that priming is related to culturally shared conceptual structures, because the main constraints stem from the affective meanings of concepts that people have acquired in socialization. The maintenance of such meanings is the cultural mechanism underlying priming. We have shown how priming can be modeled with localist constraint-satisfaction networks whose connections are grounded in empirical measurements of affective meanings. However, in the brain, the entities that compete are not unitary, local nodes but rather distributed representations that bind together multimodal representations. These representations—semantic pointers—can contribute to intentions. Intentions can interfere with priming by the same competition mechanism that governs automatic social cognition in the first place.

We have discussed the compatibility of our cognitive modeling approach with many other accounts of social priming. We hope that our theory not only contributes to a unified, mechanistic understanding of the various phenomena related to priming, but may also stimulate future empirical work that advances our understanding of social cognition.

REFERENCES

Ambrasat, J., von Scheve, C., Schauenburg, G., Conrad, M., & Schröder, T. (2014). Consensus and stratification in the affective meaning of human sociality. *Proceedings of the National Academy of Sciences of the United States of America, 111*, 8001-8006.

Bargh, J. A. (2006). What have we been priming all these years? On the development, mechanisms, and ecology of nonconscious social behavior. *European Journal of Social Psychology, 36*, 147-168.

Bargh, J. A., Chen, M., & Burrows, L. (1996). Automaticity of social behavior: Direct effects of trait construct and stereotype activation on action. *Journal of Personality and Social Psychology, 71*, 230-244.

Barsalou, L. W. (1999). Perceptual symbol systems. *Behavioral and Brain Sciences, 22*, 577-660.

Cesario, J., Plaks, J. E., Hagiwara, N., Navarrete, C. D., & Higgins, E. T. (2010). The ecology of automaticity: How situational contingencies shape action semantics and social behavior. *Psychological Science, 21*, 1311-1317.

Cesario, J., Plaks, J. E., & Higgins, E. T. (2006). Automatic social behavior as motivated preparation to interact. *Journal of Personality and Social Psychology, 90*, 893-910.

Collins, A. M., & Loftus, E. F. (1975). A spreading-activation theory of semantic processing. *Psychological Review, 82*, 407-428.

Cunningham, W. A., & Zelazo, P. D. (2007). Attitudes and evaluations: A social cognitive neuroscience perspective. *Trends in Cognitive Sciences, 11*, 97-104.

Deutsch, R., & Strack, F. (2006). Duality models in social psychology: From dual processes to interacting systems. *Psychological Inquiry, 17*, 166-172.

Eitam, B., & Higgins, E. T. (2010). Motivation in mental accessibility: Relevance of a representation (ROAR) as a new framework. *Social and Personality Psychology Compass, 4*, 951-967.

Eliasmith, C. (2013). *How to build a brain. A neural architecture for biological cognition.* New York: Oxford University Press.

Eliasmith, C., & Anderson, C. H. (2003). *Neural engineering: Computation, representation, and dynamics in neurobiological systems.* Cambridge, MA: MIT Press.

Eliasmith, C., Stewart, T. C., Choo, X., Bekolay, T., DeWolf, T., Tang, Y., & Rasmussen, D. (2012). A large-scale model of the functioning brain. *Science, 338*, 1202-1205.

Fishbein, M., & Ajzen, I. (2010). *Predicting and changing behavior: The reasoned action approach.* New York: Psychology Press (Taylor & Francis).

Fiske, S. T., Cuddy, A. J. C., & Glick, P. (2007). Universal dimensions of social cognition: Warmth and competence. *Trends in Cognitive Sciences, 11*, 77-83.

Fitzsimons, G. M., & Bargh, J. A. (2003). Thinking of you: Nonconscious pursuit of interpersonal goals associated with relationship partners. *Journal of Personality and Social Psychology, 84*, 148-164.

Fontaine, J. R. J., Scherer, K. R., Roesch, E. B., & Ellsworth, P. C. (2007). The world of emotions is not two-dimensional. *Psychological Science, 18*, 1050-1057.

Francis, C., & Heise, D. R. (2006). *Mean affective ratings of 1,500 concepts by Indiana University undergraduates in 2002-2003.* Distributed via affect control theory Internet site, program INTERACT. Retrieved January 14, 2014, from http://www.indiana.edu/~socpsy/ACT/interact.htm.

Friese, M., Hofmann, W., & Wänke, M. (2008). When impulses take over: Moderated predictive validity of explicit and implicit attitude measures in predicting food choice and consumption behavior. *British Journal of Social Psychology, 47*, 397-419.

Georgopoulos, A. P., Schwartz, A., & Kettner, R. E. (1986). Neuronal population coding of movement direction. *Science, 233*, 1416-1419.

Heider, F. (1946). Attitudes and cognitive organization. *Journal of Psychology, 21*, 107-112.

Heise, D. R. (2007). *Expressive order. Confirming sentiments in social action.* New York: Springer.

Heise, D. R. (2010). *Surveying cultures. Discovering shared conceptions and sentiments.* Hoboken, NJ: Wiley.

Hofstede, G. (2001). *Culture's consequences. Comparing values, behaviors, institutions, and organizations across nations* (2nd ed.). Thousand Oaks, CA: Sage.

Homer-Dixon, T., Leader Maynard, J., Mildenberger, M., Milkoreit, M., Mock, S. J., Quilley, S., Schröder, T., & Thagard, P. (2013). A complex systems approach to the study of ideology. Cognitive-affective structure and the dynamics of belief change. *Journal of Social and Political Psychology, 1*, 337-363.

Kervyn, N., Fiske, S. T., & Yzerbyt, V. (2013). Integrating the stereotype content model (warmth and competence) and the Osgood semantic differential (evaluation, potency, and activity). *European Journal of Social Psychology, 43*, 673-681.

Kunda, Z., & Thagard, P. (1996). Forming impressions from stereotypes, traits, and behaviors: A parallel constraint-satisfaction theory. *Psychological Review, 103*, 284-308.

Lindquist, K. A., Wager, T. D., Kober, H., Bliss-Moreau, E., & Barrett, L. F. (2012). The brain basis of emotion: A meta-analytic review. *Behavioral and Brain Sciences, 35,* 121-143.

Loersch, C., & Payne, K. B. (2011). The situated inference model: An integrative account of the effects of primes on perception, behavior, and motivation. *Perspectives on Psychological Science, 6,* 234-252.

Loersch, C., & Payne, B. K. (2014). Situated inferences and the what, who, and where of priming. This volume.

McClelland, J. L., & Rumelhart, D. E. (1981). An interactive activation model of context effects in letter perception: Part 1: An account of basic findings. *Psychological Review, 88,* 375-407.

Molden, D. C. (2014). Understanding priming effects in social psychology: An overview and integration. This volume.

Osgood, C. E., May, W. H., & Miron, M. S. (1975). *Cross-cultural universals of affective meaning.* Urbana: University of Illinois Press.

Osgood, C. E., Suci, G. J., & Tannenbaum, P. H. (1957). *The measurement of meaning.* Urbana: University of Illinois Press.

Osgood, C. E., & Tannenbaum, P. H. (1955). The principle of congruity in the prediction of attitude change. *Psychological Review, 62,* 42-55.

Plate, T. A. (2003). *Holographic reduced representations.* Stanford, CA: CSLI Publications.

Read, S. J., & Simon, D. (2012). Parallel constraint satisfaction as a mechanism for cognitive consistency. In B. Gawronski & F. Strack (Eds.), *Cognitive consistency: A fundamental principle in social cognition* (pp. 66-86). New York: Guilford.

Rogers, K. B., Schröder, T., & Scholl, W. (2013). The affective structure of stereotype content: Behavior and emotion in intergroup context. *Social Psychology Quarterly, 76,* 125-150.

Rogers, K. B., Schröder, T., & von Scheve, C. (2014). Dissecting the sociality of emotion: A multi-level approach. *Emotion Review, 6,* 124-133.

Scherer, K. R., Dan, E. S., & Flykt, A. (2006). What determines a feeling's position in affective space? A case for appraisal. *Cognition & Emotion, 20,* 92-113.

Schröder, T. (2011). A model of language-based impression formation and attribution among Germans. *Journal of Language and Social Psychology, 30,* 82-102.

Schröder, T., Netzel, J., Schermuly, C. C., & Scholl, W. (2013). Culture-constrained affective consistency of interpersonal behavior: A test of affect control theory with nonverbal expressions. *Social Psychology, 44,* 47-58.

Schröder, T., Rogers, K. B., Ike, S., Mell, J. & Scholl, W. (2013). Affective meanings of stereotyped social groups in cross-cultural comparison. *Group Processes and Intergroup Relations, 16,* 717-733.

Schröder, T., Stewart, T. C. & Thagard, P. (in press). Intention, emotion, and action: A neural theory based on semantic pointers. *Cognitive Science.*

Schröder, T., & Thagard, P. (2013). The affective meanings of automatic social behaviors: Three mechanisms that explain priming. *Psychological Review, 120,* 255-280.

Simon, D. & Holyoak, K. J. (2002). Structural dynamics of cognition: From consistency theories to constraint satisfaction. *Personality and Social Psychology Review, 6,* 649-662.

Smeesters, D., Yzerbyt, V. Y., Corneille, O., & Warlop, L. (2009). When do primes prime? The moderating role of the self-concept in individuals' susceptibility to priming effects on social behavior. *Journal of Experimental Social Psychology, 45,* 211-216.

Stewart, T. C., Bekolay, T., & Eliasmith, C. (2012). Learning to select actions with spiking neurons in the basal ganglia. *Frontiers in Decision Neuroscience, 6,* 1-4.

Stewart, T. C., & Eliasmith, C. (2012). Compositionality and biologically plausible models. In W. Hinzen, E. Machery, & M. Werning (Eds.), *Oxford handbook of compositionality.* New York: Oxford University Press.

Thagard, P. (2000). *Coherence in thought and action.* Cambridge, MA: MIT Press.

Thagard, P. (2003). Why wasn't O.J. convicted? Emotional coherence in legal inference. *Cognition and Emotion, 17,* 361-383.

Thagard, P., & Schröder, T. (in press). Emotions as semantic pointers: Constructive neural mechanisms. In L. F. Barrett & J. A.

Russell (Eds.), *The psychological construction of emotions*. New York: Guilford.

Thagard, P., & Stewart, T. C. (2013). *Two theories of consciousness: Semantic pointer competition vs. information integration.* Unpublished manuscript, University of Waterloo.

Tsakiris, M., & Haggard, P. (2010). Neural, functional, and phenomenological signatures of intentional actions. In F. Grammont, D. Legrand, & P. Livet (Eds.), *Naturalizing intention in action* (pp. 39-64). Cambridge, MA: MIT Press.

Wheeler, S. C., & DeMarree, K. G. (2009). Multiple mechanisms of prime-to-behavior effects. *Social and Personality Psychology Compass, 3*, 566-581.

Wheeler, S. C., DeMarree, K. G., & Petty, R. E. (2007). Understanding the role of the self in prime-to-behavior effects: The active-self account. *Personality and Social Psychology Review, 11*, 234-261.

CONSIDERING NEW SOURCES OF SOCIAL PRIMES

GROUNDING SOCIAL EMBODIMENT

Daniël Lakens
Eindhoven University of Technology

> Social embodiment research examines how thoughts, affect, and behavior are influenced by sensory, motor, and perceptual cues in the environment. It has repeatedly received criticism due to a focus on demonstration studies. Here, I aim to identify some of the possible reasons underlying the lack of theoretical progress. First, I warn against relying too strongly on inductive inferences due to the weak empirical support for social embodiment findings. Second, I will discuss two dominant theoretical frameworks in social embodiment research (conceptual metaphor theory and perceptual symbol systems theory) in light of their potential to inspire empirically testable hypotheses. Finally, I propose that one way to turn social embodiment research into a progressive research line is to integrate it more firmly with past theoretical work in social cognition, and to focus on understanding the contexts in which concrete cues in the environment are salient and accessible enough to influence social inferences.

> If we wish to attribute the greatest known reality to the material world which exists immediately only in our idea, we give it the reality which our own body has for each of us; for that is the most real thing for everyone.
> —*Schopenhauer, WWR 1, 105*

Sensory experiences are an important source of meaning. In recent years, researchers have examined the interrelated nature of sensory experiences, affect, behavior, and cognition in a very productive line of research, broadly referred to as embodiment. Concepts are considered *embodied* when thoughts about the meaning of mental structures depend on activity in systems also used for perception, action, and emotion (e.g., Glenberg, de Vega, & Graesser, 2008). *Social embodiment* (Barsalou, Niedenthal, Barbey, & Ruppert, 2003) is a subdiscipline of embodiment research that focuses on how people process social information. This research area

---

I would like to thank Nils Jostmann and Thomas Schubert for feedback on a previous draft of this chapter.
Address correspondence to Daniël Lakens, Human Technology Interaction Group, IPO 1.33, P.O. Box 513, 5600MB Eindhoven, The Netherlands. E-mail: D.Lakens@tue.nl.

builds on the idea that social inference processes involved in thoughts about the meanings of entities and events are influenced by sensory, motor, and perceptual cues in the environment.

It is in the context of early work on social inferences that the term *social priming* originated (see Salancik & Pfeffer, 1978; Smith, 1984), where semantic cues can activate associated concepts, which influence subsequent thoughts about social information. Researchers have drawn an analogy between the way people process social information and how a computer processes information, where input is stored in memory and translated into machine language so that a central processor can operate on the input, which is then translated back into output understandable by the user (see Wyer, 1974). Social embodiment takes a stance against this computer metaphor, and proposes that conceptual thought depends on sensorimotor information, either through conceptual metaphors (Lakoff & Johnson, 1999) or neural reactivation of sensorimotor information (Barsalou, 1999). Embodied conceptual structures have been argued to play an important role in social priming effects (Bargh, 2006).

The idea that mental representations of social concepts (e.g., *hostile*) contain sensory and affective information in addition to semantic meaning has never been questioned in social cognition research (e.g., Wyer & Srull, 1986). As Fodor (1985) notes: "No one in his right mind doubts that perception interacts with cognition somewhere. What's at issue…is the locus of this interaction" (p. 5). Social embodiment distinguishes itself from earlier work on social priming by lowering the level at which perception and cognition interact. In the work of Wyer and Srull (1986), both semantic bins (the mental dictionary) and referent bins (which can consist of visual images, episodic memories, or subjective affective responses) exist, but incoming information is first encoded into semantic concepts. Social embodiment, on the other hand, starts from the viewpoint that such a translation process is unnecessary and that sensory, motor, and affective neural states are reactivated during cognitive processes.

Reviews of embodiment research in social psychology show that embodiment effects go back at least half a century (see Barsalou et al., 2003; Meier, Schnall, Schwarz, & Bargh, 2012). In this chapter, I use the term *social embodiment* to refer to research that is most closely aligned with the social priming research that emerged from work on social inferences (e.g., Srull & Wyer, 1979). There has been some debate about whether *social embodiment* or *social priming* is a meaningful concept, and how it should be defined (see Molden, 2014, this volume). Here, I follow previous theoretical work that distinguishes between non-social and social information processing (e.g., Smith, 1984; Wyer & Srull, 1986). Of central importance in social information processing is how prior attitudes and goals influence social inferences about person impressions, judgments, affective reactions, and behaviors, whereas these types of inferences are typically ignored in cognitive models of information processing.

Social embodiment research has examined, among other things, how concrete cues such as warmth, smells, weight, brightness, roughness, elevation, body posture, or motor movements influence person perception, moral judgments, pro-social decisions, attitudes, the desirability of products, emotional states, and behaviors. It is a line of research that has repeatedly received criticism due to a focus on demonstration studies and a lack of theoretically progressive experiments (e.g., Barsalou, 2010; Meier et al., 2012; Schubert & Semin, 2009; Zwaan, 2009). Here, I will try to identify some of the reasons for this lack of theoretical progress. First, I discuss the possibility that the current empirical knowledge base in social embodiment is not strong enough to draw reliable inductive inferences. Second, I will discuss two of the dominant theoretical frameworks in social embodiment research, conceptual metaphor theory, and perceptual symbol systems theory, in light of their potential to inspire empirically testable predictions. Finally, I suggest that if we want to turn social embodiment research into a progressive research line, we need to understand the contexts in which concrete cues in the environment are salient and accessible enough to influence social inferences.

A CRITICAL LOOK AT THE EMPIRICAL DATA

As an example of how social information processing is influenced by sensory experiences, consider the finding that the physical experience of weight (manipulated by asking participants to hold either a heavy or light clipboard while filling out a questionnaire) influenced the inferred importance of issues, such as being heard in a decision-making procedure (Jostmann, Lakens, & Schubert, 2009). This study is typical for many findings in the social embodiment literature in that 1) a sensorimotor experience influences 2) social inference processes in an unrelated and often more abstract domain 3) seemingly automatically and without awareness of the individual.

Reviews of the social embodiment literature often summarize a wide range of research areas such as facial feedback (e.g., Strack, Martin, & Stepper, 1988), cross-modal stimulus response congruency effects (e.g., Lakens, 2012; Meier & Robinson, 2004; Schubert, 2005), and approach avoidance effects (e.g., Eder & Rothermund, 2008; Rotteveel & Phaf, 2004). When we turn to research that examines whether sensorimotor information influences social inferences, there are some reasons to worry about the robustness of the empirical knowledge base. Many replication studies of social embodiment effects have failed to provide support for the original hypotheses (e.g., Brandt, IJzerman, & Blanken, 2014; Earp, Everett, Madva, & Hamlin, in press; Johnson, Cheung, & Donnellan; 2014; LeBel & Campbell, 2013; LeBel & Wilbur, 2014; Lynott et al., 2014; Pashler, Coburn, & Harris, 2012). Although there might be specific reasons the hypotheses were not supported in each of these replication studies, a parsimonious explanation for such failures to replicate the original effects is that the original studies were Type 1 errors, and the null-hypothesis is true.

Due to a combination of low statistical power, publication bias, and flexibility during data analysis, the number of false positives in the literature can be much greater than desired (e.g., Ioannidis, 2005). Using p-curve analysis, we can examine whether the distribution of p-values below .05 in published research is uniformly distributed, which implies the null-hypothesis is true, or whether the distribution is right-skewed (with more p-value between .00 and .01 than between .04 and .05) which implies the alternative hypothesis is true (Simonsohn, Nelson, & Simmons, 2013). Lakens (2014) performed p-curve analyses on social embodiment findings reviewed by Meier and colleagues (2012) that examined social inferences. These analyses indicated that the social inference studies discussed in this review, taken together, lack evidential value. The findings are more likely to represent chance findings from a selection of tests from a selection of studies than a robust and reliably observed phenomenon, despite the fact that most of the reported results were statistically significant.

The reason for this lack of evidential value is that practically all studies that have examined social embodiment effects had very small sample sizes and were severely underpowered. The informational value of underpowered studies is very low, and significant published results from underpowered studies are relatively likely to be false positives (Ioannidis, 2005). Although the idea that concrete cues in the environment influence social inferences might be correct, the empirical observations we have collected so far do not yet provide strong support for this idea (despite the many studies that have reported statistically significant effects). Because of the low informational value of published research, inductive reasoning based on observed findings is less likely to turn social embodiment into a progressive research line than deductive reasoning. Instead of drawing inspiration from published research, we need theoretical work that allows researchers to make strong and empirically testable predictions. We then need to examine these predictions in larger samples, preferably using preregistered designs (e.g., Nosek & Lakens, 2014).

A CRITICAL LOOK AT THE THEORETICAL FRAMEWORKS

Two theories dominate the recent literature in social embodiment: conceptual metaphor theory (CMT; Lakoff & Johnson, 1999) and perceptual symbol systems (PSS; Barsalou, 1999). I will briefly discuss both these theories, with a special focus on their potential to allow researchers to draw strong predictions about how concrete cues influence social inferences.

CONCEPTUAL METAPHOR THEORY

It has been suggested that metaphors embody conceptual meaning (e.g., Richards, 1936; Whitney, 1875). According to Lakoff and Johnson (1999, p. 20), "An embodied concept is a neural structure that is actually part of, or makes use of, the sensorimotor system of our brains." The cognitive mechanism that underlies embodied meaning is conceptual metaphor, where concrete source domains are used to think about more abstract target domains. It is assumed that through experiential co-occurrence (e.g., feeling happy and having an upright posture), neural associations are formed through which children learn primary metaphors (e.g., "happy is up"). These primary metaphors are used in reasoning, mostly unconsciously and automatically (Lakoff, 2012). Conceptual metaphor theory (and later theoretical work such as the neural theory of thought and language) has inspired many researchers in the field of social embodiment, and some researchers have argued for a metaphor-enriched perspective on social cognition (e.g., Landau, Meier, & Keefer, 2010). I am less optimistic about the potential of such a perspective on social cognition, and believe the use of conceptual metaphors as a theoretical guide in social embodiment is one of the major reasons we are now facing a degenerative research program.

First, as has been argued repeatedly, conceptual metaphor theory lacks a description of possible psychological process models (Boroditsky, 2000; McGlone,

2007; 2011; Murphy, 1996; Schubert, Waldzus, & Seibt, 2011). This makes it difficult to deduce clearly defined novel predictions about when metaphors are used, which metaphors are used, and how metaphors influence social inferences. The discussion about these questions continues in linguistics (e.g., Gibbs, 2011; McGlone, 2011) but is rarely referred to in articles on social embodiment. Because the underlying mechanisms of conceptual metaphors are not defined a priori, conceptual metaphors can provide post-hoc explanations of almost any empirical finding that shows a relation between sensorimotor cues and social inferences, but it does not allow for strong inferences (Platt, 1964).

Further, the predictions that can be derived from conceptual metaphors can also be derived from more general cognitive theories. A prediction that has received quite some attention concerns the asymmetry between concrete source domains and more abstract target domains (Lakoff, 2008), where "results of inferences flow in one direction only, from the sensorimotor domain to the domain of subjective judgment" (Lakoff & Johnson, 1999, p. 56). However, similar predictions about asymmetric associations are made in non-metaphorical models of associative thought. For example, the fan effect (Anderson, 1974) can explain how asymmetric associations emerge because frequently encountered concepts activate many associated concepts, whereas less frequently encountered concepts activate only a few associated concepts. As a consequence, less frequently encountered concepts (e.g., burden) are more strongly associated with frequently encountered concepts (e.g., weight) than vice versa. In addition, automatic translations between domains are more likely to develop for frequently encountered concepts than for less frequently encountered concepts. Because concrete concepts are typically encountered more frequently than abstract concepts, Carlston (1994, p. 38) predicts in his associative systems theory (see below) that, "As a general rule, then, automatic translations may be more likely to proceed from concrete forms of representation to abstract forms, rather than the reverse."

Given that many aspects of conceptual metaphors can be explained by more general accounts of associative thought, the question is what unique predictions CMT provides. One of the most fundamental predictions of CMT is that experiential co-occurrences create primary metaphors (Lakoff & Johnson, 1999). For example, because children are held affectionately by their parents, people are assumed to associate affection with warmth (Lakoff, 2012). We can imagine anecdotal support for this hypothesis, and future studies that examine how experiential co-occurrences create primary metaphors might (or might not) provide support for this hypothesis. However, there are reasons to doubt that experiential co-occurrences underlie all (or even most) primary metaphors.

For example, consider the primary metaphor "bad is stinky" (Lakoff & Johnson, 1999). Disgust is not present at birth. In the first years of life, children will put anything in their mouths, and Rozin and Fallon (1987) conclude that children's concept of disgust is very limited before eight years of age, with negative responses to odors such as sweat and feces emerging somewhere after five years of age. Further, disgust reactions are learned, possibly through the facial expression of parents, and disgust responses vary across cultures. Whether smells are considered disgusting is extremely flexible even within individuals: The same smell is judged as disgusting when it is believed to originate from feces, but judged as pleasant when people believe it originates from cheese. In other words, despite the intuitive appeal that "bad is stinky" emerges through a "correlation between evaluative and olfactory experience" (Lakoff & Johnson, 1999), and notwithstanding the importance of experiential co-occurrence for learned associations, it leaves a lot to be desired as an explanation of the mechanisms underlying primary metaphors.

Social cognition is situated and context dependent (Barsalou, 1999; Mesquita, Barrett, & Smith, 2010; Schwarz, 2007), and an important question in social priming research is how this context dependency can be explained (e.g., Bargh, 2006; Blair, 2002; Loersch & Payne, 2011; Mitchell, Nosek, & Banaji, 2003). Conceptual metaphor theory has a strong focus on universal "cognitive primitives" (e.g., verticality, part-whole, balance, etc.), and these can be used to think about other concepts that we cannot understand directly. However, conceptual metaphor theory does not allow for clear predictions about which neural mapping between concrete and abstract concepts will be activated depending on the situation, and is thus less equipped to inspire research on social inferences, which are inherently contextual. Further, these cognitive primitives, which originate from work in cognitive linguistics, are not well aligned with what are considered basic dimensions of meaning in the (social) psychological literature (e.g., valence and arousal; see Osgood, Suci, & Tannenbaum, 1957). A more widely accepted viewpoint in social psychology assumes that people can directly activate psychological concepts such as valence (e.g., Wyer & Srull, 1986). An embodied theory of cognition that shares this assumption, and proposes that people partially simulate introspective states by re-activating neural systems that were also active when these introspective states were experiences, is perceptual symbol systems theory (Barsalou, 1999), to which I will turn next.

PERCEPTUAL SYMBOL SYSTEMS

In addition to work on conceptual metaphors, perceptual symbol systems theory (PSS; Barsalou, 1999) has been very influential in recent work on social embodiment (for a review, see Niedenthal, Barsalou, Winkielman, Krauth-Gruber, & Ric, 2005). The idea in perceptual theories of cognition is that both concrete and abstract conceptual processing are built on and activate sensory-motor processes. These theories are a response to views of conceptual processing that argue for a purely symbolic language of thought (e.g., Fodor, 1975; Pylyshyn, 1984). According to proponents of amodal symbol systems, computations performed on symbolic representations are the essence of mental processes. An important benefit of thought that relies on amodal symbols is that it can integrate different modal (e.g., haptic, visual, auditory) sources of information on an amodal symbolic level of representation.

A challenge for amodal symbol systems is how symbolic representations are connected to their referents, the objects in the world. This challenge is known as the symbol grounding problem (Harnad, 1990). Where do amodal symbols get their meaning from, if their only sources of meaning are other meaningless amodal symbols? Barsalou (1999) proposes a perceptual symbol system where conceptual knowledge consists of modal representations. These representations can be partially activated during language comprehension, leading to neural re-enactments (or simulations) that activate the same sensory and motor areas in our brain as were active when we directly experienced its referent. As opposed to conceptual metaphors, perceptual symbols are always context dependent, because they function as attractors in a connectionist network. Across different contexts, perceptual symbols can lead to different patterns of activation.

Perceptual symbol system theory has been embraced by emotion researchers. The idea that emotional responses have bodily components has a long history (e.g., Darwin, 1872), and there is a substantial amount of empirical data that suggests a bi-directional relationship between emotion processing and bodily states (for reviews, see Barrett & Lindquist, 2008; Niedenthal, 2007). For example, Schwarz, Weinberger, and Singer (1981) found that imagining specific emotional states changed the pattern of physiological activity in participants. In addition, the researchers found that physical activity (i.e., exercising) reduced the ability of participants to recreate as vividly as possible the feelings and physical sensations associated with states of sadness and relaxation. When it comes to emotion research, simulations that activate perceptual, motor, and introspective brain areas seem to have proven their worth.

Modal simulations are often suggested to underlie embodied social inferences (e.g., Lee & Schwarz, 2010; Meier, Hauser, Robinson, Friesen, & Schjeldahl, 2007; Schneider, Rutjens, Jostmann, & Lakens, 2011; Zhong & Liljenquist, 2006). Traditionally, thoughts about religiousness, importance, social exclusion, or moral transgressions were not thought to depend on physical experiences such as the temperature, motor activation, haptic experiences of weight, or vertical cues, but these recent studies suggest bodily experiences are closely related to higher cognitive processes. Providing unequivocal support for the idea that simulations are an essential part of social inferences is difficult, and there is a continuing debate about whether the activation of sensorimotor information simply enriches conceptual processing or is actually a necessary part of conceptual thought (see Barsalou, 2010; Mahon & Caramazza, 2008; Zwaan, 2009). Resolving these different viewpoints is anything but straightforward. The scientific debate has gone on for at least 35 years, and some researchers have expressed doubt about the possibility that this debate will lead to scientific progress (Gomilla & Calvo, 2008). In addition, the nature of mental representations might not be the most important research question for social cognition researchers.

It is widely acknowledged that not all conceptual thought is based on simulations, and that linguistic information is an efficient way to perform many cognitive tasks (e.g., Andrews, Vigliocco, & Vinson, 2009; Barsalou, Santos, Simmons, & Wilson, 2008; Louwerse, 2011). Therefore, an important question is in which situations do people rely on concrete cues during social inference processes, instead of relying solely on linguistic information. This *context challenge* (see also Barsalou, 2009; Mesquita et al., 2010; Zwaan, 2009) is not a strange concept in experimental social psychology. The contextual nature of social information processing was raised as an especially important topic in research on implicit cognition (e.g., Blair, 2002; Loersch & Payne, 2011; Mitchell et al., 2003; Schwarz, 2007), and the question of which associations between concepts are salient depending on the context has been a central research question throughout the last 30 years of research on social priming (e.g., Bargh, 2006; Higgins, 1996; Smith, 1984).

Perceptual symbols are context dependent, and they are easily integrated within situated views on cognition. Theoretical work on situated simulations provides many possibilities for social psychologists to examine contextualized social inferences (for a review, see Smith & Collins, 2010). Because past research has focused on demonstrating that concrete cues *can* influence social inferences, the question *when* people actually use these cues has not been examined in detail. To summarize, the strong focus on situated simulations in perceptual theories of cognition provides a better fit with inherently contextualized views on cognition that are prevalent in social priming research than a "metaphor-enriched" perspective on social cognition (e.g., Landau et al., 2010). For social cognition researchers, a more fruitful approach for future research might be to leave the debate between modal versus amodal representations to cognitive neuroscience, and instead focus on examining when the relationship between perceptual and conceptual information is salient and accessible enough to influence social inferences.

ONE STEP BACK, TWO STEPS FORWARD?

A critical look at recent studies that have examined whether concrete cues influence social inferences provides some reasons to doubt whether social embodiment research on social inferences has received the empirical or theoretical grounding that a progressive research line needs. Integrating social embodiment research more firmly with past theoretical work in social cognition might be one way to remedy this situation. In the following sections, I will first describe associated systems theory (Carlston, 1994), which is never used to explain social embodiment effects despite the fact that it is a dedicated theory of social concepts, and explicitly predicts interactions between perception, action, cognition, and affect. Then, I will revisit some of the central questions in early work on social inferences, and suggest that social embodiment researchers could address these questions in future research.

ASSOCIATED SYSTEMS THEORY

Associated systems theory (AST; Carlston, 1994) proposes that there are four primary mental systems that underlie representations: a visual/sensory system, a verbal/semantic system, an action system, and an affective system. It specifically tries to integrate different mental constructs into a single organized structure. Each system is hierarchically organized. At the lower level, these systems connect to highly specialized physical structures involved in perception, language, motoric behavior, and evaluation. At higher (more abstract) levels of cognition, these systems interact in *convergence zones* (a similar idea is present in PSS theory) to create secondary hybrid representations that are referred to as *categories, evaluations, behavioral observations*, and *orientations*. These initial representations can be translated into secondary forms of representation through *inferences*. Carlston (1994, p. 35) reminds us that in addition to obvious inferences (e.g., inferring a person's traits from their actions), "in principle, information in any form may be translated into any other form." He refers to Wilson's (1968) studies where the status of a person can influence judgments about the perceived height of that individual (see also Schubert, Schubert, & Topolinski, 2013).

Carlston discusses the possibility that activation in a primary processing system might be able to "warm up" that processing system and increase the likelihood that it will be used in subsequent tasks, but also notes it could interfere if the system has to be used for a second task before the first task is completed. As an example of a facilitation effect, he cites studies by Klatzky, Pellegrino, McCloskey, and Doherty (1989) that show how participants who are asked whether a particular action is plausible responded more quickly when they were primed by a hand shape than by a neutral signal. As an example of an interference effect, he mentions the studies by Engelkamp (1991) which revealed that sentences that were learned while making related movements (e.g., learning *hammering a nail* while making hammering movements) were less easily retrieved when participants had to make unrelated movements during retrieval. These studies are now often cited as examples of embodied cognition research, which highlights how social embodiment research can be effortlessly integrated with AST.

Niedenthal and colleagues (2005) discuss AST as a view related to perceptual symbol systems. They note that PSS is somewhat more radical about the modal nature of representations compared to AST, although as discussed earlier, providing unequivocal support for the nature of representations is a real challenge. Further, PSS focuses more strongly on higher cognitive functions, such as the representation of abstract concepts (e.g., *truth*, *democracy*), or the type-token distinction between a concept and the objects that are instances of the concept. The differences between PSS and AST are not irreconcilable, and the two approaches are most likely complementary. PSS provides a more a detailed account of how people think about abstract concepts such as democracy or truth, and how situated simulations influence cognition, whereas AST provides a more detailed explanation of the abstract concepts that are of focal interest to social cognition researchers (e.g., evaluations, orientations). PSS has actually faced some criticism because it explains how these abstract concepts are grounded through introspection, which is relatively poorly understood (Barsalou, 1999). Whether and how introspection contributes to the mental representation of concepts remains unclear, and AST provides a more straightforward explanation of how representations of abstract social concepts emerge through inferences. Thus, both PSS and AST have their own strengths, and social embodiment researchers should select the theoretical framework that is best suited for the questions they are trying to address.

AST (Carlston, 1994) provides a first formulation of a framework that, due to its integration of verbal, visual, behavioral, and affective representations, is perfectly suited to inspire researchers who aim to examine how concrete cues in the environment influence social inferences. In its current form, AST already provides an interesting theoretical departure point for researchers interested in the role of attention in social embodiment. The idea that different primary systems contribute to mental representations predicts that whenever attention is shifted to one of these systems, it will contribute more to the overall representation. Consider recent studies where positive and negative words are presented on the top and bottom of the screen, which shows that there is a bidirectional association between valence and vertical space (Santiago, Ouellet, Román, & Valenzuela, 2012). Valence categorizations are influenced by the vertical position of stimuli, and position categorizations are influenced by the valence of the stimuli, but only when the dimension irrelevant for the categorization was salient enough. It is surprising that social embodiment researchers have not embraced AST more enthusiastically in the last two decades by attempting to develop it further, formally refine the theory, and adapt it based on recent insights. One possible reason is that the theoretical framework is presented in books and book chapters (e.g., Carlston, 1992, 1994) which are not as accessible as journal articles.

REVISITING A FUNDAMENTAL QUESTION

Although improving the theoretical grounding of social embodiment research that examines how concrete cues in the environment influence social inferences is an important starting point, it is equally important to ask the right empirical questions. If we want to understand when and how concrete information in the environment will function as a cue that influences person perception, moral judgments, pro-social decisions, attitudes, and behaviors, we need to understand the influence of sensorimotor information on the accessibility and salience of social information (cf. Higgins, 1996). In essence, this implies examining meaning making by specifying the structure of the context in which it emerges (Bruner, 1990). These questions are not new, but revisiting them in social embodiment research might provide an important way forward.

If concrete cues can influence social inferences relatively automatically, the association between a concrete cue (e.g., weight) and an abstract concept (e.g., importance) needs to exist either due to evolutionary predispositions, Hebbian learning through repeated co-occurrences, or inferences that have become proceduralized after extensive practice. A first step is to distinguish between these different alternatives (for each social embodiment effect that can be reliably observed in replication studies). Perhaps people have repeatedly inferred that thick and heavy books contain a lot of important information, while light books are typically less important (e.g., Schneider et al., 2011). Perhaps people have come to associate warmth with affection by being (passively) held by their parents (e.g., Bowlby, 1969). Perhaps people associate darkness with negativity because we have evolved to be diurnal animals (e.g., Lakens, Semin, & Foroni, 2012). Depending on the assumptions about the origin of the relationship between physical cues and social inferences, researchers can make predictions about the accessibility of these associations, which should be more chronic in evolutionary predispositions and more goal-dependent in extensively practiced inferences (Smith, 1984).

One straightforward question is how often experiences need to co-occur to form long-lasting associations in memory. Insights from evaluative conditioning might be interesting in this respect (Hofmann, De Houwer, Perugini, Baeyens, & Crombez, 2010), such as the preliminary finding that evaluative conditioning effects are smaller in children, and evaluative conditioning effects are much greater if people are aware of the contingency between the conditioned and unconditioned stimulus. These findings speak against the idea that experiential co-occurrences create associations purely through bottom-up processes (as assumed in CMT and AST), and are more in line with simulators that rely on an integration of information through selective attention (PSS). More knowledge about how meaning is derived from experiential co-occurrences (even if they do not underlie all primary metaphors in CMT) can be gathered through developmental studies or experiments that involve learning tasks where stimuli are repeatedly presented. Researchers could examine how new associations between sensory information and social concepts are learned, or whether existing associations are flexible enough to be changed. If attentional factors indeed play a role in establishing associations through experiential co-occurrences, the question is which contextual factors direct attention to co-occurring stimuli, and which do not.

A second important question is whether there are individual differences in the way, or the extent to which, people rely on concrete cues (Meier et al., 2012). Individual differences are not only expected to exist due to differences in past experiential co-occurrences. Carlston (1994) raises the possibility that people might differ in the kind of representation (e.g., visual, verbal, affect, action) they rely on. When examining social embodiment effects, one logical prediction from AST (but not necessarily from CMT or PSS) is that inferences by people with higher sensitivity to bodily cues are especially influenced by concrete sensorimotor information. When proceduralized inferences underlie social embodiment effects (but not when they are caused by evolutionary predispositions), different contexts or goals could temporarily change the type of representations people rely on. For example, Louwerse and Jeuniaux (2010) examined when information processing makes use of perceptual simulations, and when it uses linguistic distributional information. They found that people's response times depended more strongly on linguistic information when the task was to make semantic judgments for words, but that they relied more on perceptual information when they had to perform judgments about the spatial relationship of pictures. The nature of the task people perform will almost always be a defining factor of the context.

Following the basic idea in cognition that the mind selects and seeks structure in the world (e.g., Hastie & Carlston, 1980), the *structural similarity view* (Murphy, 1996) is an alternative to CMT that proposes all concepts are directly represented, with metaphors reflecting the similarity of preexisting conceptual structures, such as when people use structural features of spatial movement to think about time (Boroditsky, 2000). Conceptual thought not only requires that the meaning content of concepts is grounded, but, especially for social relational concepts, it also requires concepts to be structured (e.g., Lakens, Semin, & Foroni, 2011; 2012). Important questions remain about when and why environmental structures are salient enough to be used as cues that influence social inferences.

There are many aspects from PSS and AST that can be used when examining contextual factors that influence the salience of concrete environmental cues and how they influence the accessibility of social information. The idea of simulators in PSS can inspire researchers to examine how people develop specific simulations of social situations or certain kinds of abstract concepts (such as democracy) in an inherently contextualized manner. AST allows researchers to derive predictions about how different primary systems might contribute to or interfere with mental representations, depending on attentional factors, individual differences, and the type of inference a person is making.

In addition, social embodiment research will show greater progress if researchers start to incorporate insights from other research areas that have addressed the context challenge. Especially social psychological work on evaluation has developed advanced models of dynamic and context dependent affective inferences (e.g., Gawronski, Rydell, Vervliet, & De Houwer, 2010; Klauer, Teige-Mocigemba, & Spruyt, 2009). These theories can be used to derive theoretical predictions about when inferences that underlie the mental representation of social concepts are influenced by activity in systems used for perception, action, or emotion. At the same time, these theories have assumptions about how valence is mentally represented, either as dedicated valence counters (Klauer et al., 2009), or a retrieved pattern of associated concepts (Gawronski et al., 2010) and developing a better understanding of the mental representation of valence might prove to be an interesting empirical question for social embodiment researchers that can in turn inspire social psychological work on evaluation.

CONCLUSION

To turn social embodiment research into a progressive research line, several challenges need to be met. Researchers need to acknowledge that practically all theories about cognition predict that cognition and perception interact. Progress can only be made by explaining how cognition depends on or is influenced by systems used for perception, action, or emotion. Existing theories of embodied cognition are either not detailed enough when it comes to the predictions they make (CMT) or have been used to examine questions about the nature of mental representations that might never be settled unequivocally. We lack a reliable empirical basis of social embodiment effects that have examined how concrete cues influence social inferences, which makes inductive inferences an unlikely source of progress. A better approach might be to try to derive hypotheses from theoretical work on the influence of sensorimotor information on the accessibility and salience of social information, which will allow us to test novel predictions about the context in which social cognition is embodied.

REFERENCES

Anderson, J. R. (1974). Retrieval of prepositional information from long-term memory. *Cognitive Psychology, 6*, 451-474.

Andrews, M., Vigliocco, G., & Vinson, D. (2009). Integrating experiential and distributional data to learn semantic representations. *Psychological Review, 116*(3), 463-498.

Bargh, J. A. (2006). What have we been priming all these years? On the development, mechanisms, and ecology of nonconscious social behavior. *European Journal of Social Psychology, 36*(2), 147-168.

Barrett, L. F., & Lindquist, K. (2008). The embodiment of emotion. In G. Semin & E. Smith (Eds.), *Embodied grounding: Social, cognitive, affective, and neuroscience approaches* (pp. 237-262). New York: Cambridge University Press.

Barsalou, L. W. (1999). Perceptual symbol systems. *Behavioral and Brain Sciences, 22*, 577-660.

Barsalou, L. W. (2009). Simulation, situated conceptualization, and prediction. *Philosophical Transactions of the Royal Society of London: Biological Sciences, 364*, 1281-1289.

Barsalou, L. W. (2010). Grounded cognition: Past, present, and future. *Topics in Cognitive Science, 2*, 716-724.

Barsalou, L. W., Niedenthal, P. M., Barbey, A. K., & Ruppert, J. A. (2003). Social embodiment. *Psychology of Learning and Motivation, 43*, 43-92.

Barsalou, L. W., Santos, A., Simmons, W. K., & Wilson, C. D. (2008). Language and simulation in conceptual processing. In M. de Vega, A. M. Glenberg, & A. C. Graesser (Eds.), *Symbols, embodiment, and meaning* (pp. 245-283). Oxford: Oxford University Press.

Blair, I. V. (2002). The malleability of automatic stereotypes and prejudice. *Personality and Social Psychology Review, 6*(3), 242-261.

Boroditsky, L. (2000). Metaphoric structuring: Understanding time through spatial metaphors. *Cognition, 75*, 1-28.

Bowlby, J. (1969). *Attachment and loss: Vol. 1. Attachment*. New York: Basic Books.

Brandt, M. J., IJzerman, H., & Blanken, I. (2014). Does recalling moral behavior change the perception of brightness? A replication and meta-analysis of Banerjee, Chatterjee, and Sinha (2012). *Social Psychology, 45*(3), 246-252.

Bruner, J. (1990). *Acts of meaning*. Cambridge: Harvard University Press.

Bruner, J. S., Goodnow, J., & Austin, G. A. (1956). *A study of thinking*. New York: Wiley.

Carlston, D. E. (1992). Impression formation and the modular mind: The associated systems theory. In L. L. Martin & A. Tesser (Eds.), *The construction of social judgments* (pp. 301-341). Hillsdale, NJ: Erlbaum.

Carlston, D. E. (1994). Associated systems theory: A systematic approach to the cognitive representation of persons and events. In R. S. Wyer (Ed.), *Advances in Social Cognition, Vol. 7: Associated Systems Theory* (pp. 1-78). Hillsdale, NJ: Erlbaum.

Carlston, D. E. (2010). Models of implicit and explicit mental representation. In B. Gawronski & B. Keith Payne (Eds.), *Handbook of implicit social cognition: Measurement, theory, and applications* (pp. 38-61). New York: Guilford.

Darwin, C. (1872). *The expression of the emotions in man and animals*. London: John Murray.

Earp, B. D., Everett, J. A. C., Madva, E. N., & Hamlin, J. K. (in press). Out, damned spot: Can the "Macbeth effect" be replicated? *Basic and Applied Social Psychology*.

Eder, A. B., & Rothermund, K. (2008). When do motor behaviors (mis)match affective stimuli? An evaluative coding view of approach and avoidance reactions. *Journal of Experimental Psychology: General, 137*(2), 262-281.

Engelkamp, J. (1991). Memory of action events: Some implications for memory theory and for imagery. In C. Cornoldi & M.A. McDaniel (Eds.), *Imagery and cognition* (pp. 183-219). New York: Springer-Verlag.

Fodor, J. A. (1975). *The language of thought*. Cambridge, MA: Harvard University Press.

Fodor, J. A. (1985). Précis of the modularity of mind. *Behavioral and Brain Sciences, 8,* 1-42.

Gawronski, B. Rydell, R. J., Vervliet, B., & De Houwer, J. (2010). Generalization versus contextualization in automatic evaluation. *Journal of Experimental Psychology: General, 139,* 683-701. doi:10.1037/a0020315

Gibbs Jr., R. W. (2011). Evaluating conceptual metaphor theory. *Discourse Processes, 48,* 529-562.

Glenberg, A., de Vega, M., & Graesser, A. C. (2008). Framing the debate. In M. de Vega, A. Glenberg, & A. C. Graesser (Eds.), *Symbols and embodiment: Debates on meaning and cognition* (pp. 1-10). Oxford, UK: Oxford University Press.

Gomila, A., & Calvo, F. (2008) Directions for an embodied cognitive science: Towards an integrated approach. In F. Calvo & A. Gomila (Eds.), *Handbook of cognitive science: An embodied approach* (pp. 1-25). San Diego, CA: Elsevier.

Harnad, S. (1990). The symbol grounding problem. *Physica D, 42,* 335-346.

Hastie, R., & Carlston, D. (1980).Theoretical issues in person memory. In R. Hastie et al. (Eds.), *Person memory* (pp. 1-53). Hillsdale, NJ: Erlbaum.

Higgins, E. T. (1996). Knowledge activation: Accessibility, applicability, and salience. In E. T. Higgins & A. W. Kruglanski (Eds.), *Social psychology: Handbook of basic principles* (pp. 133-168). New York: Guilford.

Hofmann, W., De Houwer, J., Perugini, M., Baeyens, F., & Crombez, G. (2010). Evaluative conditioning in humans: A meta-analysis. *Psychological Bulletin, 136,* 390-421.

Ioannidis, J. P. A. (2005). Why most published research findings are false. *PLoS Medicine, 2, e124.* doi:10.1371/journal.pmed.0020124

Johnson, D. J., Cheung, F., & Donnellan, M. B. (2014). Does cleanliness influence moral judgments? A direct replication of Schnall, Benton, and Harvey (2008). *Social Psychology, 45,* 209-215.

Jostmann, N. B., Lakens, D., & Schubert, T. W. (2009). Weight as an embodiment of importance. *Psychological Science, 20,* 1169-1174. doi:10.1111/j.1467-9280.2009.02426.x

Klatzky, R. L., Pellegrino, J. W., McCloskey, B. P., & Doherty, S. (1989). Can you squeeze a tomato? The role of motor representations in semantic sensibility judgments. *Journal of Memory and Language, 28*, 56-77. doi:10.1016/0749-596X(89)90028-4

Klauer, K. C., Teige-Mocigemba, S., & Spruyt, A. (2009). Contrast effects in spontaneous evaluations: A psychophysical account. *Journal of Personality and Social Psychology, 96*(2), 265-287.

Lakens, D. (2011). High skies and oceans deep: Polarity benefits or mental simulation? *Frontiers in Psychology, 2*, 21. doi:10.3389/fpsyg.2011.00021

Lakens, D. (2012). Polarity correspondence in metaphor congruency effects: Structural overlap predicts categorization times for bi-polar concepts presented in vertical space. *Journal of Experimental Psychology: Learning, Memory, and Cognition, 38*, 726-723. doi:10.1037/a0024955

Lakens, D. (2014). Effects of sensorimotor information on thoughts, attitudes, and behavior lack evidential value. Manuscript in preparation. A working paper can be retrieved from https://dl.dropboxusercontent.com/u/133567/Lakens%20-%20Pcurve.pdf

Lakens, D., Semin, G. R., & Foroni, F. (2011). Why your highness needs the people: Comparing the absolute and relative representation of power in vertical space. *Social Psychology, 42*, 205-213. doi:10.1027/1864-9335/a000064

Lakens, D., Semin, G. R., & Foroni, F. (2012). But for the bad, there would not be good: Grounding valence in brightness through structural similarity. *Journal of Experiment Psychology: General, 141*, 584-594

Lakoff, G. (2008). The neural theory of metaphor. In: R. W. Gibbs (Ed.), *Cambridge handbook of metaphor and thought* (pp. 17-38). Cambridge, MA, Cambridge University Press.

Lakoff, G. (2012). Explaining embodied cognition results. *Topics in Cognitive Science, 4*, 773-785.

Lakoff, G., & Johnson, M. (1999). *Philosophy in the flesh: The embodied mind and its challenge to Western thought*. Chicago: University of Chicago Press.

Landau, M. J., Meier, B. P., & Keefer, L. A. (2010). A metaphor-enriched social cognition. *Psychological Bulletin, 136*, 1045-1067.

LeBel, E. P., & Campbell, L. (2013). Heightened sensitivity to temperature cues in highly anxiously attached individuals: Real or elusive phenomenon? *Psychological Science, 24*(10), 2128-2130.

LeBel, E. P., & Wilbur, C. J. (2014). Big secrets do not necessarily cause hills to appear steeper. *Psychonomic Bulletin & Review, 21*, 696-700.

Lee, S. W., & Schwarz, N. (2010). Dirty hands and dirty mouths: Embodiment of the moral-purity metaphor is specific to the motor modality involved in moral transgression. *Psychological Science, 21*(10), 1423-1425.

Loersch, C., & Payne, B. K. (2011). The situated inference model: An integrative account of the effects of primes on perception, behavior, and motivation. *Perspectives on Psychological Science, 6*(3), 234-252.

Louwerse, M. M. (2011). Symbol interdependency in symbolic and embodied cognition. *Topics in Cognitive Science, 3*(2), 273-302.

Louwerse, M. M., & Jeuniaux, P. (2010). The linguistic and embodied nature of conceptual processing. *Cognition, 114*, 96-104.

Lynott, D., Corker, K. S., Wortman, J., Connell, L., Donnellan, M. J., Lucas, R. E., &, O'Brien, K. (2014). Replication of "Experiencing physical warmth promotes interpersonal warmth" by Williams & Bargh (2008, *Science*). *Social Psychology, 45*, 216-222.

Mahon, B. Z., & Caramazza, A. (2008). A critical look at the embodied cognition hypothesis and a new proposal for grounding conceptual content. *Journal of Physiology-Paris, 102*, 59-70.

McGlone, M.S. (2007). What is the explanatory value of a conceptual metaphor? *Language & Communication, 27*, 109-126.

McGlone, M. S. (2011). Hyperbole, homunculi, and hindsight bias: An alternative evaluation of conceptual metaphor theory. *Discourse Processes, 48*, 563-574.

Meier, B. P., Hauser, D. J., Robinson, M. D., Friesen, C. K., & Schjeldahl, K. (2007). What's "up" with God? Vertical space as a representation of the divine. *Journal of Personality and Social Psychology, 93*(5), 699-710.

Meier, B. P., & Robinson, M. D. (2004). Why the sunny side is up: Associations between affect and vertical position. *Psychological Science, 15*(4), 243-247.

Meier, B. P., Schnall, S., Schwarz, N., & Bargh, J. A. (2012). Embodiment in social psychology. *Topics in Cognitive Science, 4,* 705-716.

Mesquita, B. Barrett, L. F., & Smith, E. R. (Eds.). (2010). *The mind in context*. New York: Guilford.

Mitchell, J. P., Nosek, B. A., & Banaji, M. R. (2003). Contextual variations in implicit evaluation. *Journal of Experimental Psychology: General, 132*(3), 455-469.

Molden, D. (2014). Understanding priming effects in social psychology: What is "social priming" and how does it occur? This volume.

Murphy, G. L. (1996). On metaphoric representation. *Cognition, 60,* 173-204.

Murphy, G. L. (2004). *The big book of concepts*. Cambridge, MA: MIT Press.Niedenthal, P. M. (2007). Embodying emotion. *Science, 316*(5827), 1002-1005.

Niedenthal, P. M., Barsalou, L., Winkielman, P., Krauth-Gruber, S., & Ric, F. (2005). Embodiment in attitudes, social perception, and emotion. *Personality and Social Psychology Review, 9,* 184-211.

Nosek, B. A., & Lakens, D. (2014). Registered reports: A method to increase the credibility of published results. *Social Psychology, 43,* 137-141.

Osgood, C. E., Suci, G. J., & Tannenbaum, P. H. (1957). *The measurement of meaning*. Urbana: University of Illinois Press.

Pashler, H., Coburn, N., & Harris, C. R. (2012). Priming of social distance? Failure to replicate effects on social and food judgments. *PLOS ONE, 7*(8), e42510.

Platt, J. R. (1964). Strong inference. *Science, 146*(3642), 347-353.

Pylyshyn, Z. W. (1984). *Computation and cognition*. Cambridge, MA: MIT Press.

Richards, I. A. (1936). *The philosophy of rhetoric*. Oxford, UK: Oxford University Press.

Rotteveel, M., & Phaf, R. H. (2004). Automatic affective evaluation does not automatically predispose for arm flexion and extension. *Emotion, 4*(2), 156-172.

Rozin, P., & Fallon, A. E. (1987). A perspective on disgust. *Psychological Review, 94,* 23-41. doi:10.1037/0033-295X.94.1.23

Salancik, G. R., & Pfeffer, J. (1978). A social information processing approach to job attitudes and task design. *Administrative Science Quarterly, 23,* 224-253.

Santiago, J., Ouellet, M., Román, A., & Valenzuela, J. (2012). Attentional factors in conceptual congruency. *Cognitive Science, 36*(6), 1051-1077.

Schneider, I. K., Rutjens, B., Jostmann, N. B., & Lakens, D. (2011). Weighty matters: Importance literally feels heavy. *Social Psychological and Personality Science, 2,* 474-478. doi:10.1177/1948550610397895

Schubert, L., Schubert, T. W., & Topolinski, S. (2013). The effect of spatial elevation on respect depends on merit and medium. *Social Psychology, 44,* 147-159. doi:10.1027/1864-9335/a000134

Schubert, T. W. (2005). Your highness: Vertical positions as perceptual symbols of power. *Journal of Personality and Social Psychology, 89*(1), 1-21.

Schubert, T. W., & Semin, G. R. (2009). Embodiment as a unifying perspective for psychology. *European Journal of Social Psychology, 39*(7), 1135-1141.

Schubert, T. W., Waldzus, S., & Seibt, B. (2011). More than a metaphor: How the understanding of power is grounded in experience. In T. W. Schubert & A. Maass (Eds.), *Spatial dimensions of social thought* (pp. 153-185). Berlin: Mouton de Gruyter.

Schwartz, G. E., Weinberger, D. A., & Singer, J. A. (1981). Cardiovascular differentiation of happiness, sadness, anger, and fear following imagery and exercise. *Psychosomatic Medicine, 43*(4), 343-364.

Schwarz, N. (2007). Attitude construction: Evaluation in context. *Social Cognition, 25,* 638-656.

Simonsohn, U., Nelson, L., & Simmons, J. (2013). P-curve: A key to the file drawer. *Journal of Experimental Psychology: General, 143*(2), 534-547.

Smith, E. R. (1984). Model of social inference processes. *Psychological Review, 91*(3), 392-413.

Smith, E. R., & Collins, E. C. (2010). Situated cognition. In B. Mesquita, L. F. Barrett, & E. R. Smith (Eds.), *The mind in context* (pp. 126-145). New York: Guilford.

Srull, T. K., & Wyer, R. S. (1979). The role of category accessibility in the interpretation of information about persons: Some determinants and implications. *Journal of Personality and Social Psychology, 37,* 1660-1672

Strack, F., Martin, L. L., & Stepper, S. (1988). Inhibiting and facilitating conditions of the human smile: A nonobtrusive test of the facial feedback hypothesis. *Journal of Personality and Social Psychology, 54*(5), 768-777.

Wilson, P. R. (1968). Perceptual distortion of height as a function of ascribed academic status. *Journal of Social Psychology, 74,* 97-102.

Whitney, W. D. (1875). *The life and growth of language: An outline of linguistic science.* New York: Appleton.

Wyer, R. S. (1974). *Cognitive organization and change: An information processing approach.* Potomac, MD: Erlbaum.

Wyer, R. S., & Srull, T. K. (1986). Human cognition in its social context. *Psychological Review, 93,* 322-359. doi:10.1037/0033-295X.93.3.322

Zhong, C. B., & Liljenquist, K. (2006). Washing away your sins: Threatened morality and physical cleansing. *Science, 313*(5792), 1451-1452.

Zwaan, R. A. (2009). Mental simulation in language comprehension and social cognition. *European Journal of Social Psychology, 39,* 1142-1150.

PRIMING FROM OTHERS' OBSERVED OR SIMULATED RESPONSES

Eliot R. Smith
Indiana University, Bloomington

Diane M. Mackie
University of California, Santa Barbara

>We discuss a novel form of priming that (a) involves the activation of embodied as well as mental representations in the perceiver and (b) is caused by the observation or simulation of the belief, attitude, emotion, or behavior of one or more other people. As in any form of priming, the representation, once activated, may have effects on the perceiver's own responses. We focus on effects of simulating another person's or group's responses, which give rise to a form of priming that can occur without observation of or communication from the other. Theoretical considerations predict that this type of priming will be moderated by self–other overlap between the perceiver and the other, and will have greater effects on implicit or time-pressured responses than on more explicit, deliberative responses. Laboratory findings offer preliminary evidence for this form of priming, and recent thinking in cultural psychology converges by proposing that an individual's judgments and behavior are often driven not by that individual's beliefs, attitudes, or values, but by those that are assumed to be held by many people in the culture. Several implications of this novel form of priming are discussed.

At its core, priming refers to the activation or increased accessibility of a representation within a perceiver, which then influences or becomes incorporated into the individual's later judgment, behavior, or other response. The activation can be caused by many different sources, from attending to a brief flash of a prime word or image on a screen, to answering a previous question on a survey. The activated representation can be of many different types, including goals, semantic knowledge, affective reactions, or behavioral plans. And the effects of the activated con-

---

Address correspondence to Eliot Smith, Department of Psychological and Brain Sciences, 1101 E. Tenth St., Bloomington, IN 47405; E-mail: esmith4@indiana.edu.

tent can be diverse, including assimilation, as when an affective response to an image spills over into pleasantness judgments regarding subsequently presented neutral stimuli (Payne, Cheng, Govorun, & Stewart, 2005), or contrast, as when exposure to an extreme exemplar moderates judgments on the same dimension about subsequently encountered exemplars (Herr, Sherman, & Fazio, 1983).

We wish to focus on two areas within this wide-ranging definition, areas that are relatively novel although they have been considered in scattered existing work. First, we consider situations where the source of the priming activation is a response of another individual or group, whether a belief or attitude, an emotion, or an overt behavior. Learning another's attitude may influence your subsequently reported attitude, or observing another's emotional expression may influence your own emotion. Observing behaviors that imply that others have a specific goal can cause you to adopt the same goal (Aarts, Gollwitzer, & Hassin, 2004). This can occur, of course, if you deliberately shape your own response accordingly, but also may occur because (like any activated representation) the other person's response can unintentionally influence your feelings, judgments, or behavior. Because another person's or group's response influences the individual's later response, this form of priming goes beyond a single individual.

Second, we expand consideration of the types of representations that can be activated beyond the traditional assumptions about mental representations (stereotypes, attitudes, goals, etc.) to include *embodied* representations as well. So observing someone else's emotional reaction may cause the perceiver to automatically imitate the facial expression and experience the same emotion (termed "emotion contagion," Hatfield, Cacioppo, & Rapson, 1994). Observing someone's behavior may cause the perceiver to mimic that behavior (Chartrand & van Baaren, 2009; Heyes, 2011). These effects involve the activation of embodied (not merely mental) representations of the other's response.

Because the form of priming on which we focus involves effects of others on the individual, one notable implication is that the relationship between the perceiver and the other(s) will have a powerful effect on the process. Responses of friends or fellow ingroup members—with whom the perceiver experiences self-other overlap (Aron, Aron, Tudor, & Nelson, 1991; Smith & Henry, 1996)—will have the largest effects. This is because self–other overlap involves a psychological merging of self and other, resulting in application of the self's attributes to the other and vice versa. High self–other overlap will therefore make it more difficult for perceivers to separate the other's response from their own. Evidence supports this assumption. For example, people mimic the emotions of ingroup members but not outgroup members (Weisbuch & Ambady, 2008), and imitate the behaviors of liked individuals, but not disliked individuals (Miles, Griffiths, Richardson, & Macrae, 2010).

PRIMING FROM ANOTHER'S UNOBSERVED BUT SIMULATED RESPONSES

Existing theory and research just described makes clear that another's responses (expressed beliefs or attitudes, or observed emotional or behavioral responses) can induce similar responses in the perceiver, in a form of priming. Our major goal in this chapter is to lay out a theoretical argument, and describe supporting evidence, that the same process can occur when another's response is not observed but merely *simulated*. As an example of the type of situation we will be considering, imagine someone who sees a hated politician making distasteful comments on a news show. If this perceiver knows that her father regularly watches this news show and admires this politician, she may mentally simulate his favorable reactions to the politician's comments. As with any instance of priming, that activated material (favorable evaluations) may influence the perceiver's own response, perhaps making it less unfavorable. Such an effect would represent a novel type of priming, and indeed social influence, that occurs without any direct observation of, or communication from, the other person.

Several points can be made using this example. First, in most demonstrations of attitudinal conformity, emotion contagion, or behavioral mimicry, the other person is physically salient (for example, the perceiver is in a conversation with the other or directly observes them). In this case, however, the perceiver's father is not physically present, but his response is simulated because she knows that he likes this politician. This observation raises important research questions regarding whose opinions people are likely to simulate. Second, it is of course possible for people to intentionally simulate relevant others' opinions—you might simulate your boss's reactions to the arguments you are incorporating in a presentation you will make, or your friend the camera buff's reactions to a new camera you are considering purchasing. But in the example, we intend to suggest that the simulation of another person's opinion is unintended. Third, as has been demonstrated in existing research on influence by others' directly observed responses (e.g., Weisbuch & Ambady, 2008), the relationship of the individual to the person whose reaction is simulated should be expected to determine the magnitude and perhaps even the direction of effects. In our example, despite the father's differing political views, we believe that self–other overlap with one's parent should create an assimilative influence of the parent's reaction. Evidence supporting this conjecture comes from a study by Jost, Ledgerwood, and Hardin (2008), whose participants were students who reported that their parents had opposite political views. The students were randomly assigned to think about a recent interaction with either their father or mother, and then complete a measure of their own political attitudes. The attitudes they endorsed were influenced by whichever parent they had thought about.

THEORETICAL CONSIDERATIONS

It is probably uncontroversial to argue that perceivers will generally form representations of the responses of others they encounter or observe. Knowing others' beliefs, attitudes, emotions, and behaviors facilitates interaction, cooperation, and adaptive action in general. Our novel claim is that perceivers will automatically simulate the probable responses of others even when they do not directly observe those responses. This can occur either when a person or group is salient in the environment, or when they are automatically called to mind (e.g., because they are associated with the particular topic of interest, or because they are interpersonally close, sharing high self–other overlap). Thus, in this first stage of the process we postulate, salience of another person or group leads to simulation of the other's relevant response.

In the second stage, the other's simulated response influences the perceiver's own response. The mechanism here is the same as in any priming paradigm (Loersch & Payne, 2011), in which previously activated material becomes incorporated into the perceiver's response, or (using different language) is misattributed as the perceiver's response. The effect may be to alter the content of the response, as in the Affect Misattribution Procedure (AMP) (Payne et al., 2005), where positive or negative responses to a prime influence the pleasantness rating given to a neutral target stimulus. Or it may be to alter the speed of a response, as in evaluative priming (Fazio & Olson, 2003) where responses are faster when the evaluation of the prime is similar to the evaluation of the target, compared to trials where they mismatch.

At this second stage, being influenced by the other's simulated response, self–other overlap exerts a moderating influence. Self–other overlap not only makes it more likely that a close other's response will be simulated, but also makes it more difficult to identify the other's response as separate from one's own, and thus more difficult to avoid being influenced by it. When influence is successfully avoided, it can only be through thoughtful, deliberative processing. As a consequence, we hypothesize that these effects will be observed more often on implicit or time-pressured responses than on thoughtful, explicit responses.

To summarize our model, we postulate two stages. First, people represent the relevant responses of salient individuals or groups, without any conscious intention. Our novel claim is that they may simulate a salient other's responses even when they do not directly observe them. Second, those responses are likely to influence the individual's own response, through the same processes that occur in any priming paradigm (Loersch & Payne, 2011). This will again happen more often when the perceiver and other have high self–other overlap, and more often for implicit or time-pressured responses. This is because both of these conditions make it more difficult for perceivers to effortfully separate the other's response from their own, avoiding influence.

PRELIMINARY EVIDENCE

Existing evidence shows that people automatically simulate another's perceptual viewpoint even when that other is merely a cartoon, symbolic representation of a person. Samson and colleagues (2010, experiment 3) had participants view scenes in which an image of an agent stood in the middle of a room, facing right or left (see Figure 1). On each trial, large dots appeared on the right and left walls of the room, so the agent could be inferred to see the dots in front of him/her but not behind. Participants viewed such a scene followed by a number, and pressed a yes or no key to indicate whether that was the total number of dots in the scene. Although the agent's perspective was irrelevant to the task, response time patterns showed that participants simulated the agent's viewpoint. For example, "no" responses to an incorrect number were slowed when the number matched what the agent could be inferred to see, such as "no" responses to the number 1 for the scene on the right.

This paradigm provides evidence for several aspects of the automaticity of the simulation of the other's viewpoint. The agent's inferred belief is not informationally useful; in fact, it is obviously limited and incorrect, detracting from

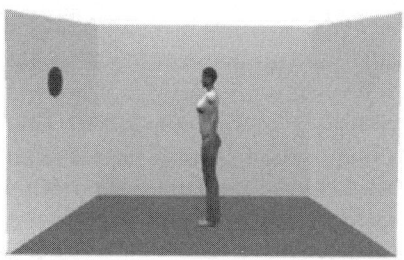 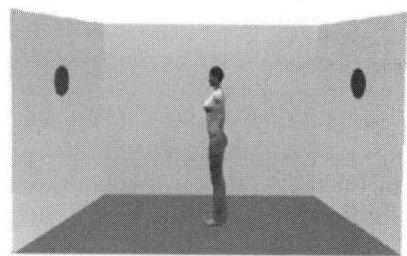

FIGURE 1. Example of stimulus displays from Samson, Apperly, Braithwaite, Andrews, & Bodley Scott (2010). Reprinted from Samson et al., "Seeing it their way: Evidence for rapid and involuntary computation of what other people see." *Journal of Experimental Psychology: Human Perception and Performance, 36,* 1255-1266, published in 2010 by the American Psychological Association. Reprinted with permission.

the perceiver's goal of answering quickly and correctly. In addition, because the agent is merely a cartoon, normative motives to conform (e.g., to strengthen social relationships) are also absent. Still, participants simulated the other's view even though doing so interfered with their explicit goals to respond quickly and accurately, supporting the unintended nature of the process. This evidence also suggests (although not conclusively) that the process is uncontrollable, because presumably participants would try to control a process that interferes with their task performance. Additional studies in related paradigms (e.g., Kovacs, Teglas, & Endress, 2010) support these conclusions, and show that children less than a year old also spontaneously simulate the perceptual viewpoint of a cartoon agent.

A recent study obtains a conceptually parallel finding in the area of impression formation, and shows that others' simulated responses can influence the content of a perceiver's response as well as just response times. Waggoner Denton (2012) recruited participants for a study of group–person perception. Seated in separate cubicles, participants in each experimental session first performed a group cohesion-building task. Then in the main person perception task, they all first received initial positive or negative behavioral information about a target. They rated their initial impressions of the target and saw what they thought were the other participants' ratings (actually constructed by the researchers). They then received further information about the target, which was either consistent or inconsistent in valence with the initial information. The crucial manipulation was that participants believed either that they alone saw this additional information or that all participants in the session saw it. They then recorded their final impressions and rated their confidence.

Our model predicts that when perceivers believe others are also seeing the later information, they will simulate the others' responses to it, which will then spill over and influence their own final ratings (amplifying the impact of the later information). When perceivers believe that others do not receive the later information, the simulation will of course not occur. Results were consistent with these predictions. Final liking ratings were influenced in the obvious way by the valence of the later information, but more strongly for participants who believed that all saw that information (compared to those who believed that only they saw it; interaction $F(1, 175) = 59.79, p < .001$). Similarly, judgmental confidence was increased, not surprisingly, when the later information was consistent with the initial information. This effect was also stronger when the later information was believed to have been seen by all (interaction $F(1, 175) = 17.49, p < .001$).

Thus, existing evidence from several laboratory paradigms supports the idea that people automatically simulate and are influenced by the unobserved responses of others. Additional, converging support comes from a very different area, cultural psychology. Research in this area usually compares samples drawn from different cultural contexts and typically has a substantive focus on values such as individualism/collectivism. However, a strikingly similar set of ideas has recently emerged in this literature: The effects of culture on an individual's emotions, judgments, or behavior may be mediated not by the individual's own internalization of cultural values, but by the individual's perceptions of the values that are endorsed by other members of the culture.

One type of evidence on this point comes from work by Shteynberg, Gelfand, & Kim (2009), who measured both personal endorsement of collectivist values (with items like "I will sacrifice for the benefit of the group") and perceptions of the values endorsed by most members of the culture ("Most Americans will sacrifice..."). In both American and Korean samples, perceptions of others' values but not personal endorsement of those values influenced judgments related to harm and blame. Zou and colleagues (2009) used similar methods and obtained parallel results. Using a different methodological approach, Becker and colleagues (2012) obtained samples from many different cultural contexts and applied a multilevel analysis that allowed estimation of separate effects of each *individual's* level of individualism/collectivism and of the *mean* levels within each sample—in other words, the consensual level of individualism/collectivism within each cultural context. The researchers found strong effects of the cultural consensus, but generally trivial individual-level effects. They conclude, "The differences we found ... cannot be attributed to individuals' internalization of cultural beliefs and values—instead, they appeared to be effects of living in a particular cultural context where certain things are believed and valued" (p. 850).

Many recent articles in cultural psychology contain explicit statements of the view that effects of others' beliefs, attitudes, or values often outweigh the individual's own. Shteynberg and colleagues (2009, p. 48) state that, "[T]o thrive in a social environment, people must not only be keenly aware of the thoughts and intentions of others in that social environment but also allow such social cognitions a unique status in their behavioral decisions." Zou and colleagues (2009, p. 580) similarly observe, "As we strive to see the world 'through the eyes of others' to be 'objective' and reach epistemically sound judgments, we think and act on ideas perceived to be consensual with little reservation." Chiu and colleagues (2010, pp. 482-483) review work in this area and conclude that, "[R]ather than acting on their personal beliefs and values, people sometimes act on the beliefs and values they perceive to be widespread in their culture. That is, what individuals see inside themselves (internalized cultural beliefs and values) does not always channel psychological processes; what the individuals see when looking outward at their social environments can also direct behaviors." Evidence obtained by these and other researchers in cultural psychology therefore supports the idea that people are often strongly influenced by the simulated views of ingroup others—in this case, by their assumptions about the values held by other members of their culture—even more than by their own personally endorsed values.

SIMILARITIES AND DIFFERENCES FROM OTHER FORMS OF PRIMING

Our conception shares with all mainstream models of priming the assumption that a priming event (in this case, observing or simulating another's response) activates representations that then influence the perceiver's later responses (e.g., Loersch & Payne, 2011). However, there are also some meaningful differences in our thinking.

Most standard models of priming have assumed that the representations that are activated by a prime (influencing later judgments or behavior) are mental representations. One difference from most classic models is that we believe that embodied as well as mental representational systems may be involved in priming. Much evidence shows that when we perceive others' emotions and behaviors, we represent them not only mentally but by using our own bodies. Findings of automatic mimicry of others' emotional expressions (Niedenthal, 2007) or behaviors (Heyes, 2011) support this idea. The latter has often been studied in tightly controlled paradigms. For example, participants are instructed to close or open their hands cued by a visual signal, while observing a video of a hand making a task-irrelevant opening or closing movement. Responses are facilitated or inhibited by the observed hand movement. Notably, this effect is enhanced by priming participants with prosocial words such as *friend* or *cooperate*, and reduced by priming antisocial words such as *selfish* (Leighton et al., 2010). And the effect is reduced when participants see the identical video of movements by a gloved hand described as the movements of a wooden hand, compared to when it is believed to be a human hand (Liepelt & Brass, 2010). These findings show that even low-level imitation effects depend on one's orientation toward the other, such as ingroup membership and the resulting self–other overlap. To explain behavioral imitation, some have postulated mirror neuron systems, which are supposed to display similar activations when one perceives another's action and when one performs the action (Gallese, Keysers, & Rizzolatti, 2004; Brass, Ruby, & Spengler, 2009). This specific proposal is somewhat controversial, but our theoretical ideas do not depend on any specific proposed neural mechanism.

Another important difference is that the relational aspect of priming in our model brings in a new set of moderators of priming effects. We have emphasized the role of self–other overlap, with the responses of close or ingroup others having more influence compared to distant others (e.g., Weisbuch & Ambady, 2008). But other variables may shape perceived closeness or similarity to others, also moderating priming effects. For example, the perceiver's power relative to the other will be relevant. High power makes people see others as more socially distant (Magee & Smith, 2011). As a consequence, it should be easier for high- than for low-power people to distinguish themselves from others, leading to less susceptibility to influence by others' simulated responses among those with high power. Even a momentary or trivial experience of similarity or interpersonal connection with another person may create self–other overlap and enable these effects. Something as simple as learning that one shares a birthday with another individual has been shown to cause the individual to take on the other's attitudes (Cheung, Noel, & Hardin, 2011). Or a brief experience of being mimicked by another can cause people to share the other's emotions (Stel & Vonk, 2010).

DISCUSSION AND IMPLICATIONS

In this paper, we have outlined a novel type of priming, driven by the simulation of others' responses, that can occur without communicating with or observing the other. We outlined theoretical hypotheses about the conditions under which this process would occur, and gave an overview of some preliminary evidence supporting it. Nevertheless, many important research questions remain open.

One intriguing possibility is that we may simulate not only others' overt responses such as beliefs or behaviors, but also their metacognitive experiences such as feelings of fluency. In fact, fluency-based processes may contribute to the unintended influence of others' responses on the perceiver's own, because after perceiving or simulating another's specific response, such as an attitude or behavior, generating a similar response oneself is likely to be more fluent. As we know, that feeling of fluency then may be misattributed, taken as evidence for the validity of the information or its appropriateness as a personal response (Reber & Schwarz, 1999).

Recent work supports the plausibility of this hypothesized process by demonstrating the opposite direction of misattribution (misattribution to an observed other of fluency that is actually based on one's own responses). In this study (Tipper & Bach, 2008), participants saw photos of two different individuals performing activities, and pressed a left or right key to indicate which person appeared in each photo. The photos were presented on the left or right side of the screen. In a condition where the photos were presented on the same side as the required response, spatial response compatibility made the key-press responses more fluent. And in that condition, the pictured individuals were rated as more competent in the activities they were performing: For example, a person shown performing athletic activities was rated as more athletic. This presumably occurred because the fluency of the participant's response was misattributed so the stimulus person's behavior seemed more fluent. The authors suggest that we represent both our own and others' actions, including not only specific motor acts but also higher-order appraisals (such as the experience of fluency). This idea supports our proposal that fluency due to having simulated another person's judgment or behavior may cause us to experience fluency when we consider making the same response ourselves, leading to a "feeling" that it is correct and appropriate.

The process outlined in this paper may have a range of potential effects. For example, suppose a White person who has a Latino friend encounters another White making anti-Latino comments in a social setting. Might this individual simulate his or her friend's potential reactions to the comments? Simulation of the friend's anger could make the individual feel angry, potentially motivating confrontation of the prejudiced individual. This would be a novel mechanism that differs from prior conceptualizations such as activating a nonprejudiced or egalitarian identity.

Another interesting possibility regards potential effects on the self-concept. Suppose an individual engages in several performances that reveal aspects of his or her ability (athletic competitions, academic tests, etc.). Knowing that a friend or ingroup will learn the results of a specific performance may lead to simulation of the other's view of the self—potentially increasing the impact of that particular performance on the self-concept (compared to an otherwise equivalent performance that is not witnessed by the other). There is a finding in the literature somewhat like this example. Kelly and Rodriguez (2006) asked participants to present themselves as introverted and extraverted (respectively) in two videotaped segments they believed would be viewed by others. They were then told that only one of the tapes was necessary, and they watched the other tape being erased. If the introversion tape was erased so that the participant believed only the extroversion tape would be seen by others, the participant subsequently displayed more extroverted behavior, compared to those whose extroversion tape was erased. Thus, when others are anticipated to view subsets of one's behavior, simulation of their beliefs about the self can alter self-perceptions and even overt behavior.

It is also worth speculating about the potential role of the process described in this paper in contributing to the power of stereotypes and prejudice, and the difficulty of changing them, which has been a major theme in social psychology over the past few decades. Theorists have advanced several plausible reasons for their power. It has been argued that we rely on stereotypes because they constitute easily applied general knowledge (compared to a more specific and detailed body of individuating information), and that we are "cognitive misers" who prefer such easily applicable information. It is also postulated that stereotypes and prejudice are learned early in life and therefore take precedence over beliefs or attitudes that are learned later (Wilson, Lindsey, & Schooler, 2000). The analysis advanced here foregrounds a very different type of reason: Stereotypes and prejudice are widely shared in society. It is even likely that the perceived sharedness of stereotypes and prejudiced views is greater than their actual sharedness—and as Zou and colleagues (2009) have argued, perceptions of cultural consensus are often biased in the direction of perceiving others to hold more traditional, conservative views than they actually do. In short, the tendency to draw on what one perceives as consensual views may contribute to the perpetuation of stereotyped beliefs and prejudiced attitudes. This idea is related to the claim (e.g., Fazio & Olson, 2003) that some implicit measures such as the IAT are sensitive to cultural learning rather than to individual attitudes. However, we strongly disagree with any implication that as a result, such implicit measures have little predictive power over the individual's judgments and behavior. As we have argued throughout, other people's perceived attitudes have pervasive, though unintended effects on our own responses (e.g, Chiu et al., 2010).

We conclude with a brief consideration of the functionality of priming. Barsalou, Breazeal, & Smith (2007) argue that priming is fundamentally for anticipation (allowing the organism to prepare for what is likely to come next). So if the word "doctor" is encountered in text, the representation of the word "nurse" becomes more active, enabling the reader to recognize that word more quickly should it appear (as is statistically likely). We agree that anticipation is one function of priming, but find this perspective overly individualistic. Another function of priming—the type of priming from others' responses we describe here—is social coordination, enabling convergence of beliefs, attitudes, emotions, and behavior within a dyadic relationship or ingroup. Others have also argued that behavior priming often serves as preparation for adaptive interpersonal behavior (e.g., Cesario, Plaks, & Higgins, 2006). This type of social coordination may well contribute to the convergence of emotions within an ingroup, a topic to which we have devoted much study (Mackie, Smith, & Ray, 2008).

Social coordination in turn is a major part of the answer to a question that some may have about our theory: Is acting on others' beliefs, emotions, or behaviors adaptive? Should people not act on their own personal beliefs, emotional appraisals, and action plans, rather than those of other people? Chiu and colleagues (2010), working in the cultural psychology tradition described earlier, offer three reasons why influence by others' thoughts, emotions, and behavior is indeed generally adaptive. One is the point just noted, that adopting the same beliefs, emotions, and behaviors as ingroup others eases coordination and interaction. A second reason is that opinions or behaviors favored by many ingroup others are likely to be correct, valid, and useful—because they have been tested by many people, not just you. Third, shared beliefs, attitudes, and so forth promote the communicability of information. People prefer to and find it easier to communicate information that is shared rather than unique or idiosyncratic (Kashima, 2000), a process that also helps maintain and reinforce cultural norms (Fast, Heath, & Wu, 2009).

By advancing these theoretical ideas, we hope to promote convergence among detailed laboratory studies of the underlying mechanisms of priming, work on embodied representations and their effects such as automatic imitation (Heyes, 2011), and even work in cultural psychology stressing the powerful effects of others' perceived attitudes and values (Chiu et al., 2010). Conceptualizing all these phenomena under the umbrella of a novel form of priming from others' responses should allow productive interchanges among researchers and open new and exciting research questions.

REFERENCES

Aarts, H., Gollwitzer, P. M., & Hassin, R. R. (2004). Goal contagion: Perceiving is for pursuing. *Journal of Personality and Social Psychology*, 87(1), 23-37. doi:10.1037/0022-3514.87.1.23

Aron, A., Aron, E. N., Tudor, M., & Nelson, G. (1991). Close relationships as including other in the self. *Journal of Personality and Social Psychology*, 60, 241-253.

Barsalou, L. W., Breazeal, C., & Smith, L. B. (2007). Cognition as coordinated non-cognition. *Cognitive Processing*, 8(2), 79-91. doi:10.1007/s10339-007-0163-1

Becker, M., Vignoles, V. L., Owe, E., Brown, R., Smith, P. B., Easterbrook, M., et al. (2012). Culture and the distinctiveness motive: Constructing identity in individualistic and collectivistic contexts. *Journal of Personality and Social Psychology*, 102(4), 833-855. doi:10.1037/a0026853

Brass, M., Ruby, P., & Spengler, S. (2009). Inhibition of imitative behaviour and social cognition. *Philosophical Transactions of the Royal Society B: Biological Sciences*, 364(1528), 2359-2367. doi:10.1098/rstb.2009.0066

Cesario, J., Plaks, J. E., & Higgins, E. T. (2006). Automatic social behavior as motivated preparation to interact. *Journal of Personality and Social Psychology*, 90(6), 893-910. doi:10.1037/0022-3514.90.6.893

Chartrand, T. L., & Van Baaren, R. B. (2009). Human mimicry. *Advances in Experimental Social Psychology*, 41, 219-274. doi:10.1016/S0065-2601(08)00405-X

Cheung, R. M., Noel, S., & Hardin, C. D. (2011). Adopting the system-justifying attitudes of others: Effects of trivial interpersonal connections in the context of social inclusion and exclusion. *Social Cognition*, 29(3), 1-15.

Chiu, C., Gelfand, M. J., Yamagishi, T., Shteynberg, G., & Wan, C. (2010). Intersubjective culture: The role of intersubjective perceptions in cross-cultural research. *Perspectives on Psychological Science, 5*(4), 482-493. doi:10.1177/1745691610375562

Fast, N. J., Heath, C., & Wu, G. (2009). Common ground and cultural prominence: How conversation reinforces culture. *Psychological Science, 20*(7), 904-911.

Fazio, R. H., & Olson, M. A. (2003). Implicit measures in social cognition research: Their meaning and use. *Annual Review of Psychology, 54*(1), 297-327. doi:10.1146/psych.2003.54.issue-1

Gallese, V., Keysers, C., & Rizzolatti, G. (2004). A unifying view of the basis of social cognition. *Trends in Cognitive Sciences, 8*(9), 396-403.

Hatfield, J. T., Cacioppo, J. C., & Rapson, R. L. (1994). *Emotional contagion.* Cambridge, England: Cambridge University Press.

Herr, P. M., Sherman, S. J., & Fazio, R. H. (1983). On the consequences of priming: Assimilation and contrast effects. *Journal of Experimental Social Psychology, 19,* 323-340.

Heyes, C. (2011). Automatic imitation. *Psychological Bulletin, 137*(3), 463-483. doi:10.1037/a0022288

Jost, J. T., Ledgerwood, A., & Hardin, C. D. (2008). Shared reality, system justification, and the relational basis of ideological beliefs. *Social and Personality Psychology Compass, 2,* 171-186.

Kashima, Y. (2000). Maintaining cultural stereotypes in the serial reproduction of narratives. *Personality and Social Psychology Bulletin, 26*(5), 594-604. doi:10.1177/0146167200267007

Kelly, A. E., & Rodriguez, R. R. (2006). Publicly committing oneself to an identity. *Basic and Applied Social Psychology, 28,* 185-191.

Kovacs, A. M., Teglas, E., & Endress, A. D. (2010). The social sense: Susceptibility to others' beliefs in human infants and adults. *Science, 330*(6012), 1830-1834. doi:10.1126/science.1190792

Leighton, J., Bird, G., Orsini, C., & Heyes, C. (2010). Social attitudes modulate automatic imitation. *Journal of Experimental Social Psychology, 46*(6), 905-910. doi:10.1016/j.jesp.2010.07.001

Liepelt, R., & Brass, M. (2010). Top-down modulation of motor priming by belief about animacy. *Experimental Psychology, 57,* 221-227. doi: 10.1027/1618-3169/a000028

Loersch, C., & Payne, B. K. (2011). The situated inference model: An integrative account of the effects of primes on perception, behavior, and motivation. *Perspectives on Psychological Science, 6*(3), 234-252. doi:10.1177/1745691611406921

Mackie, D. M., Smith, E., & Ray, D. G. (2008). Intergroup emotions and intergroup relations. *Social and Personality Psychology Compass, 2*(5), 1866-1880. doi:10.1111/j.1751-9004.2008.00130.x

Magee, J. C., & Smith, P. K. (2011). Social distance theory of power. Unpublished.

Miles, L. K., Griffiths, J. L., Richardson, M. J., & Macrae, C. N. (2010). Too late to coordinate: Contextual influences on behavioral synchrony. *European Journal of Social Psychology, 40,* 52-60. doi:10.1002/ejsp.721

Niedenthal, P. M. (2007). Embodying emotion. *Science, 316,* 1002-1005. doi:10.1126/science.1136930

Payne, B. K., Cheng, C. M., Govorun, O., & Stewart, B. D. (2005). An inkblot for attitudes: Affect misattribution as implicit measurement. *Journal of Personality and Social Psychology, 89*(3), 277-293. doi:10.1037/0022-3514.89.3.277

Reber, R. L., & Schwarz, N. (1999). Effects of perceptual fluency on judgments of truth. *Consciousness and Cognition, 8,* 338-342.

Samson, D., Apperly, I. A., Braithwaite, J. J., Andrews, B. J., & Bodley Scott, S. E. (2010). Seeing it their way: Evidence for rapid and involuntary computation of what other people see. *Journal of Experimental Psychology: Human Perception and Performance, 36*(5), 1255-1266. doi:10.1037/a0018729

Shteynberg, G., Gelfand, M. J., & Kim, K. (2009). Peering into the "magnum mysterium" of culture: The explanatory power of descriptive norms. *Journal of Cross-Cultural Psychology, 40,* 46-69.

Smith, E., & Henry, S. (1996). An in-group becomes part of the self: Response time evidence. *Personality and Social Psychology Bulletin, 22*(6), 635-642. doi:10.1177/0146167296226008

Stel, M., & Vonk, R. (2010). Mimicry in social interaction: Benefits for mimickers, mimickees, and their interaction. *Bri-*

tish *Journal of Psychology, 101*(2), 311-323. doi:10.1348/000712609X465424

Tipper, S., & Bach, P. (2008). Your own actions influence how you perceive other people: A misattribution of action appraisals. *Journal of Experimental Social Psychology, 44*(4), 1082-1090. doi:10.1016/j.jesp.2007.11.005

Waggoner Denton, A. (2012). *Impression formation in a social network context.* Unpublished doctoral dissertation, Indiana University.

Weisbuch, M., & Ambady, N. (2008). Affective divergence: Automatic responses to others' emotions depend on group membership. *Journal of Personality and Social Psychology, 95*(5), 1063-1079. doi:10.1037/a0011993

Wilson, T. D., Lindsey, S., & Schooler, T. Y. (2000). A model of dual attitudes. *Psychological Review, 107*(1), 101-126. doi:10.1037//0033-295X.107.1.101

Zou, X., Tam, K., Morris, M. W., Lee, S., Lau, I. Y. M., & Chiu, C. (2009). Culture as common sense: Perceived consensus versus personal beliefs as mechanisms of cultural influence. *Journal of Personality and Social Psychology, 97*(4), 579-597.

FROM THE PAST OF SOCIAL PRIMING TO ITS FUTURE

EVALUATING BEHAVIOR PRIMING RESEARCH: THREE OBSERVATIONS AND A RECOMMENDATION

Ap Dijksterhuis, Ad van Knippenberg, and Rob W. Holland
Radboud University Nijmegen

We discuss three observations about the state of the field of behavior priming. The first is that there are many more empirical demonstrations of behavior priming than may be apparant at first sight. The second is that some people doubt the validity of behavior priming effects because they are "counterintuitive," and we argue that this reasoning is subjective, often circular, and sometimes based on an underappreciation of relevant theories. The third is that we concede that—just as in many other areas—publication bias and the use of researchers' degrees of freedom have presumably led to a somewhat distorted literature because they caused what we call "information leakage." Because of some of the habits in response to publication bias, our field knows much less about moderators and boundary conditions than we could have known. We conclude that although replication efforts can be very useful, the only true solution to further improve our field is to stop practices, such as the liberal use of researchers' degrees of freedom, that scientists have adopted in response to the pressure to publish only statistically significant results.

Recently, one of the authors of this paper watched a documentary on Eddy Merckx, widely regarded as the most successful professional cyclist ever. Merckx won more than 500 races in his career, an astounding number. His nickname was "the cannibal," as Merckx wanted to win every single race he participated in, ranging from the Tour de France to the most insignificant local race (which is quite unusual, as most great riders are known to "delegate" the unimportant races to their lieutenants). The next morning, the author cycled to work—which he does every day—and he suddenly realized that he was cycling extremely fast. He fanatically overtook other cyclists, as he was indeed racing. He then remembered that he had glanced at the Merckx DVD that was still lying around while he was having breakfast.

This is priming at work. A concept—such as a stereotype, or trait, or state, or person—is activated, and it affects, generally without the actor being aware of it,

---

Address correspondence to Ap Dijksterhuis, Department of Social Psychology, Behavioural Science Institute, Radboud University Nijmegen, Montessorilaan 3, P.O. Box 9104, 6500 HE, Nijmegen, the Netherlands. E-mail: a.dijksterhuis@psych.ru.nl.

overt behavior. In the example above, the concept of speed, or of speedy cycling, is activated, and one indeed starts to cycle much faster. The effects of priming on behavior have been studied widely and quite happily for many years (e.g., Bargh, Chen & Burrows, 1996; Dijksterhuis & van Knippenberg, 1998; Loersch & Payne, 2011), but in the past year, the research area of social priming had to endure more than its fair share of criticism and skepticism.

We do not want to try to precisely characterize the causes of the headwind the field of social priming is facing. The fraud (Stapel) and presumed fraud (Smeesters) of two researchers we thought had contributed (a little) to priming research, a few well-publicized non-replications of key findings (Doyen, Klein, Pichon, & Cleeremans, 2012; Shanks et al., 2013), and a famous letter may all have landed on the fertile soil of colleagues who were already quite skeptical about priming research, but there is no point in speculating about the past and in generalizing across many different people's views. Rather, we acknowledge that the area is under siege, and we would like to articulate our personal view on what exactly we think the problems are. At least as important, we would also like to discuss issues we know some regard as problems that we think should not be seen as such.

In the remainder of this paper, we want to convey three messages before we end with conclusions and a recommendation. However, before we move on, it should be noted that the current paper is about behavior priming, an area we see as part of the broader area of social priming that most people now see as encompassing effects of priming on other dependent variables, such as impressions or choices.

The first message is that there are many more empirical demonstrations of behavior priming than most researchers think. This pertains not only to skeptics; people who study behavior priming themselves sometimes seem to underestimate the sheer number of relevant studies reporting behavior priming results. The second is that although we deem it understandable that some colleagues doubt the validity of behavior priming effects because the effects are seen as "counterintuitive," this reasoning is subjective and often circular. Moreover, it may be based on an underappreciation of relevant theories. The third is that we argue that—and this we see as the only "real" problem—publication bias and the use of researchers' degrees of freedom have led to a somewhat distorted literature because they caused what we call "information leakage." The effects of behavior priming are more fragile than a naive observer may conclude on the basis of the current evidence, and there simply are many more moderators and boundary conditions than the ones that have been documented properly. We conclude that although replication efforts can be very useful, the only true solution is for researchers to stop (ab)using researchers' degrees of freedom (which from now on we will call p-hacking; Simmons, Nelson, & Simonsohn, 2011) and for scientists in general, but especially journals, to stop practices that encourage publication bias.

A LARGE AMOUNT OF EVIDENCE

In their original behavior priming paper, Bargh, Chen, and Burrows (1996) showed behavior priming effects in two broad domains. The most famous experiment (or actually experiments, as the authors showed the initial effect again in an immediate replication) showed an effect of priming on motor behavior: Participants primed with the elderly walked more slowly down the hallway than control participants.

In two other experiments, Bargh, Chen, and Burrows demonstrated that primes could also affect social behavior. Priming participants with rudeness or politeness affected the time it took participants to interrupt a conversation between the experimenter and a confederate, and priming participants with African Americans increased their aggression after an annoying request by the experimenter.

A little later, Dijksterhuis and van Knippenberg (1998) published the first conceptual replication in the domain of intellectual performance. They showed that participants primed with professors performed better on a general knowledge test than control participants, whereas participants primed with hooligans performed worse. In the following years, effects in all three domains—motor, social, and intellectual—were conceptually replicated in independent labs. For instance, Kawakami, Young, and Dovidio (2002) demonstrated that priming people with the elderly led to slower reaction times. Macrae and Johnston (1998) found that priming helpfulness led people to help a confederate pick up pens she had "accidently" dropped. Finally, Wheeler, Jarvis, and Petty (2001) primed people with African Americans and showed a deterioration in their performance on a math test, while Shih and colleagues (Shih, Ambady, Richeson, Fujita & Gray, 2002) improved people's performance on a math test by priming them with Asian Americans.

In turn, all these replications have been replicated, and especially the work on priming social behavior expanded rapidly. Priming African Americans has been shown to decrease cooperation among highly prejudiced individuals (Brown, Croizet, Bohner, Fournet & Payne, 2003), priming loyalty affects people's choices in a minimal group paradigm (Hertel & Kerr, 2003), and priming cooperation and competition led to corresponding behavior in a Prisoners' Dilemma game (Kay & Ross, 2003). Priming conformity (as opposed to non-conformity) made participants agree more with a confederate, and participants primed with a punk (!) conformed less in a classic Asch paradigm than participants primed with an accountant (Pendry & Carrick, 2001).

In recent years, behavior priming has also become part of the toolkit of researchers in various related research domains. Justice researchers have primed people with concepts such as justice and morality (e.g., Callan, Kay, Olson, Brar & Whitefield, 2010), researchers on terror management theory primed participants with thoughts of death (see Vail et al., 2012, for a recent review), colleagues interested in religion primed people with God (e.g., Gervais & Norenzayan, 2012), psychologists interested in group behavior primed identity (e.g., Levine, Cassidy, & Jentzsch, 2010), and literally dozens of papers have reported effects of priming people with power (e.g., Galinsky, Gruenfeld, & Magee, 2003; Smith & Trope, 2006; Yap, Mason, & Ames, 2012). Many people may not classify this research as examples of behavior priming, but in our view they are. And importantly, they show that behavior priming is not just an interesting research area in its own right, but that it is also a useful methodology—sometimes the dominant methodology—in other areas.

Finally, the techniques developed by behavior priming researchers have been used in various applied domains or settings. Branaghan and Gray (2010) showed that people who were primed with the elderly drove more slowly in a driving simulator, and Latham and colleagues published a wealth of research on how priming can change the behavior of employees in call centers (e.g., Latham & Piccolo, 2012; Shantz & Latham, 2011). Perhaps needless to say, we do not have the space to refer to every single relevant article, but the total number of empirical papers demonstrating behavior priming effects must be in the hundreds right now (in a review written in 2005, we counted around 80; see Dijksterhuis, Chartrand, & Aarts, 2007).

In our view, it is essential to appreciate the sheer amount of evidence, because not doing so may lead to inappropriate conclusions. Shanks and colleagues (2013) aimed to replicate the Dijksterhuis and van Knippenberg (1998) experiments in which participants were primed with professors or soccer hooligans, and they did not find the primes to have changed intellectual performance. These results are highly interesting for various reasons—hopefully they will point us toward a moderator—but not because we should now believe that priming intelligence does not affect intellectual performance after all. We should not, in other words, believe that the initial findings were false positives. This is simply extremely unlikely. The effect of intelligence- or stupidity-related primes on intellectual performance have been obtained in many different published experiments (Bry, Follenfant, & Meyer, 2008; Dijksterhuis, Spears et al., 1998; Dijksterhuis & van Knippenberg, 1998; Dijksterhuis & van Knippenberg, 2000; Galinsky, Wang, & Ku, 2008; Haddock, Macrae, & Fleck, 2002; Hansen & Wänke, 2009; LeBoeuf & Estes, 2004; Lowery, Eisenberger, Hardin, & Sinclair, 2007; Nussinson, Seibt, Häfner, & Strack, 2010; Schubert & Häfner, 2003, Webb, Sheeran, Gollwitzer & Trötschel, 2012). Two more working papers reached us recently (Chen & Latham, 2013; Stel, Zeelenberg, van Dijk, & Kutsal, 2012), adding up to a total number of 28 experiments in 13 different labs in 8 different countries. These experiments are not all exact replications of the original paper (though many of them are close), but they all showed, in one way or another, that priming people with concepts related to intelligence (often the stereotype of professors) or stupidity changes people's intellectual performance.

On top of the sheer number of replications, throughout the years we also gained an improved understanding of the underlying mechanism. For instance, Hansen and Wänke (2009) showed that self-efficacy mediates the effects, whereas Galinsky and colleagues (2008) showed that self-perceived intelligence mediates the effects. Recently, the first paper on neural correlates was published demonstrating increased (after an intelligent prime) or decreased (after a stupid prime) activity in the anterior cingulate cortex (Bengtsson, Dolan, & Passingham, 2011).

Now, not all these individual experiments or sets of experiments are perfect, but the conclusion that there is insufficient evidence that primes can affect intellectual performance is clearly unwarranted. And if one really wants to draw this conclusion, one would do well to realize that if we all decide to only teach our students findings that have been conceptually replicated in more than 12 different labs, our academic year would end around late October rather than in June.

ARE BEHAVIOR PRIMING FINDINGS COUNTERINTUITIVE?

An often-heard complaint about behavior priming (and automaticity research in general) is that the effects are counterintuitive. Although we concede that intuition is a wonderful psychological tool and, indeed, that many important scientific discoveries started with someone having a profound intuition, it can also be counterproductive. While intuition can help us to raise hypotheses, giving it a major role in assessing the evidence for a hypothesis can lead us astray, especially when it is used to judge a large set of homogeneous phenomena rather than a single finding. In science, intuition often reflects long-standing beliefs concerning the order of things. The history of science is replete with examples of new insights (e.g., Galileo, Darwin) having a hard time overcoming resistance from orthodoxy. Intuition is not a good substitute for hard empirical facts.[1]

Not trusting an effect because it is counterintuitive is often essentially a form of circular reasoning. Research on issues such as free will, unconscious processes, and automaticity is sometimes, unavoidably so it seems, ideological. Some researchers are skeptical about the sophistication of the operations people can do without conscious guidance, and hence, they think priming effects on intelligence or cooperation are counterintuitive. Of course, the prononents of behavior priming research run similar risks. For the authors of this paper, the idea that one needs consciousness for each and every higher order cognitive process is counterintuitive, and indeed, they would probably be quite critical of a paper reporting empirical findings suggesting that consciousness always mediates such higher cognitive processes.

Using intuition as a tool to assess the validity of research findings may be an even greater problem in psychology than in the natural sciences. Intuition in the domain of psychological processes is most likely fueled by the scientists' own subjective experiences concerning the causes of their behavior. As many behaviors are subjectively experienced as consciously caused (Wegner, 2002), the "intuition argument" should be used only with utmost restraint or, better yet, not at all. Intuition is for coming up with hypotheses, not for testing them.

That being said, we would like to argue that behavior priming effects should not be all that counterintuitive in the first place. The findings on automaticity that have become an essential part of the theories of social psychologists are in line with a burgeoning neurocognitive literature on the relation between higher cognition, attention, and consciousness. When a mental representation—say that of an elderly person—is activated, the default consequence is that it affects downstream behavior. This general notion is consistent with several broad theoretical approaches, such as embodied cognition (e.g., Barsalou, 1999) and perception-action and common coding theories (Prinz, 1997). The idea that people first need some kind of express conscious fiat can perhaps not be ruled out, but there is no neurocognitive theory we know of that claims such a conscious intervention is necessary. Instead, an influential perspective that started to emerge ten years ago was that the amount of attention—that is, the amount of effort we pay to process a stimulus—is crucial for almost all behavior and, importantly, that attention and consciousness are theoretically best seen as orthogonal (Dehaene, Changeux, Naccache, Sackur, & Sergent, 2006; Dijksterhuis & Aarts, 2010; Koch & Tsuchiya, 2007; Lamme, 2003).

Recently, various papers have been published arguing that attention and consciousness are indeed dissociable (Berridge, 2011; Van Gaal, Lamme, Fahrenfort, & Ridderinkhof, 2011). Such claims are not without controversy, but there seems to be wide agreement among the researchers in this area that we routinely attend to stimuli (that then affect our actions) without becoming consciously aware of them (Naccache, Blandin, & Dehaene, 2002; Tsuchiya, Block, & Koch, 2012). Such attended-to-but-unconscious effects are not restricted to low-level cognition. For instance, reward processing (Pessiglione et al., 2007) and inhibitory control processes (Van Gaal et al., 2008) can be initiated unconsciously. In fact, the question

---

1. One of the authors recently came across an extreme example. He likes to travel in less developed countries, and recently found himself in Papua. During an evening conversation with a village chief and some of his men, it dawned on him that people who rely on intuition rather than on scientific fact (in this case because they did not have access to the latter) still firmly believe that the earth is flat.

whether consciousness without attention is possible elicits a lively discussion in this area. The converse, that is, the fact that attention without consciousness is possible, is seen as a given. We believe this is essential for someone who wants to understand behavior priming research.

A second reason for why some may see behavior priming as counterintuitive is that the effects are, presumably, not embedded in (social) psychological theory. Notwithstanding the fact that theorizing is obviously an ongoing process, this is simply not true. The area of behavior priming is already in its third stage of theorizing and went from initial, rather straightforward mechanistic explanations (Bargh et al., 1996; Dijksterhuis & Bargh, 2001), via more active, self-related and motivational theories (Cesario, Higgins, & Plaks, 2006; Wheeler & Petty, 2001), to recently published models (Klatzky & Creswell, 2014; Loersch & Payne, 2011; Schröder & Thagard, 2013) that successfully explain and integrate a host of (behavior) priming findings, including its moderators. In fact, the work of people such as Wyer, Srull, and Higgins from the 1970s and 1980s who started the larger area of social priming is highly theoretically driven. Finally, behavior priming research is also given its place in more general (social) psychological perspectives (Kahneman, 2011: Strack & Deutsch, 2004).

The bottom line is that an appreciation of the neurocognitive literature on attention and (un)conscious processes as well as the social psychological theorizing of social and behavior priming effects may lead to the conclusion that behavior priming effects are really not that counterintuitive.

MODERATORS, MODERATORS, MODERATORS...

At least part of the current turmoil has been caused by unsuccessful but highly publicized replication attempts (e.g., Doyen et al., 2012; Pashler, Coburn, & Harris, 2012; Shanks et al., 2013). Such non-replications can evoke many different, interesting reactions—and indeed they did, also by some of us—but seen in perspective, by far the most likely explanation is that the researchers stumbled on one or more new moderators or boundary conditions. We realize that pointing at yet-to-be-identified moderators is tricky. Skeptics of priming research may accuse proponents of hiding behind this reasoning whenever a non-replication is published, and this reaction is understandable. That being said, many moderators of behavior priming research are already documented quite extensively, and they can be explained in meaningful ways (e.g., Dijksterhuis et al., 2007: Loersch & Payne, 2011). Two such examples are assimilation versus contrast effects (e.g., Dijksterhuis, Spears et al., 1998) and the role of self-relevance of the primed concept (Schubert & Häfner, 2003; Shih et al., 2002).

Obviously, the fact that there are many moderators is in itself not a problem. However, they can become a problem when researchers trying to replicate findings of others fail to take such moderators into account. Indeed, some—not all—of the recent replication projects overlooked moderating variables that were both well-known at the time and were quite obviously relevant. This is a shame. For example, when one uses a priming stimulus that evokes contrast among some participants and assimilation among others, for instance because they do or do not identify with it, this moderator should be taken into account, as not doing so can lead to misleading results.

More important, moderators enrich our understanding of a phenomenon, especially when these moderators can be accommodated by theory. In addition, most psychological phenomena tend to have many moderators (including factors that cannot always be easily controlled in a lab. One example is mood, which is in part dependent on such things as the weather, lighting, and other athmospherics in a lab). When one delves into the literature of a new phenomenon, one often starts with the naive idea that the phenomenon can be found under (almost) all circumtances, only to then find out there are an astounding number of moderators.

One well-known example is loss aversion. People are more aversive to losses than they are attracted to gains of similar magnitude. And, because of this, people fall prey to the endowment effect, the finding that they demand more for an object they already possess than they would be willing to pay to obtain it in the first place. This effect has been shown numerous times (Kahneman, Knetsch, & Thaler, 1991), and an incomplete grasp of the literature may lead to the conclusion that this effect always shows up. One manifestation of loss aversion is that people are often reluctant to trade an object for something of comparable value; indeed, people who are given a bottle of Bulgarian (or Spanish) wine are immediately reluctant to trade it for a bottle of comparable quality from Spain (or Bulgaria). However, when the two bottles are more similar because they are from the same country (i.e., people either trading a Spanish bottle for another Spanish bottle or a Bulgarian bottle for another Bulgarian bottle), no loss aversion occurs (van Dijk & van Knippenberg, 1998; the willingness to trade a bottle of wine is also dependent on the knowledge of wine; van Dijk and van Knippenberg, 2005).

Another example is that goods that are intended to be given up are not subject to loss aversion. We may, under some circumstances, be hesitant to trade our bottle of wine, but our local wine salesman is not, as he always intended to part with it. Indeed, there are quite a number of moderators or boundary conditions of the endowment effect (see e.g., Ariely, Huber, & Wertenbroch, 2005; Novemsky & Kahneman, 2005).

The same is true for areas related to behavior priming, such as semantic priming. Anyone who has ever taken the trouble to tinker with the parameters (such as the SOA, or the duration of the prime, or the length and frequency of prime and target words, etc.) of a lexical decision paradigm knows that semantic priming effects are not exactly rock-solid. Some of the boundary conditions are straightfoward (such as semantic relatedness itself); others less so. For instance, the way the primes are processed is important. If we intend to process the meaning of the word, we find semantic priming, but if we process some phonological aspect (does the word start with a vowel?), we do not (Adams & Kiefer, 2012).

In sum, the fact that phenomena have all kinds of moderators or boundary conditions is the nature of our field. However, as we said earlier, the skeptics' accusation of the proponents' use of the "there must be another moderator out there" argument as an excuse has some merit. We believe that there may be quite a number of moderators out there that could have already been documented but were not, because they were withheld from publication. In our view, there are two related causes why researchers, collectively, know more than what is published. The first is p-hacking, the second is publication bias. We think that p-hacking, combined with journals' pressure to publish only significant results, has led to what one may call "information leakage." In the process of doing research, we lose information we should not have lost.

INFORMATION LEAKAGE

Simmons and colleagues (2011) have given a vivid and engaging example of how p-hacking, or the use of researchers' degree of freedom, can lead to idiotic results. Their example is quite extreme, but the liberal use of researchers' degrees of freedom can make research areas look brighter and indeed much more straightforward than they really are. In fact, it is likely that this is true for many areas of psychology. Behavior priming is just an example.

Let's go through a hypothetical example of how p-hacking can lead to information leakage, or witholding the field meaningful information on moderators. It's purely hypothetical. Say you want to study whether priming participants with Nelson Mandela makes their behavior more moral. You show participants a few photographs of Mandela, and you administer a morality questionnaire and a task that measures cheating. And, contrary to your expectations, you find no statistically significant differences between conditions. Then someone tells you that priming a single person (an "examplar") is tricky in that it usually leads to behavioral contrast rather than behavioral assimilation. You decide to prime your participants with pictures of Mandela, but also with photos of Desmond Tutu, the Dalai Lama, Martin Luther King, and Gandhi. Still, you do not find a priming effect. Then you remember two participants telling you, during the debriefing, how humble they felt after the experiment. Did you still cause contrast among some participants because the photo images were too vivid? You decide to ask people to imagine what it would be like to be someone like Mandela, Desmond Tutu, the Dalai Lama, Martin Luther King, or Gandhi. And yes, you find a marginally significant effect on your cheating task in the predicted direction. You didn't find effects on your questionnaire which was administered before the cheating task though. But the study isn't all that strong anyway, as your effect only had a p-value of .07, after using religion as a covariate. Perhaps the weakness of the effect also has to do with the fact that the first-year students who participated in your experiment know your cheating task too well by now. After all, it was your third priming study this academic year. In September, you repeat your experiment again with new students and with only the cheating task and BINGO! There it is. Your effects turns up beautifully. Study 1 of your paper.

No, actually that was Study 4. It could be Study 1, but then at least it should be Study 1 of a paper with an extensive supplement or appendix with three "pilot studies." Though extreme, the above example shows that the combined effects of publication bias and p-hacking can easily lead a researcher to inadvertently prevent knowledge on three useful moderators (one versus multiple stimuli; processing photographs versus imagining something; and a behavioral measure versus a questionnaire) from entering the literature, not realizing that she or he could have saved a beginning graduate student—who ambitiously started her project three years later by priming participants with a photo of Gandhi—quite some time, resources, and frustration. In this example, research habits have led to unnecessary and potentially harmful information leakage.

Ironically, the current trend toward preregistering experiments—although laudable—may make this information leakage worse, as researchers may be tempted to do even more experiments ("pilots") that will never be published in order to get all the parameters exactly right, before an experiment is preregistered. We are not arguing against preregistration, far from it, but it provides an extra reason to take information leakage into account.

The point we are making here was recently made very eloquently by McGuire (2013). John Jost compiled a paper in which he introduces a draft paper originally written by McGuire in 1978. In Jost's words, McGuire argues that "it would benefit psychological scientists to be more forthright and communicative not only about those research discoveries that 'worked,' but also the entire process of insight and theoretical and empirical refinement, which might involve pilot studies, multiple revisions of materials and procedures, and more than a few 'dead ends'" (p. 414).

To some extent, experimentation, especially in certain areas, is craftmanship. It may be useful for journals to adopt a policy whereby researchers publish not just the beautiful experiments that resulted from months or years of finetuning, but also failures, pilots, reports on how they wrestled with certain parameters, or, in other words, the rocky road that led to the smooth endproduct.

WHERE DO WE GO FROM HERE?

We hope readers will not interpret the above as criticism of the area of behavior priming. We think that our analysis is applicable to the vast majority of research areas in psychology (and probably many outside). It's not simply a problem of behavior priming; it's also not simply a problem of social psychology. It may be tempting to criticize other areas for their research practices while thinking you're doing just fine, but at some point you might find your area lagging behind to those areas that improved their research practices while complacency prevented you from doing the same.

In our view, replication efforts are useful. More replications of an experiment (perhaps by different labs) before it is published will improve our field. In addition, replications shed light on the robustness and the generalizability of effects, whereas nonreplications are often the first step toward the discovery of new moderators. Obviously, it is essential that replications be executed properly and with enough statistical power, and when original effects are not replicated, the "oh-they-must-have-reported-false-positives" heuristic should be used with utmost caution. Just as p-hacking can demotivate young colleagues as it makes them wonder why they cannot replicate the findings of others, so are easily made allusions to false positives potentially degrading and indeed sure ways to suppress the creativity and courage of those colleagues in their endeavors to study new phenomena. Skepticism is helpful, but a fanatical hunt for false positives based on mistrust sucks the life out of our field.

We are convinced that we can improve psychological science more fruitfully when editors and reviewers are open to publishing experiments on the basis of their inherent quality rather than on their p-levels, and when researchers stop leaking inconvenient information away. If we all follow McGuire's (2013) advice to freely disclose failures and dead ends, we will soon talk about theory again rather than about stats. And while individual research progress may become a little slower, progress of the field as a whole will become much faster.

REFERENCES

Adams, S. C., & Kiefer, M. (2012). Testing the attentional boundary conditions of subliminal semantic priming: The influence of semantic and phonological tasks sets. *Frontiers in Human Neuroscience, 6,* 241. doi:10.3389/fnhum.2012.00241

Ariely, D., Huber, J., & Wertenbroch, K. (2005). When do losses loom larger than gains? *Journal of Marketing Research, XLII,* 134-138.

Bargh, J. A., Chen, M., & Burrows, L. (1996). Automaticity of social behavior: Direct effects of trait construct and stereotype activation on action. *Journal of Personality and Social Psychology, 71,* 230-244.

Barsalou, L. W. (1999). Perceptual symbol systems. *Behavioral and Brain Sciences, 22,* 577-660.

Bengtsson, S. L., Dolan, R. J., & Passingham, R. E. (2011). Priming for self-esteem influences the monitoring of one's own performance. *Social Cognitive and Affective Neuroscience, 6,* 417-425.

Berridge, K. C. (2011). Limbic generators of reward liking and wanting versus aversive motivations. *Behavioral Pharmacology, 22,* E1.

Branaghan, R. J., & Gray, R. (2010). Nonconscious activation of an elderly stereotype and speed of driving. *Perceptual and Motor Skills, 110,* 580-592. doi:0.2466/PMS.110.2.580-592

Brown, R., Croizet, J. C., Bohner, G., Fournet, M., & Payne, A. (2003). Automatic category activation and social behavior: The moderating role of prejudiced beliefs. *Social Cognition, 21,* 167-193.

Bry, C., Follenfant, A., & Meyer, T. (2008). Blonde like me: When self-construals moderate stereotype priming effects on intellectual performance. *Journal of Experimental Social Psychology, 44,* 751-757.

Callan, M. J., Kay, A. C., Olson, J. M., Brar, N., & Whitefield, N. (2010). The effects of priming legal concepts on perceived trust and competitiveness, self-interested attitudes, and competitive behavior. *Journal of Experimental Social Psychology, 46,* 325-335. doi:10.1016/j.jesp.2009.12.005

Cesario, J., Higgins, E. T., & Plaks, J. E. (2006). Automatic social behavior as motivation to interact. *Journal of Personality and Social Psychology, 90,* 893-910.

Chen, X., & Latham, G. P. (2013). *The effects of subconscious learning vs. performance goals on performance on a complex task.* Manuscript submitted for publication.

Dehaene, S., Changeux, J., Naccache, L., Sackur, J., & Sergent, C. (2006). Conscious, preconscious, and subliminal processing: A testable taxonomy. *Trends in Cognitive Sciences, 10,* 204-211.

Dijksterhuis, A., & Aarts, H. (2010). Goals, attention, and (un)consciousness. *Annual Review of Psychology, 61,* 467-490.

Dijksterhuis, A., & Bargh, J. A. (2001). The perception-behavior expressway: Automatic effects of social perception on social behavior. In M. P. Zanna (Ed.), *Advances in experimental social psychology,* Vol. 33 (pp. 1-40). San Diego: Academic Press.

Dijksterhuis, A., Chartrand, T. L., & Aarts, H. (2007). Effects of priming and perception on social behavior and goal pursuit. In J. A. Bargh (Ed.), *Social psychology and the unconscious* (pp. 51-132). New York: Psychology Press.

Dijksterhuis, A., Spears, R., Postmes, T., Stapel, D. A., Koomen, W., van Knippenberg, A. & Scheepers, D. (1998). Seeing one thing and doing another: Contrast effects in automatic behavior. *Journal of Personality and Social Psychology, 75,* 862-871.

Dijksterhuis, A., & van Knippenberg, A. (1998). The relation between perception and behavior or how to win a game of Trivial Pursuit. *Journal of Personality and Social Psychology, 74,* 865-877.

Dijksterhuis, A., & van Knippenberg, A. (2000). Behavioral indecision: Effects of self-focus on automatic behavior. *Social Cognition, 18,* 55-74.

Doyen, S., Klein, O., Pichon, C. L., & Cleeremans, A. (2012). Behavioral priming: It's all in the mind, but whose mind? *PLOS ONE, 7,* doi:10.371/journal.pone.0029081

Galinsky, A. D., Gruenfeld, D. H., & Magee, J. C. (2003). From power to action. *Journal* of Personality and Social Psychology, 85, 453-466. doi:10.1037/022-3514.85.3.453

Galinsky, A. D., Wang, C. S., & Ku, G. (2008). Perspective-takers behave more stereotypically. Journal of Personality and Social Psychology, 95, 404-419.

Gervais, W. M., & Norenzayan, A. (2012). Reminders of secular authority reduce believers' distrust of atheists. Psychological Science, 23, 483-491. doi:10.1177/0956797611429711

Haddock, G., Macrae, C. N., & Fleck, S. (2002). Syrian science and smart supermodels: On the when and how of perception-behavior effects. Social Cognition, 20(6), 461-479.

Hansen, J., & Wänke, M., (2009). Think of capable others and you can make it! Self-efficacy mediates the effect of stereotype activation on behavior. Social Cognition, 27, 76-88.

Hertel, G., & Kerr, N. L. (2003). Priming ingroup favoritism: The impact of normative scripts in the minimal group paradigm. Journal of Experimental Social Psychology, 37, 316-324.

Kahneman, D. (2011). Thinking fast and slow. New York: Farrar, Straus and Giroux.

Kahneman, D., Knetsch, J. L., & Thaler, R. H. (1991). Anomalies—The endowment effect, loss aversion, and status-quo bias. Journal of Economic Perspectives, 5, 193-206.

Kawakami, K., Young, H., & Dovidio, J. F. (2002). Automatic stereotyping: Category, trait, and behavioral activations. Personality and Social Psychology Bulletin, 28, 3-15.

Kay, A. C., & Ross, L. (2003). The perceptual push: The interplay of implicit cues and explicit situational construals on behavioral intentions in the Prisoner's Dilemma. Journal of Experimental Social Psychology, 39, 634-643.

Klatzky, R. L., & Creswell, J. D. (2014). An Intersensory interaction account of priming effects-and their absence. Perspectives on Psychological Science, 9, 49-58.

Koch, C., & Tsuchiya, N. (2007). Attention and consciousness: Two distinct brain processes. Trends in Cognitive Sciences, 11, 16-22.

Lamme, V. A. F. (2003). Why visual attention and awareness are different. Trends in Cognitive Sciences, 7, 12-18.

Latham, G. P., & Piccolo, R. F. (2012). The effect of context-specific versus nonspecific subconscious goals on employee performance. Human Resource Management, 51, 511-523. doi:10.1002/hrm.21486

LeBoeuf, R. A., & Estes, Z. (2004). "Fortunately, I'm no Einstein": Comparison relevance as a determinant of behavioral assimilation and contrast. Social Cognition, 22, 607-636.

Levine, M., Cassidy, C., & Jentzsch, I. (2010). The implicit identity effect: Identity primes, group size, and helping. Britisch Journal of Social Psychology, 49, 785-802. doi:10.1348/014466609X480426

Loersch, C., & Payne, B. K. (2011). The situated inference model: An integrative account of the effects of primes on perception, behavior, and motivation. Perspectives on Psychological Science, 6, 234-252.

Lowery, B. S., Eisenberger, N. I., Hardin, C. D., & Sinclair, S. (2007). Long-term effects of subliminal priming on academic performance. Basic and Applied Social Psychology, 29, 151-157.

Macrae, C. N., & Johnston, L. (1998). Help, I need somebody: Automatic action and inaction. Social Cognition, 16, 400-417.

McGuire, W. (2013). An additional future for psychological science. Perspectives on Psychological Science, 8, 414-423. doi:10.1177/1745691613491270

Naccache, L., Blandin, E., & Dehaene, S. (2002). Unconscious masked priming depends on temporal attention. Psychological Science, 13, 416-424. doi:10.1111/1467-9280.00474

Novemsky, N., & Kahneman, D. (2005). The boundaries of loss aversion. Journal of Marketing Research, XLII, 119-128.

Nussinson, R., Seibt, B., Häfner, M., & Strack, F. (2010). Come a bit closer: Approach motor actions lead to feeling similar and behavioral assimilation. Social Cognition, 28, 40-58.

Pashler, H., Coburn, N., & Harris, C. R. (2012). Priming of social distance? Failure to replicate effects of social and food judgments. PLOS ONE, 7(8), e42510. doi:10.1371/journal.pone.0042510

Pendry, L., & Carrick, R. (2001). Doing what the mob do: Priming effects on conformity. *European Journal of Social Psychology, 31*, 83-92.

Pessiglione, M., Schmidt, L., Drganski, B., Kalisch, R., Lau, H., Dolan, R. J., & Frith, C. D. (2007). How the brain translates money into force: A neuroimaging study of subliminal motivation. *Science, 316* (5826), 904-906. doi:10.1126/science.1140459

Prinz, W. (1997). Perception and action planning. *European Journal of Cognitive Psychology, 9*, 129-154.

Schröder, T., & Thagard, P. (2013). The affective meanings of automatic social behaviors: Three mechanisms that explain priming. *Psychological Review, 120*, 255-280.

Schubert, T. W., & Häfner, M. (2003). Contrast from social stereotypes in automatic behavior. *Journal of Experimental Social Psychology, 39*, 577-584.

Shanks, D. R., Newell, B. R., Lee, E. H., Balakrishnan, D., Ekelund, L., Cenac, Z., et al. (2013). Priming intelligent behavior: An elusive phenomenon. *PLOS ONE, 8*, e56515. doi:10.1371/journal.pone.0056515

Shantz, A., & Latham, G. (2011). The effects of primed goals on employee performance: Implications for human resource management. *Human Resource Management, 50*, 289-299. doi:10.1002/hrm.20418

Shih, M., Ambady, N., Richeson, J. A., Fujita, K., & Gray, H. (2002). Stereotype performance boosts: The impact of self-relevance and the manner of stereotype-activation. *Journal of Personality and Social Psychology, 83*, 638-647.

Simmons, J. P., Nelson, L. D., & Simonsohn, U. (2011). False-positive psychology: Undisclosed flexibility in data collection and analysis allows presenting anything as significant. *Psychological Science, 22*, 1359-1366. doi:10.1177/0956797611417632

Smith, P. K., & Trope, Y. (2006). You focus on the forest when you're in charge of the trees: Power priming and abstract information processing. *Journal of Personality and Social Psychology, 90*, 578-596.

Stel, M., Zeelenberg, M., van Dijk, W., & Kutsal, Z. (2012). Imitating a professor makes you act smart! The influence of mimicry on behavioral effects of stereotype activation. Presentation at the 12th ESCON conference in Estoril, Portugal.

Strack, F., & Deutsch, R. (2004). Reflective and impulsive determinants of social behavior. *Personality and Social Psychology Review, 8*, 220-247. doi:10.1207/s15327957pspr0803_1

Tsuchiya, N., Block, N., & Koch, C. (2012). Top-down attention and consciousness: A comment on Cohen et al. *Trends in Cognitive Sciences, 16*, 527-527. doi:10.1016/j.tics.2012.09.004

Vail III, K. E., Juhl, J., Arndt, J., Vess, M., Routledge, C., & Rutjens, B. T. (2012). When death is good for life: Considering the positive trajectories of terror management. *Personality and Social Psychology Review, 16*, 303-329. doi:10.1177/1088868312440046

van Dijk, E., & van Knippenberg, D. (1998). Trading wine: On the endowment effect, loss aversion, and the comparability of consumer goods. *Journal of Economic Psychology, 19*, 485-495.

van Dijk, E., & van Knippenberg, D. (2005). Wanna trade? Product knowledge and the perceived differences between the gains and losses of trade. *European Journal of Social Psychology, 35*, 23-34. doi:10.1002/ejsp.230

van Gaal, S., Lamme, V. A. F., Fahrenfort, J. J., & Ridderinkhof, K. R. (2011). Dissociable brain mechanisms underlying the conscious and unconscious control of behavior. *Journal of Cognitive Neuroscience, 23*, 91-105. doi:10.1162/jocn.2010.21431

van Gaal, S., Ridderinkhof, K. R., Fahrenfort, J. J., Scholte, H. S., & Lamme, V. A. F. (2008). Frontal cortex mediates unconsciously triggered inhibitory control. *Journal of Neuroscience, 28*, 8053-8062. doi:10.1523/JNEUROSCI.1278-08.2008

Webb, T. L., Sheeran, P., Gollwitzer, P. M., & Trötschel, R. (2012). Strategic control of unconscious social influences on behavior. *Zeitschrift für Psychologie, 220*, 187-193.

Wegner, D. M. (2002). *The illusion of conscious will*. Cambridge, MA: MIT Press.

Wheeler, S. C., Jarvis, W. B. G., & Petty, R. E. (2001). Think unto others: The self-destructive impact of negative racial stereotypes. *Journal of Experimental Social Psychology, 37*(2), 173-180.

Wheeler, S. C., & Petty, R. E. (2001). The effects of stereotype-activation on behavior: A review of possible mechanisms. *Psychological Bulletin, 127,* 797-826.

Yap, A. J., Mason, M. F., & Ames, D. R. (2013). The powerful size others down: The link between power and estimates of others' size. *Journal of Experimental Social Psychology, 49,* 591-594. doi:10.1016/j.jesp.2012.10.003

THE HISTORICAL ORIGINS OF PRIMING AS THE PREPARATION OF BEHAVIORAL RESPONSES: UNCONSCIOUS CARRYOVER AND CONTEXTUAL INFLUENCES OF REAL-WORLD IMPORTANCE

John A. Bargh
Yale University

Contrary to the recent assertions of skeptics of behavioral priming effects, the concept of priming was not introduced by the Meyer and Schvaneveldt (M-S, 1971) study of brief semantic spreading activation effects (perceptual-interpretation priming); it was originally introduced by Karl Lashley (1951) as a mechanism to increase the probability of a behavioral response (behavioral priming). The priming of the response was Lashley's solution to the problem of smooth behavioral response sequencing. Moreover, the initial priming demonstrations in experimental psychology, which predated M-S by many years, were of carryover effects from one experimental task to another—the same priming paradigm commonly employed in social psychology since the pioneering study of Higgins, Rholes, and Jones (1977). These priming effects were thus of considerably longer duration than the fleeting spreading activation effects obtained by M-S in the lexical decision task. Priming and accessibility effects of which the individual is unaware are commonplace in tasks involving higher mental processes, across diverse areas of psychological research, and often take the original form of carryover effects of task or emotional state to an unrelated subsequent context. In addition, behavioral priming is a natural and ecological phenomenon, as imitation and mimicry effects of perceiving another's behavior on one's own behavioral tendencies are clear manifestations of behavioral priming effects in the real world. These and other natural priming effects have now been demonstrated to have practical and applied importance in everyday life, such as in therapeutic interventions for addictions, increasing production in the workplace, and providing useful and effective "nudges" to a happier and healthier life.

Address correspondence to John A. Bargh, Department of Psychology, Yale University, 2 Hillhouse Ave., New Haven, CT 06520; E-mail: john.bargh@yale.edu

Priming effects are driven by the natural contact of external environmental stimulation with internal mental representations of those environments, part of the process by which sensation is turned into perception. In an initial "preattentive" or "preconscious" information analysis stage, incoming external stimulation is massively reduced and simplified, and imbued with categorical meaning, prior to one's becoming consciously aware of the products of this analysis (e.g., Bargh, 1989; Bruner, 1957; Neisser, 1967; Norretranders, 1998). By early childhood, an individual has had enough experience with the physical and social worlds that these analyses, reductions, and categorizations are made automatically, so that the perceptual analyses are experienced directly, without subjective feelings of effort after meaning. The process of sensation thus comes to proceed seamlessly into that of perception, and the results of the effortless analysis experienced, and trusted, as if it were all sensory and "out there," and the perceiver unaware of the important role played by the internal processing (Jones & Nisbett, 1971).

Understood this way, priming as a psychological principle should be noncontroversial. It occurs constantly and reflects the natural way a human mind keeps in touch with its current environment. What appears to be controversial is the effect of such priming on action, and this may reflect a disagreement over larger issues—the purpose and function of cognition itself. That the mental representations activated (as by primes) in the natural course of perception could also influence ongoing behavior has long been a basic guiding assumption of the research program of Wolfgang Prinz (1997) and colleagues (e.g., Knuf, Aschersleben, & Prinz, 2001). Today, the "pragmatic" movement in cognitive science that he and his students helped to found argues that cognition is not so much for the purpose of making models of the world as it is to subserve action; thus, brain states are not so much representations of the world as functional directives that guide action (Clark, 1998; Engel, Mare, Kurthen, & Koenig, 2013). In social psychology thirty years ago, McArthur and Baron (1983) advanced a similar ecological theory of social perception, based on Gibson's (1979) ecological theory of visual perception, with its basic premise that "perceiving is for doing," emphasizing the functional nature of social perception in the service of action preparation. The hypothesis then that behavioral priming, or the temporary activation of schemas containing social behavioral information, can lead directly to action tendencies is in harmony with this pragmatic or "enactive" movement within cognitive science (for more, see Engel et al., 2013; Morsella, Bargh, & Gollwitzer, 2009) although it might be more difficult to reconcile with the more traditional "mental models" meta-view.

Skeptics of behavioral priming effects (e.g., Harris, Coburn, Rohrer, & Pashler, 2013) question the validity of behavioral priming effects in part because the semantic priming studies of Meyer and Schvaneveldt (1971) using a lexical decision task showed only fleeting accessibility effects lasting less than a second (e.g., DOCTOR primes NURSE, OCEAN primes WATER). How then, they argue, can the effects of social or behavioral priming manipulations last so much longer (5 or 10 minutes or so)? In commenting on the behavioral priming effects in social psychology, Harris and colleagues (2013) question whether any priming more complex than that found by Meyer and Schevaneveldt (1971) is possible or even likely:

> The function and mechanism of the perceptual priming effects described in the previous paragraph seem relatively straightforward. Signal detection analysis shows that these priming effects reflect a perceptual bias toward assuming that

target information is consistent with the prime . . . Whereas the function of perceptual priming seems easy to understand, as mentioned above, the functional purpose achieved by higher-level priming effects is less obvious. (pp. 1–2)

In an effort to reconcile studies that find versus do not find behavioral priming effects, Klatzky and Creswell (in press) also point to the Meyer and Schvaneveldt (1971) studies as the standard or typical priming effect; in support of this premise, they state at the outset that Meyer and Schvaneveldt were the originators of priming research: "The term *priming* has its origins in research concerned with the spread of activation from one concept or neural site to another (e.g., Meyer & Schvaneveldt, 1971; Dehaene, Naccache, Cohen, et al., 2001). Priming has further been extended to effects on complex behaviors that are often quite distal or remote to the primed concept" (Klatzky & Creswell, in press).

But in fact Meyer and Schvaneveldt (1971) were *not* the originators of the priming concept or priming research. It was Karl Lashley (1951) who originated the concept, and tellingly, he invoked it to explain how *behavioral responses* were prepared by the mind. Moreover, Meyer and Schvaneveldt (1971) did not do the original priming research. The original priming studies used the same carryover (unrelated) task paradigms as did the social priming studies that came later (e.g., Higgins, Rholes, & Jones, 1977) and have the same time scale of priming effect durations as well, with effects lasting 5 or 10 minutes or more, not milliseconds.

In contrast to the pragmatic view of cognition as in the service of preparing adaptive behavioral responses, many cognitive scientists instead assume that the basic, evolved function of cognition is to understand the world and to form accurate mental models of it. This assumption is reflected in the above quote from Harris and colleagues (2013) and is a basis for their contention that longer-term social or behavioral priming effects are implausible. But as the actual history of the priming concept and of priming research in experimental psychology shows, the concept of priming did not originate with Meyer and Schvaneveldt (1971; hereafter "M-S") and it did not originate in demonstrations of rapid perceptual interpretations of the world.

KARL LASHLEY AND THE ORIGINS OF PRIMING RESEARCH

The term *priming* was first used by Karl Lashley in his 1951 chapter, "The problem of serial order in behavior." Lashley was dealing with the problem of how serial response sequences, as in speech production, flow so quickly and apparently effortlessly. He argued that there had to be a mediating state intervening between the act of will or intention (to perform an action, to speak a given sentence) and the production of the intended behavior, which assembled the action into the proper serial sequence. This he called the *priming* of the response. In this remarkable paper, Lashley (himself a behaviorist) rejected the then-dominant behaviorist reflex chaining accounts of the sequencing of behavior (ridiculed even more savagely by Koestler, 1967), and argued instead for a more mentalistic account in which behavioral sequences are typically controlled with central (executive) plans. The plans operated through first *priming* the behavioral steps in advance, so that they could roll off smoothly upon production, as in the spontaneous and fluent utterance of a complex, grammatically correct sentence in unrehearsed conversation with another person.

The idea of priming thus entered the experimental psychological literature to refer to a preparedness of mental representations to serve a response function. It did not refer initially to the very rapid and fleeting spread of activation from one mental representation to another. Moreover, the original priming demonstrations were of task carryover effects that lasted a matter of several minutes (similar to those of the original social priming study of Higgins et al., 1977), not a matter of milliseconds.

The discovery of carryover priming effects was actually quite serendipitous. Storms (1958) first gave his participants a list of words to memorize, and then had them free associate to a series of stimulus words. Unexpectedly, Storms found that the words presented in the memory task became more likely than usual to be given as associates (compared to standard free associate norms). Storms reported this effect but could not explain it, concluding that "the mechanisms of this recency effect remain unexplored" (p. 394).

It was Segal and Cofer (1960) who should be credited with the first use of the term *priming* to refer to this effect: the recent use of a concept in one task on the probability of its usage in a subsequent, unrelated task. Segal and Cofer replicated Storms' finding but, critically, without the use of explicit recall instructions—instead, merely exposing participants to the list of words was shown to have the effect of increasing the probability that those words would be used in the subsequent free association task.

Following this initial demonstration, priming began to be used as an experimental technique, especially to show how information had been stored in memory despite the individual's inability to recall it (Grand & Segal, 1966; Koriat & Feuerstein, 1976; Segal, 1967). That is, words presented in a first task still were more likely than usual to show up as free associates in a subsequent task, even though participants had failed to recall them at the end of the first task. Thus, these early priming studies were the forerunners of the important contemporary distinction between implicit and explicit forms and uses of memory (e.g., Schacter, 1987).

This is the model priming study that Higgins, Rholes, and Jones (1977) followed in their groundbreaking study of carryover effects in impression formation (not the M-S type of priming). They showed that personality trait concepts such as *adventurous* or *independent* could be primed by recent use. Using the same unrelated studies paradigm as had Segal and his colleagues, Higgins and colleagues (1977) exposed participants to synonyms of certain personality traits as part of a first, memory experiment. Next, in what participants believed to be an unrelated experiment, they read about a target person named Donald who behaved in ways ambiguously related to the primed traits, such as sailing across the ocean alone or preferring to study by himself instead of with classmates. Those participants who had been exposed to words such as *adventurous* and *independent* formed more positive impressions of Donald than did participants who had been previously exposed to relevant terms such as *reckless* and *aloof*. Importantly, participants evidenced no awareness of having been influenced by their prior exposure to trait terms in the earlier "memory experiment."

The advance beyond the previous priming studies was that the responses of the Higgins and colleagues' participants did not involve using the prime words themselves, as in the free association studies by Segal and colleagues; instead, they gave an overall impression or evaluation of Donald. What had been primed was not just the single, concrete lexical memory locations corresponding to the stimulus words, but also the abstract trait concepts themselves. These in turn, because they were primed and more accessible for use in perception (Bruner, 1957), became more likely to capture the relevant but ambiguous behavioral information about Donald, thus slanting final impressions in the positive or negative direction.

The Higgins and colleagues' (1977) study revealed for the first time how an individual's recent experience could affect, in a passive and unintended manner, his or her perceptual interpretation of another person's behavior. In their study, all participants read about the same target person doing the same things, yet they came away from their reading with markedly different impressions of that person, differences that were only accountable by reference to the experimentally manipulated differences in their recent use of different trait concepts.

In all of these studies, and in most of the behavioral priming studies discussed below, priming manipulations involved the recent use of mental concepts in one context that carried over to influence responses in an unrelated context, often several minutes later. This *unrelated-studies paradigm* has been used in many other domains of psychological research to demonstrate carryover effects of one situation or type of experience into subsequent contexts, with the individual unaware of the carryover effect of their recent experience. For example, classic work by Zillman (1978) and associates on "excitation transfer" showed that arousal caused by one context (e.g., a scary movie) could be misattributed in a subsequent context (one's degree of attraction to one's movie date). More recently, Lerner and associates (Lerner & Keltner, 2001; Lerner, Small, & Loewenstein, 2004) have demonstrated carryover effects of emotional states from one context into an unrelated one. In the case of carryover sadness emotional experiences, the priming effect is strong enough to reverse the usual endowment effect (Kahneman, Knetsch, & Thaler, 1991) on one's valuation of a commodity (Lerner et al., 2004). In both the Zillman and the Lerner research paradigms, the arousal or emotion experienced earlier in the experimental session continues to influence the participant but without his or her awareness of that continuing influence; many minutes later, this influence is demonstrated, compared to control conditions, on the second task.

Given the historical precedence and the many and varied demonstrations of carryover priming effects in the psychological literature, there is no logical reason for invoking the Meyer-Schvaneveldt type of priming, and its short duration, as a kind of litmus test for the plausibility of other forms of priming effects. There is also no logical basis in historical precedence or the overall research evidence base to restrict plausible priming effects to perceptual interpretation or to be skeptical that priming could influence higher-order cognition; the latter has been demonstrated many times in many areas of psychological research in addition to social-behavioral priming.

IMITATION AND MIMICRY: THE PERCEPTION-BEHAVIOR LINK

There is a second historical basis for behavioral priming effects in social psychology. Historically, social as well as developmental psychology have long focused on how the perceived behavior of others influences one's own behavioral tendencies. The study of *imitation and mimicry* tendencies (starting with the early Gestalt psychologists Koffka and Koehler in the 1920s) documented how social perceptual activity naturally creates tendencies to physically behave in the same manner, in young children as well as adults. This "perception-behavior link" (Chartrand & Bargh, 1999) exists in humans as in many other animals (e.g., birds, fish, antelope; see review in Dijksterhuis & Bargh, 2001). Moreover, the fact that perceiving another's behavior automatically activates tendencies to behave similarly oneself is in harmony with long-standing social psychological research that focuses on conformity and group coordination, and behavioral and emotional contagion effects, as well as imitation and mimicry.

Imitation and mimicry based on the perceived physical behavior of another person is present starting in infancy and toddlerhood and has been amply demonstrated in imitation and behavioral mimicry tendencies in adult humans (see Chartrand & Lakin, 2013 for a review; Chartrand & Bargh, 1999; Hatfield, Cacioppo, & Rapson, 1993; Kohler, 1925; Meltzoff, 1985; Meltzoff & Moore, 1977, 1983). Yet behavioral priming, which in its semantic form has engendered such skepticism and controversy recently, is the same phenomenon as imitation and mimicry, because whether the priming vehicle is semantic (e.g., action verbs) or the physical behavior of others, internal social-perceptual representations are activated that increase the probability of behaving the same way oneself (Chartrand, Maddux, & Lakin, 2005; Dijksterhuis & Bargh, 2001). Pointing out that these were the same basic phenomena, Chartrand and colleagues (2005) identified two sources of perception-behavior effect: *observables* and *abstract representations* and argued that both of these had their effect through the activation of related behavioral tendencies.

Social network studies (Christakis & Fowler, 2009) have shown how important forms of social behavior spread in a social network, typically to three degrees of separation or more between the individuals, so that the chain of our influence on others extends to many people we do not know and have never met. Obesity, cooperation, and others spread this way, as well as physical health problems such as diseases spread by germs. The perception-behavior link—the natural priming of behavioral tendencies by the perceived state or behavior of others—is very likely one important mechanism by which this spread occurs, unless one wants to insist—against the dictates of Occam's razor—that in each node of the network the individual is consciously thinking and deciding to behave the same way as the person they are interacting with. On that point, we already know from the chameleon effect (Chartrand & Bargh, 1999) and extensive subsequent imitation and mimicry research (reviewed in Chartrand & Lakin, 2013) that this additional conscious decision step is not necessary for behavioral contagion effects to occur.

Prinz's (e.g., 1997) notion of a representational overlap between perception and behavior was the forerunner of neuroscience research on "mirror neurons." Rizzolatti and colleagues (e.g., Rizzolatti & Sinigaglia, 2008) revealed shared regions of activation (in premotor cortex) when primates (including humans) observed another's action compared to when they performed the action themselves. Moreover, validating the equivalency of semantic and direct-perceptual vehicles for behavioral priming effects as argued by Chartrand and colleagues (2005), several of the mirror-neuron studies revealed effects of semantic priming on behavioral dispositions. Perani and colleagues (1999) showed that merely hearing action verbs activates implicit motor representations, as well as working memory structures such as the dorsolateral prefrontal cortex, the anterior cingulate, and premotor and parietal cortices, all of which are needed to carry out that behavior in an uncertain environment. Jeannerod (1999) showed that this link works in the other direction as well: observation of a meaningful action caused the activation of the same brain area (Brodmann 45) as did the generation of action verbs by the participant, or his or her active retrieval of verbs from memory. Grezes and Decety (2001, p. 12) concluded from a review of the verb-motor program research that, "motor programs can be seen as part of the meaning of verbal items that represent action."

Although words standing for these types of behavior have been used in laboratory studies as symbolic equivalents (and it is these original demonstrations involving verbal stimuli that have tended to be the focus of the recent replication attempts), the underlying and natural priming mechanism is the social perception of others' behavior. In line with this assumption, as noted in the previous section, factors that enhance or attenuate social-behavior priming effects, such as our liking versus disliking for the stereotyped group that is primed are also moderators of whether we will imitate the physical behavior of others (see Chartrand & Lakin, 2013, for a review).

Smith and Mackie (2014, this volume) similarly argue that the degree of self-other overlap will be an important moderator of interpersonal priming effects. As they point out, the cognitive psychology account of the function of priming as for perceptual anticipations only is "overly individualistic." Another function of priming "is social coordination, enabling convergence of beliefs, attitudes, emotions, and behavior within a dyadic relationship or ingroup." Smith and Mackie have extended the sources of these interpersonal priming effects to include one's simulations of others' likely responses in a given situation, based on that other person's presumed beliefs, attitudes, emotions or behavior.

Other chapters in this volume (Loersch & Payne, 2014; Wheeler, DeMarree, & Petty, 2014) also argue that an important moderator of the perception-behavior effect is the inclusion of the primed content into the active self-concept. Indeed, in the first published set of studies replicating the elderly-walking effect (Bargh, Chen, & Burrows, 1996), Hull, Slone, Meteyer, and Matthews (2002) published five studies in which stereotypes, emotional faces, and achievement-related primes were presented either subliminally or supraliminally. In two studies, implicit elderly-stereotype primes caused participants subsequently to walk more slowly, replicating the original effect, but only for dispositionally high self-conscious individuals.

That the primed trait construct needs to be included in the active self-concept for behavioral priming to occur is also consistent with research on "stereotype threat" effects (Steele & Aronson, 1995) in which the trait construct is *chronically* part of the person's identity already, as the group membership (to which the stereotype applies) is part of that person's self-concept. For example, Ambady, Shih, Kim, and Pittinsky (2001) showed stereotype threat on math task performance in girls as young as 5 years. In line with the stereotype contents, their task performance was better if the Asian identity had been primed but worse, compared to a control condition, if the female identity had been primed; the primes were drawings of children with Asian features or of non-Asian female children.

PRIMING EFFECTS IN REAL-WORLD CONTEXTS

As evidenced by the behavioral priming effects demonstrated by Ambady and colleagues (2001) in 5-year-old children (see Over & Carpenter, 2009, for similar behavior priming effects in 18-month-old infants), social priming effects likely reflect the operation of a natural, evolved mechanism. Therefore, they should be more likely to occur the more that the priming stimuli resemble the natural kinds corresponding to evolved adaptations. As argued above, for social behavioral priming the main natural prime is the behavior of other people (Chartrand & Bargh, 1999), including nonverbal emotional expressions and body posture. Another type of naturalistic prime is using real-life situational contexts as primes instead of verbal material, such as actual television shows containing actual food advertising (Harris, Bargh, & Brownell, 2009), or sitting in the professor's versus the student's office chair in order to fill out some questionnaires (to prime power: Chen, Lee-Chai, & Bargh, 2001). While verbal stimuli have often been used as convenient priming vehicles, the focus of the research was never on words per se or the effects they can produce but on generalizing the priming effect to natural real world contexts.

Real-life contexts are more natural, complete, and richer sources of primes than the artificial and simple lab environments required to demonstrate and disentangle them. Recent field studies have in fact confirmed the real world importance and influence of priming effects for important *in vivo* social behaviors, such as following norms (versus antisocial behavior) and voting in actual elections as well as the impulsivity of financial decision making.

1. Berger, Meredith, and Wheeler (2008) studied patterns of actual voting behavior for ballot referenda and showed that the situational context in which votes were cast influenced the outcome of the election within the same election district (town, region of the country): If the precinct's polling location was in a church, religion-related issues on the ballot received more votes than otherwise; if the location was in a school, education-related issues (e.g., school bond referenda) received more votes compared to other polling locations in the same locality.
2. In a set of field experiments, Keizer, Lindenberg, and Steg (2008) showed that people were more likely to behave in unscrupulous ways, such as littering, stealing, or disobeying posted signs, in contexts where there was evidence of past disorder (e.g., graffiti, litter). Behavior priming thus has real social consequences and can occur even in the absence of the original actors and the actual behavior being mimicked—when only vestiges of the relevant behavior remain. Simply perceiving evidence that social norm violations have been committed in the recent past—such as when viewing graffiti scrawled on city walls or litter on the streets—leads to the general spreading of disorder and crime.
3. Papies and colleagues (2013) conducted a field experiment in which overweight and obese customers in a grocery store were handed either a recipe flier containing healthy and diet-related primes or a control flier. Then, at checkout, those in the healthy/diet prime condition were found to have purchased nearly 75% fewer snacks at the store than did those in the control condition. When participants were debriefed after leaving the store, information on their purchases was obtained from their receipts. Questions were also asked about how much they had thought about the recipe flyer during shopping, and no effects of amount of thought about the flyer on purchasing were found; the authors concluded that

"the effects of the health prime on purchasing behavior were independent of whether participants consciously thought about it during shopping." Moreover, only a tiny minority of the participants could recall whether the recipe was either low in calories or contained diet-related words, and none of the participants showed awareness of the hypothesis of the study.

Of course, in any field study it is difficult to control for factors that can be controlled much better in laboratory settings. Thus, it is important to note that in their prior laboratory studies in which such control was possible, Papies and colleagues showed similar unconscious operation of the weight control goal using subliminal priming methods. For example, dieters who were primed subliminally with their weight control goal paid reduced attention to hedonic food cues compared with dieters who had not been primed (Papies, Stroebe, & Aarts, 2008).

4. DeVoe, House, and Zhong (2013) in a correlational study showed that the number of fast food restaurants located in an online study participant's zip code region predicted the speed and impulsivity with which the participant made financial decisions. The more fast food restaurants in the participants' natural ecology (very visible on the streets and roads), the faster and more impulsive were his or her financial decisions across several studies. Households saved less when living in neighborhoods with a higher concentration of fast food restaurants relative to full service restaurants. On a direct measure of individuals' delay discounting preferences, a higher concentration of fast food restaurants within one's neighborhood was associated with greater financial impatience. In an experimental test, having participants recall a recent fast food, as opposed to full service, dining experience at restaurants within the same neighborhood induced greater delay discounting tendencies (financial impatience). Finally, pedestrians walking down the same city street manifested greater delay discounting in their choices of financial reward if they were surveyed in front of a fast food restaurant, compared to a full service restaurant. The researchers concluded that the pervasiveness of organizational cues in the everyday social ecology can have a far-ranging influence on an individual's important decisions and behaviors.

5. Zaval, Keenan, Johnson, and Weber (in press) showed how contextual effects of the current general ambient temperature (i.e., hot weather vs. cold weather over a period of time) strongly influence the public's concern over the global warming or climate change problem. In general, when the current weather is hot, public opinion holds that global warming is occurring, and when the current weather is cold, people believe less that global warming is a general problem. This contextual influence on belief in a long-term problem is akin to Schwarz and Clore's (1983) demonstration that the current weather (sunny vs. cloudy) influenced the survey respondents' opinions about their overall life satisfaction.

In one of a series of studies to get at the underlying reasons why current weather influenced opinions about long-term climate change patterns, Zaval and colleagues used scrambled sentence priming of heat, cold, or neutral related topic sentences to show that it is the accessibility of similar (to the current day's weather) hot or cold days in memory that produced the effect on global warming opinions (i.e., the availability heuristic in operation). Those primed with heat-related concepts were more concerned about global warming as a problem than were other participants, and in further studies, those who believed the current weather was unusually hot also believed that more days over the past year had been hotter than average, compared to the estimate of other participants. Because public opinion strongly shapes public policy on climate change, this natural weather-priming effect has high practical importance.

6. Just as the perceived behavior of others is the natural behavioral prime, the perceived goal of others is a natural prime for one's own unconsciously instigated goal pursuits. Thus, Aarts, Gollwitzer, and Hassin (2004) showed *goal-contagion* effects such that the perceived goal pursuits of another person caused the perceiver to be more likely to pursue that same goal. Friedman and colleagues (2010) also showed that motivational orientations could be primed with observations of others' behavior, creating what they called "motivational synchrony" between the interactants. Moreover, Hamlin, Hallinan, and Woodward (2008) demonstrated these same types of goal-contagion effects in infants as young as 7 months.

Consistent with the present hypothesis that more realistic stimuli produce more reliable priming effects, Latham and colleagues, in a series of studies, used a photographic high-performance manipulation to consistently produce higher workplace task performance. Using a photograph of a woman winning a long-distance road race, the researchers successfully primed achievement motivation, as classically assessed by free responses on the projective Thematic Apperception Test (TAT). Then, Shantz and Latham (2009) found that working adults who were primed by that same photograph wrote significantly more ideas for a brainstorming task than people who had been given a blank sheet of paper, and in a subsequent field study (Shantz & Latham, 2011), the presence of that prime resulted in significantly higher amounts of money solicited for charities by telephone call center employees. This result was replicated in two additional call centers, and the TAT and call center fundraising results were again replicated in additional studies by Latham and Piccolo (2012), who showed further that the increase in fund-raising held across the entire subsequent work week.

7. One large class of motivational behavioral priming effects are automatic approach or avoidance arm and hand (finger) movement tendencies in response to positive versus negative stimuli, respectively (Cacioppo, Priester, & Berntson, 1993; Chen & Bargh, 1999). Although space limitations preclude a more complete review of the replications of this effect, as with the behavior and goal priming domains discussed above, the original Chen and Bargh research has been a) both exactly and conceptually replicated, b) extended by further discovery of important contextual moderating variables, and c) shown to have important practical consequences and applications. Its ecological validity was demonstrated by Slepian and colleagues (2012) who found that participants were faster to make approach movements to trustworthy faces and avoidance movements to untrustworthy faces, even though their task was merely to classify face versus house pictures and no explicit evaluation instructions were given. Its practical importance was shown by its success as a means to reduce alcohol cravings and reverse positive implicit attitudes toward alcohol to negative attitudes in a series of studies by Wiers and colleagues (2010, 2011). Compared to a control group, participants trained to make implicit avoidance movements (push) to alcohol-related and control stimuli, merely by classifying the presented photos as either landscape or portrait orientation, had their automatic positive attitudes toward alcohol change to negative, and were found a year later to have substantially lower drinking relapse rates (59 to 46%).

EMERGING FMRI STUDIES OF SOCIAL PRIMING EFFECTS

Before closing, it is important to note that an emerging research literature involving fMRI brain region imaging during priming manipulations is both replicating the original social behavioral and judgmental priming effects and revealing further details as to the brain regions involved in producing them. Brain imaging of priming effects furnishes a more sensitive form of measurement of the effects of primes on mental processes, compared to collection of the behavioral dependent variable alone, as the latter is subject to considerable variability from many other simultaneous influences. Space constraints do not permit a full description and review of these new studies, but here are a few examples.

1. Inagaki and Eisenberger (in press), using fMRI methods, compared brain regions activated while the participant read socially warm as well as socially neutral messages from close others, on the one hand, to those brain regions activated when the participant held physically warm as well as neutral temperature objects. Replicating previous research (e.g., Williams & Bargh, 2008), Inagaki and Eisenberger observed an overlap in subjective experience following manipulations of social versus physical warmth: participants felt physically warmer after reading the socially warm messages (compared to the neutral messages), and they also felt more connected to their close others after holding the physically warm stimulus (compared to the neutral temperature stimulus). They also found that neural activity during social warmth overlapped with neural activity during physical warmth in the ventral striatum and middle insula, but neural activity did not overlap during a control task (soft touch). The authors concluded that "together, these results suggest that a common neural mechanism underlies physical and social warmth."
2. Schaefer, Heinze, and Rotte (in press), in a within-participant design, replicated the behavioral priming findings of Ackerman, Nocera, and Bargh (2010), with rough physical primes causing social judgments that social interactions were less smooth and coordinated (across 96 different interaction scenarios). Simultaneous fMRI imaging revealed a significant involvement of the somatosensory cortex in making the coordination but not the control relationship-quality judgments. Using a within-participant design, each participant received a smooth versus a rough versus no physical prime before reading each given scenario. Significant correlations were obtained between primary somatosensory cortex activation and the extremity of not-smooth (rough) judgments of interaction coordination. Thus, physical primes influence more abstract social judgments through the involvement of sensory brain regions at the time of judgment.
3. Bengtsson, Dolan, and Passingham (2011) in an fMRI study primed participants to "be clever" or to "be stupid" (in a replication of Dijksterhuis & van Knippenberg, 1998) and assessed the priming's effect on the n-back task. Activating the representation of "clever" caused participants to slow their reaction times after errors on the working memory task, while the reverse pattern was seen for participants primed with "stupid." Critically, these behavioral effects were absent in control conditions. The fMRI data showed that the neural basis of this effect involves the anterior paracingulate cortex (area 32) where activity tracked the observed behavioral pattern, increasing its activity during error monitoring in the "clever" condition and decreasing in the "stupid" condition. The research-

ers concluded that implicit cues, which specifically target a person's self-concept, influence the way people react to their own behavior, in harmony with the emerging conclusion of how behavioral priming effects operate via involvement of the self-concept (see above).

CONCLUSIONS

Here, I have argued that it is both misleading and historically inaccurate to use the Meyer and Schvaneveldt (M-S; 1971) semantic priming paradigm as a standard against which to assess the plausibility of social and behavioral priming effects. The short time course of the M-S form of priming is likely because of the very short duration of the priming stimulus and the minimal deliberative processing given that prime in the lexical decision task (indeed participants are instructed not to respond to the prime stimulus at all and only to the target stimulus that follows on each trial). The actual origins of the priming concept and of priming research itself are instead much more in harmony with the social psychological tradition of priming studies. Lashley (1951) originated the concept as a theoretical vehicle to approach the problem of response or behavior preparation, especially in speech production. Thus, the concept of priming originated as a proposed mechanism for the activation of behavioral tendencies. Research after Lashley (1951), but well before the M-S studies, used the same "carryover effect" or "unrelated studies" paradigm that first Higgins and colleagues (1977) and then most other social judgment and behavior priming effects emulated. In those carryover priming studies, effects lasted many minutes, not merely the brief milliseconds duration of the M-S studies. Thus, the M-S paradigm should not be used as a litmus test for the plausibility of other priming studies, either for the nature of their effects on behavior and higher-order forms of cognition (as compared to perceptual interpretation) or for the duration of their priming effects.

The duration of a priming effect appears to be a function of the extent of the deliberate or effortful processing of the priming stimuli as required by the priming task. Clearly, the semantic priming stimulus in the M-S type of priming is very fleeting and short lived, and participants are not attending to it but rather to the target stimulus that comes next. When a greater degree of processing of the priming stimuli is required, priming effects last longer. And when physiological arousal-based priming occurs, as in excitation transfer and emotional priming carryover effects, the effect can last even longer (see Srull & Wyer, 1980, for an experimental demonstration).

Second, semantic behavioral priming effects are of the same class of phenomena as imitation and mimicry effects (perception-behavior effects), which are established beyond doubt. If one chooses not to believe in the reality of behavioral priming, then they also do not believe in the reality of imitation and mimicry effects. If skeptics of behavioral priming studies do not wish to include imitation and mimicry effects as examples of behavioral priming, then they should explicitly restrict their skepticism to semantic priming effects (or those that do not involve the physical behavior of others or natural contexts and carryover effects, as in arousal and emotional priming), not of behavioral priming per se (in which the most common naturally occurring prime is the behavior of other people). Unlike cognitive psychology, social psychology's history has focused on behavioral contagion, conformity, and imitation effects and is not as concerned with the effects of more artificial verbal and symbolic stimuli as is cognitive psychology. Social psychology has instead striven to use more naturally occurring stimuli as primes that then produce behavioral tendencies as well as influences on social judgments and other higher mental processes. This is because our goal has been to establish the ecological validity of our procedures and to be able to generalize to real-world stimuli and situations.

Thus, it is of high importance that studies of social priming effects have successfully demonstrated real-life priming effects. Whether or not every researcher can successfully reproduce the behavioral priming effects in the laboratory, these effects are being demonstrated to have real-world impact and importance, such as in the spread of social disorder, contextual effects of the polling place on election outcomes, and job performance in actual workplaces. The behavior priming effects first demonstrated in the laboratory are now being successfully translated into effective real-world applications, such as decreasing the purchase of unhealthy snacks in grocery stores by overweight individuals, increasing the amount of money raised for charities, and therapeutic interventions that significantly reduce cravings and relapse rates among addicts. These successful practical uses of behavioral priming effects to reduce the suffering and improve the lives of real individuals would not be possible unless the effects were real in the first place, as well as robust enough for practical application.

REFERENCES

Aarts, H., Gollwitzer, P. M., & Hassin, R. R. (2004). Goal contagion: Perceiving is for pursuing. *Journal of Personality and Social Psychology, 87,* 23-37.

Ackerman, J. M., Nocera, C. C., & Bargh, J. A. (2010, 25 June). Incidental haptic sensations influence social judgments and decisions. *Science, 328,* 1712-1715.

Ambady, N., Shih, M., Kim, A., & Pittinsky, T. L. (2001). Stereotype susceptibility in children: Effects of identity activation on quantitative performance. *Psychological Science, 12,* 385-390.

Bargh, J. A. (1989). Conditional automaticity: Varieties of automatic influence in social perception and cognition. In J. S. Uleman & J. A. Bargh (Eds.), *Unintended thought* (pp. 3-51). New York: Guilford.

Bargh, J. A., Chen, M., & Burrows, L. (1996). Automaticity of social behavior: Direct effects of trait construct and stereotype priming on action. *Journal of Personality and Social Psychology, 71,* 230-244.

Bengtsson, S. L., Dolan, R. J., & Passingham, R. E. (2011). Priming for self-esteem influences the monitoring of one's own performance. *Social Cognitive and Affective Neuroscience, 6,* 417-425.

Berger, J., Meredith, M., & Wheeler, S. C. (2008). Contextual priming: The influence of polling location type on voting behavior. *Proceedings of the National Academy of Sciences, 105,* 8846-8849.

Bruner, J. S. (1957). On perceptual readiness. *Psychological Review, 64,* 123-152.

Cacioppo, J. T., Priester, J. R., & Berntson, G. G. (1993). Rudimentary determinants of attitudes. II: Arm flexion and extension have differential effects on attitudes. *Journal of Personality and Social Psychology, 65,* 5-17.

Chartrand, T. L. & Bargh, J. A. (1999) The chameleon effect: The perception-behavior link and social interaction. *Journal of Personality and Social Psychology, 76,* 893-910.

Chartrand, T. L. & Lakin, J. (2013). The antecedents and consequences of human behavioral mimicry. *Annual Review of Psychology. 64,* 285-308.

Chartrand, T. L., Maddux, W. W., & Lakin, J. L. (2005). Beyond the perception-behavior link: The ubiquitous utility and motivational moderators of nonconscious mimicry. In R. R. Hassin, J. S. Uleman, & J. A. Bargh (Eds.), *The new unconscious* (pp. 334-361). New York: Oxford University Press.

Chen, M., & Bargh, J. A. (1999). Consequences of automatic evaluation: Immediate behavioral predispositions to approach or avoid the stimulus. *Personality and Social Psychology Bulletin, 25,* 215-224.

Chen, S., Lee-Chai, A. Y., & Bargh, J. A. (2001). Relationship orientation as a moderator of the effects of social power. *Journal of Personality and Social Psychology, 80,* 173-187.

Christakis, N. A., & Fowler, J. H. (2009). *Connected: The surprising power of our social networks and how they shape our lives.* New York: Little Brown.

Clark, A. (1998). *Being there: Putting brain, body, and world together again.* Cambridge, MA: MIT Press.

DeVoe, S. E., House, J., & Zhong, C. (2013) Fast food and financial impatience: A socioecological approach. *Journal of Personality and Social Psychology, 105,* 476-494.

Dijksterhuis, A., & Bargh, J.A. (2001). The perception-behavior expressway: Automatic effects of social perception on social behavior. *Advances in Experimental Social Psychology, 33,* 1-40.

Dijksterhuis, A., & van Knippenberg, A. (1998). The relation between perception and behavior, or how to win a game of Trivial Pursuit. *Journal of Personality and Social Psychology, 74,* 865-877.

Engel, A. K., Mare, A., Kurthen, M., & Koenig, P. (2013). Where's the action? The pragmatic turn in cognitive science. *Trends in Cognitive Science, 17,* 8-15.

Friedman, R., Deci, E. L., Elliot, A., Moller, A., & Aarts, H. (2010). Motivation synchronicity: Priming motivational orientations with observations of others' behavior. *Motivation and Emotion, 34,* 34-38.

Gibson, J. J. (1979). *The ecological approach to visual perception.* Boston: Houghton Mifflin.

Grand, S., & Segal, S. J. (1966). Recovery in the absence of recall. *Journal of Experimental Psychology, 72,* 138-144.

Grezes, I., & Decety, J. (2001). Functional anatomy of execution, mental simulation, observation, and verb generation of actions: A meta-analysis. *Human Brain Mapping, 12,* 1-19.

Hamlin, J. K., Hallinan, E. V., & Woodward, A. L. (2008). Do as I do: 7-month-old infants selectively reproduce others' goals. *Developmental Science, 11,* 487-494.

Harris, C. R., Coburn, N., Rohrer, D., & Pashler, H. (2013). High-performance-goal priming? Two failures to replicate. *PLOS ONE, 8*(8), e72467.

Harris, J. L., Bargh, J. A., & Brownell, K. D. (2009). Priming effects of television food advertising on eating behavior. *Health Psychology, 28,* 404-413.

Hatfield, E., Cacioppo, J. T., & Rapson, R. L. (1993). Emotional contagion. *Current Directions in Psychological Science, 2,* 96-100.

Higgins, E. T., Rholes, W. S., & Jones, C. R. (1977). Category accessibility and impression formation. *Journal of Experimental Social Psychology, 13,* 141-154.

Hull, J. G., Slone, L. B., Meteyer, K. B., & Matthews, A. R. (2002). The nonconsciousness of self-consciousness. *Journal of Personality and Social Psychology, 83,* 406-424.

Inagaki, T. K., & Eisenberger, N. I. (in press). Shared neural mechanisms underlying social warmth and physical warmth. *Psychological Science.* doi:10.1177/0956797613492773

Jeannerod, M. (1999). To act or not to act: Perspectives on the representation of actions. *Quarterly Journal of Experimental Psychology, 52A,* 1-29.

Jones, E. E., & Nisbett, R. E. (1971). The actor and the observer: Divergent perceptions of the causes of behavior. In E. E. Jones, D. E. Kanouse, H. H. Kelly, R. E. Nisbett, S. Valins, & B. Weiner (Eds.), *Attribution: Perceiving the causes of behavior.* New York: General Learning Press.

Kahneman, D., Knetsch, J. L., & Thaler, R. H. (1991). Anomalies: The endowment effect, loss aversion, and status quo bias. *Journal of Economic Perspectives, 5,* 193-206.

Keizer, K., Lindenberg, S., & Steg, L. (2008, 12 December). The spreading of disorder. *Science, 322,* 1681-1685.

Klatzky, R. L., & Creswell, J. D. (in press). An inter-sensory interaction account of priming effects – and their absence. *Perspectives on Psychological Science*.

Knuf, L., Aschersleben, G., & Prinz, W. (2001). An analysis of ideomotor action. *Journal of Experimental Psychology: General, 130*, 779-798.

Koestler, A. (1967). *The ghost in the machine*. New York: Macmillan.

Kohler, W. (1925). *The mentality of apes*. New York: Harcourt, Brace & Co.

Koriat, A., & Feuerstein, N. (1976). The recovery of incidentally acquired information. *Acta Psychologica, 40*, 463-464.

Lashley, K. S. (1951). The problem of serial order in behavior. In L. A. Jeffress (Ed.), *Cerebral mechanisms in behavior* (pp. 112-131). New York: Wiley.

Latham, G. P., & Piccolo, R. F. (2012). The effect of context specific versus nonspecific subconscious goals on employee performance. *Human Resources Management, 51*, 535-548.

Lerner, J. S., & Keltner, D. (2001). Fear, anger, and risk. *Journal of Personality and Social Psychology, 81*, 146-159.

Lerner, J. S., Small, D. A., & Loewenstein, G. (2004). Heart strings and purse strings: Carryover effects of emotions on economic decisions. *Psychological Science, 15*, 337-341.

Loersch, C., & Payne, B. K. (2014). Situated inferences and the what, who, and where of priming. This volume.

McArthur, L. Z., & Baron, R. S. (1983). Toward an ecological theory of social perception. *Psychological Review, 90*, 215-238.

Meltzoff, A. N. (1985). Immediate and deferred imitation in fourteen- and twenty-month-old infants. *Child Development, 56*, 62-72.

Meltzoff, A. N., & Moore, M. K. (1977). Imitation of facial and manual gestures by human neonates. *Science, 198*, 75-78.

Meltzoff, A. N., & Moore, M. K. (1983). Newborn infants imitate adult facial gestures. *Child Development, 54*, 702-709.

Meyer, D. E., & Schvaneveldt, R. W. (1971). Facilitation in recognizing pairs of words: Evidence of a dependence between retrieval operations. *Journal of Experimental Psychology, 90*, 227-234.

Morsella, E., Bargh, J., & Gollwitzer, P. (Eds., 2009). *Oxford handbook of human action*. New York: Oxford University Press.

Neisser, U. (1967). *Cognitive psychology*. New York: Appleton-Century-Crofts.

Norretranders, T. (1998). *The user illusion*. New York: Viking.

Over, H., & Carpenter, M. (2009) Eighteen-month-old infants show increased helping following priming with affiliation. *Psychological Science, 20*, 1189-1193.

Papies, E. K., Potjes, I., Keesman, M., Schwinghammer, S., & van Koningsbruggen, G. M. (2013). Using health primes to reduce unhealthy snack purchases among overweight consumers in a grocery store. *International Journal of Obesity*, 1-6.

Papies E. K., Stroebe, W., & Aarts, H. (2008). The allure of forbidden food: On the role of attention in self-regulation. *Journal of Experimental Social Psychology, 44*, 1283-1292.

Perani, D., Cappa, S. F., Schnur, T., Tettamanti, M., Collina, S., Rosa, M. M., & Fazio, F. (1999). The neural correlates of verb and noun processing: A PET study. *Brain, 122*, 2337-2344.

Prinz, W. (1997). Perception and action planning. *European Journal of Cognitive Psychology, 9*, 129-154.

Rizzolatti, G., & Sinigaglia, C. (2008). *Mirrors in the brain: How our minds share actions and emotions*. New York: Oxford University Press.

Schacter, D. L. (1987). Implicit memory: History and current status. *Journal of Experimental Psychology: Learning, Memory, and Cognition, 13*, 501-518.

Schaefer, M., Heinze, H.-J., & Rotte, M. (in press). Rough primes and rough conversations: Evidence for a modality-specific basis to mental metaphors. *Social Cognitive and Affective Neuroscience*.

Schwarz, N., & Clore, G. L. (1983). Mood, misattribution, and judgments of well-being: Informative and directive functions of affective states. *Journal of Personality and Social Psychology, 45*, 513-523.

Segal, S. J. (1967). The priming of association test responses. *Journal of Verbal Learning and Verbal Behavior, 6*, 216-221.

Segal, S. J., & Cofer, C. N. (1960). The effect of recency and recall on word association. *American Psychologist, 15*, 451.

Shantz, A., & Latham, G. P. (2009). An exploratory field experiment of the effect of subconscious and conscious goals on employee performance. *Organizational Behavior and Human Decision Processes, 109*, 9-17.

Shantz, A., & Latham, G. P. (2011). The effect of primed goals on employee performance: Implications for human resource management. *Human Resource Management, 50,* 1-11.

Slepian, M. L., Young, S. G., Rule, N. O., Weisbuch, M., & Ambady, N. (2012). Embodied impression formation: Social judgments and motor cues to approach and avoidance. *Social Cognition, 30,* 232-240.

Smith, E. R., & Mackie, D. M. (2014). Taking priming interpersonal: Priming from other's observed or simulated responses. This volume.

Srull, T. K., & Wyer, R. S., Jr. (1980). The role of category accessibility in the interpretation of information about persons: Some determinants and implications. *Journal of Personality and Social Psychology, 37,* 1660-1667.

Steele, C. M., & Aronson, J. (1995). Stereotype threat and the intellectual test performance of African Americans. *Journal of Personality and Social Psychology, 69,* 797-811.

Storms, L. H. (1958). Apparent backward association: A situational effect. *Journal of Experimental Psychology, 55,* 390-395.

Wheeler, S. C., DeMarree, K. G., & Petty, R. E. (2014). Understanding prime-to-behavior effects: Insights from the active-self account. This volume.

Wiers, R. W., Rinck, M., Kordts, R., Houben, K., & Strack, F. (2010). Retraining automatic action-tendencies to approach alcohol in hazardous drinkers. *Addiction, 105,* 279-287.

Wiers, R. W., Eberl, C., Rinck, M., Becker, E. S., & Lindenmeyer, J. (2011). Re-training automatic action tendencies changes alcoholic patients' approach bias for alcohol and improves treatment outcome. *Psychological Science, 22,* 490-497.

Williams, L. E., & Bargh, J. A. (2008, 24 October). Experiencing physical warmth influences interpersonal warmth. *Science, 322,* 606-607.

Zaval, L., Keenan, E. A., Johnson, E. J., & Weber, E. U. (in press). How warm days increase belief in global warming. *Nature: Climate Change.* doi:10.1038/nclimate2093

Zillman, D. (1978). Attribution and misattribution of excitatory reactions. In J. H. Harvey, W. J. Ickes, & R. F. Kidd (Eds.), *New directions in attribution research* (Vol. 2, pp. 335-368). Hillsdale, NJ: Erlbaum.

PRIMING... SHMIMING: IT'S ABOUT KNOWING *WHEN* AND *WHY* STIMULATED MEMORY REPRESENTATIONS BECOME ACTIVE

E. Tory Higgins
Columbia University

Baruch Eitam
University of Haifa

A funny thing happened along the way of researchers using priming techniques to study psychological questions. Rather than priming being just a tool to study mind—dealing with questions like the nature of and the mechanisms underlying mental representation, semantic organization and judgment—priming became *the* object of study. In other words, it morphed from being a stagehand to being the star of the show. People began to talk about, and currently worry about, the nature of "priming effects." We selectively review some of this history and emphasize the importance of returning to trying to understand the psychological mechanisms that underlie what priming "does." Adopting our own suggestion, we focus on *accessibility* and present a recent framework that links understanding of how accessibility (and priming) works. Further, we demonstrate how a focus on mechanism both unlocks and enables adding to a large body of knowledge; namely, research on human memory.

Research involving so-called "social priming" is taking a beating. Some knew it all along: How could it even be possible that being exposed to a few words related to achievement (or cooperation, or a stereotype, or a trait) would affect people's thought and action?

Intuitions aside, it must be recognized that the possibility of faulty experimentation, data "beautifying," and even fraud have affected both scientists' and lay peoples' perception of the strength, nature, and meaning of social priming effects. While this is definitely disconcerting, it does not entail the blanket faulting of stud-

---

Both authors contributed equally to this manuscript and order of authorship was determined by the flip of a coin. This research was supported by the Israel Science Foundation (ISF) Grant 277/12 to Baruch Eitam.

Address correspondence to Baruch Eitam at beitam@psy.haifa.ac.il or E. Tory Higgins at tory@psych.columbia.edu

ies that use priming methods to address issues that are of interest to social psychologists. In fact, the phenomena and methods associated with priming studies and, importantly the mental mechanisms that are assumed to support them, such as accessibility, represent some of the most fundamental contributions to psychology over recent decades. Hence, as a scientific field, we are not in a position to simply disengage from this line of research even through it has come under attack. This is the context for the current paper.

To begin with, we wish to emphasize that we believe that one of the problems with the current discussion is that it emphasizes priming per se and particular phenomena that were found in priming studies rather than emphasizing the *mechanisms* that underlie such phenomena. Because of this emphasis, when a study is conducted and a priming phenomenon is not replicated, there is currently a tendency to question the experimental rigor or statistical reliability of the research rather than asking how this failure contributes to our understanding of the mechanism that makes the phenomenon appear or *disappear*. Let us begin by considering how the same tendency might have played out 30 years ago when social-psychological priming studies first began as a way for us to distinguish between emphasizing phenomena versus emphasizing underlying mechanisms.

FROM PHENOMENA TO BOUNDARY CONDITIONS TO MECHANISMS

The first social priming phenomenon can be characterized as follows: After exposure to a trait-related word (verbal priming), subsequent memory and judgment of a target person's behavior will be assimilated to the word-related representation in memory. The results of many priming studies have demonstrated this phenomenon (for an early review, see Higgins, 1996). The first evidence was provided by Higgins, Rholes, and Jones (1977). The participants in this study were initially exposed to one or another set of trait-related constructs as an incidental aspect of a study on perception. They then participated in a supposedly unrelated study on reading comprehension where they were asked to characterize the ambiguous behaviors of a target person. For example, they read the following ambiguous behavior: Once Donald made up his mind to do something it was as good as done no matter how long it might take or how difficult the going might be. Only rarely did he change his mind, even when it might well have been better if he had. Pilot testing had indicated that this behavior was equally likely to be characterized as "stubborn" or as "persistent." In the earlier perception task, half of the subjects had been exposed to the word "stubborn" as an incidental part of a Stroop task (i.e., a supposed memory load to make the task more difficult) whereas the other half of the subjects had been exposed to the word "persistent." The study found that the participants were significantly more likely to use the trait-related constructs primed in the initial perception task to categorize the target person's behaviors in the second reading comprehension task than to use the equally applicable alternative construct.

After early replications of this priming phenomenon (e.g., Srull & Wyer, 1979, 1980), it wasn't long before studies appeared where this phenomenon *disappeared* (e.g., Martin, 1986; cf. Herr, Sherman, & Fazio, 1983). In fact, under specific conditions not only did verbal priming fail to produce assimilation of the judgment to the word-related representation in memory that had been primed earlier, these studies found an opposite *contrast* effect! In a study by Martin (1986), for example, when "persistent" was verbally primed, participants later categorized ambiguous persistent-stubborn behaviors as "stubborn" rather than as "persistent"—a contrast effect rather than an assimilation effect. What happened then? Were the earlier studies showing an assimilation effect criticized for their rigor or validity? Fortunately not. Instead, social psychologists began conducting new research to determine *when* verbal priming produced assimilation effects on judgment and when it produced contrast effects (Zanna & Fazio's [1982] second-generation *When?* question) as well as research to try to understand the underlying mechanisms or processes that produced either assimilation or contrast under different conditions (Zanna & Fazio's [1982] third-generation *How?* or *Why?* questions).

The first clue to what was going on was the recognition that the verbal priming in studies that found a contrast effect was much more blatant or salient than the verbal priming used in the previous studies that had found assimilation: *when* the verbal priming is relatively subtle, an assimilation effect is likely to occur; *when* the verbal priming is relatively blatant, a contrast effect is likely to occur. Subsequent research operationalized this in terms of whether participants at the time of judging the target's behaviors were or were not aware of the earlier verbal priming as an event they still remembered: *when* the priming event itself is not remembered at the time of categorization, an assimilation effect is likely to occur; *when* the priming event itself is remembered at the time of categorization, a contrast effect is likely to occur (see, for example, Lombardi, Higgins, & Bargh, 1987; Newman & Uleman, 1990; Strack, Schwarz, Bless, Kübler, and Wänke, 1993).

These studies helped to clarify when to expect either the contrast or assimilation phenomenon to replicate. Apparently, when people are aware of or remember the priming event at the time of judging the target, recent verbal priming will produce a contrast effect; if not, then an assimilation effect. But hold on. In one of the conditions in a study by Martin (1986), the participants were prepared to respond to 12 phrases, but they were *interrupted* and told to proceed to the next task after completing only 8. The priming in this condition was also blatant, but it produced an assimilation effect on subjects' subsequent judgments rather than a contrast effect. Lombardi and colleagues (1987) also found that when the priming task was interrupted, an assimilation effect of increased accessibility from priming was obtained even for subjects who later remembered the priming events. Thus, the usual contrast effect of priming when participants are aware of or remember the priming event *disappeared* in these studies. Instead, an assimilation effect was found.

What is the moral of this story? First, even if we devised a paradigm that reliably produces a medium-sized effect (phenomenon), we should not expect that it will replicate across all conditions, *and* we don't know which conditions matter ahead of time. As a heuristic, it is also worth noting that the cognitively higher the phenomenon, the more sensitive it will be to changing contexts.[1] Once we have discovered an effect, we need to do more research to discover the conditions for *when* the phenomenon will appear or disappear (the second-generation question). Second, trying to answer just the *when* question (e.g., looking for moderators) merely sets

---

1. An interesting case is Asch's (1951; 1956) classic conformity studies that were argued to be "unreplicable" (Lalancette & Standing, 1990; Perin & Spencer, 1981). A large meta-analysis uncovered both a time-related decline in the size of the effect and cross-cultural differences (Bond & Smith, 1996).

the stage for the next phase of research. We now need to uncover what generates the phenomenon—why it happens. An efficient way to do so is by investigating the mechanisms and processes that explain when the phenomenon—in this case the two phenomena of assimilation and contrast—will appear or disappear.

In the case of assimilation versus contrast from verbal priming, it became clear that mechanisms other than just accessibility played a role, including *judged usability* where the judged relevance or appropriateness of using the primed representation affected whether assimilation or contrast occurred (Higgins, 1996). When the primed representation was judged not to be relevant or appropriate to use, suppression or inhibition of the primed representation was likely to produce a contrast effect. And there are other mechanisms as well that determine when these phenomena will appear or disappear, including the relation between the specific content of the prime and the content of the stimulus information (Smith, 1989; Smith & Branscombe, 1987) and whether participants have a global versus local processing style (Förster, Liberman, & Kuschel, 2008) that impacts inclusion/exclusion processes underlying assimilation and contrast (see Schwarz & Bless, 1992).

The bottom line is that it is not priming per se that matters—it is just a tool after all—nor even a particular phenomenon that is discovered from a priming study, although some phenomena can be important in themselves as effects worth noting (e.g., Asch's demonstration of social influence). Again, it is not even discovering when a phenomenon appears or disappears that is most important (i.e., the *moderators*). All these are merely precursors; what matters most is determining *mediators*: the mechanisms and processes underlying a phenomenon. What underlying perceptual processes produce the Muller-Lyer illusion? What mechanisms underlie the cluster of symptoms (the syndrome) that is associated with someone who has an obsessive-compulsive personality? And, in this case, what mechanisms determine whether stimulation of a representation in memory from priming will increase the likelihood that it will be used to categorize subsequent input?

One issue, however, needs to be addressed. In the early history of trying to understand assimilation effects from priming, when the initial assimilation phenomenon disappeared in a later study, why did researchers not conclude that this was a failure to replicate and that this meant the phenomenon was unreliable and not worth studying further? This is an important and difficult question. One of us (Higgins) knows that he and others at the time (e.g., John Bargh; Bob Wyer) believed that the basic priming phenomenon was an assimilation effect whose underlying mechanism was increased accessibility of the primed representation (making it temporarily more accessible than alternative representations), and thus its disappearance must be due to some other mechanism or mechanisms. This inspired a search for that other mechanism. Without this strong initial belief in a basic mechanism that underlay the initial assimilation effect, a subsequent failure to replicate could indeed cause researchers to consider a phenomenon unreliable and not worth further study.

What makes things challenging is that we often do not know initially what mechanism beyond the one we believe we are investigating is also necessary for the phenomenon to appear—a mechanism that just happens to be present in a particular form (e.g., high judged usability) that has allowed the initial phenomenon to appear. Once a study has this other mechanism in a different form (i.e., low judged usability) the initial phenomenon can disappear. But this does *not* mean that the original *mechanism* that inspired the initial research (i.e., accessibility) has disappeared. It remains and works with this other mechanism, and together they produce a resultant effect that can vary with different forms of the moderating mechanism. The goal should be to identify different relevant mechanisms and learn how they work together to produce different effects. Who said it was going to be easy? But you do have to believe in the original mechanism—not the initial phenomenon per se.

PRIMING AS THE MANIFESTATION OF INCIDENTALLY RELEVANT STIMULATION

Moving away from the content-specific nature of a specific study or even a body of work (e.g., "social priming") enables the abstraction of basic mechanisms. Interestingly, social cognition was born by applying basic mental processes discovered by cognitive psychologists to the specific content of social judgments and memory. More than 30 years have passed since that time, and the body of research generated by the social-cognitive movement enables psychologists now to move in the opposite direction—propose mechanisms that underlie how basic mental processes work, such as knowledge activation and accessibility changes over time.

The focus of the remainder of this paper is to address this last issue; namely, to answer what mechanisms underlie mental activation. We begin by establishing some common ground (for extensive reviews, see Förster and Liberman, 2007; Higgins, 1996; see also Eitam & Higgins, 2010) and then set two additional aims for the remainder of this paper. One additional aim is to introduce the importance of informational relevance for priming and spell out some of the implications of understanding this mechanism. Another additional aim is to *re*establish a somewhat forgotten understanding—that priming is a form of incidental memory activation (Roediger, 1990; Smith & Branscombe, 1987). Through establishing the role relevance plays in both priming and other forms of memory, we hope that we can place research on social priming within a still somewhat crude but more coherent framework—one that will facilitate "cross talk" with related fields of research while emphasizing the benefits of a more mechanism-oriented focus.

ESTABLISHING COMMON GROUND ON PRIMING

In their essence, the ideas underlying priming are as ancient as they are simple and are tightly bound to the notion of mental representation. In Latin, the notion of mental representations apparently dates back to the 12th century, but the idea of their activation by appropriate external stimulation dates back much earlier, to the early Greek philosophers (Lagerlund, 2011). Leaping forward to 20th-century psychology, this notion of mind developed into an experimental paradigm by cognitive-era psychologists interested in how the mind processes language—with classic demonstrations, such as presenting the word "bank" after the word "money" influencing people's tendency to interpret the meaning of a word (i.e., activate one versus another specific meaning; Mackay, 1973). Priming was also used as a tool by researchers examining human memory and its organization (e.g., Tulving & Pearlstone, 1966; for reviews, see Roediger, 1990; Tulving & Schacter, 1990).

After the idea of semantic (meaning carrying) mental representations and their dynamics took hold in cognitive psychology and was investigated using the methodology of priming,[2] social psychologists who were interested in how the mind performs judgments of social input modified the cognitive *method* of priming (i.e., pre-activating specific meaning) in their research in order to understand better how people form impressions of others' behaviors (e.g., Bargh & Pietromonaco, 1982; Higgins et al., 1977; Srull & Wyer, 1979, 1980). Notably, the early social psychologists who used priming methods were not interested in priming per se but were instead interested in what it meant for person perception to increase the accessibility of trait constructs in memory, including its implications for automatic or unintentional ("passive") interpretation of ambiguous target person behaviors. This is evident from these papers referring to "accessibility" or "automaticity" in their titles rather than "priming." Nonetheless, this new use of priming methods by social psychologists demonstrated a much broader range of priming effects.

At the time within cognitive psychology, the effects of priming were considered to be limited to basic linguistic and memorial processes, such as recalling a second exemplar from a category (Loftus, 1973), the production of verbal associations (Cramer, 1964; Storms, 1958), and affecting the interpretation of homonyms (Mackay, 1973). In contrast, social psychologists have shown that priming may influence what is thought to be highly complex judgments, such as *forming an impression* of a protagonist based on ambiguous (e.g., Higgins et al., 1977) or vague (e.g., Higgins & Brendl, 1995) descriptions of a target person's behaviors.[3] The use of priming continued to break new ground in its new (social) home and was shown to influence a large variety of seemingly complex forms of thinking—from stereotyping (Banaji, & Hardin, 1996) to problem solving (e.g., Higgins & Chaires, 1980).

In the last two decades, the use of priming in social cognition increasingly shifted from demonstrating the effects of priming on thought to demonstrating the effects of priming on observable action.[4] Importantly, in the great majority of these later studies the methodology of priming was used for demonstrating that the "automatic" (i.e., unconscious, unintentional or both) mind plans, initiates and modifies actions—operations traditionally considered to be markers of the conscious mind (i.e., requiring consciousness). For example, researchers set out to show that norms (Aarts & Dijksterhuis, 2003), ideologically driven action (Hassin, Ferguson, Shidlovski, & Gross, 2007), planned behavior (Bargh et al., 2001), allocation of effort

---

2. Priming is a method for activating representations, and not only semantic ones. For example "repetition priming" is argued to be a "perceptual" form of priming in which only the superficial (i.e., perceptual) features of a stimulus are activated (Tulving & Schacter, 1990). In this paper, we refer to what is often called "conceptual" or semantic priming.

3. These effects were/are often interpreted as evidence for priming of traits, just as later priming effects on thought and action were/are interpreted to reflect priming of stereotypes, behaviors, and goals. It is worth noting that observing that priming affects an outcome (e.g., how a certain task is performed) doesn't entail that a behavior or a goal was primed or that knowledge about goals or behaviors is any different from ordinary semantic knowledge (e.g., Loersch & Payne, 2011).

4. Notably, failures to replicate key (non-fraudulent) priming effects predominantly come from this domain. Thus, at this stage we consider the question of semantic priming *directly* affecting behavior as open, consistent with the difference between a direction expression account of walking slowly (Bargh, Chen, & Burrows, 1996) and a preparation for interaction account that introduces an additional moderating mechanism (Cesario et al., 2006). This is apparently less the case for semantic priming assimilation effects on judgments which have been considered to be sufficiently established (see DeCoster & Claypool, 2004).

and mental resources (Bijleveld, Custers, & Aarts, 2012), goal-directed adaptation to a rule-governed environment (Eitam, Hassin, & Schul, 2008), and even conflict between goals (Kleiman, & Hassin, 2011) can all occur without awareness. Interestingly, and regardless of what outcome of priming was measured (thought or action), priming has thrived as a paradigm and as a phenomenon-generating tool. This held throughout changes in theorizing about the structure of the mind—from spread of activation through semantic nodes (Collins, & Loftus, 1975), to "mentalese" (Fodor, 1975), to parallel distributed processing (PDP; Rumelhart, & McClelland, 1986) and other associative network models.

We speculate that one of the reasons this new kind of priming effect studied by social cognition researchers in the late 1970s and early 1980s grabbed the experimental-psychological community's attention is that they defied (and still defy) a number of features thought to define priming. One of these is the duration of priming effects. In such (let's call them "lexical priming") studies, an ambiguous word is interpreted as a function of a prior priming context or the speed of reading a word is affected as a function of whether it is preceded by a semantic associate versus a string of meaningless letters. Such effects were theoretically understood as reflecting a first brief "automatic" priming effect (up to 2 seconds) followed by a "controlled" (i.e., expectancy driven) process (Neely, 1977; see also Bruner, 1957). As these were the kind of automatic semantic priming effects that cognitive psychologists recognized, it was (and still is) surprising for them to learn that social psychologists argue for *automatic* semantic priming effects *minutes* after the prime event. At the bottom of this bewilderment lies the necessity for finding the mechanism(s) that would support such long term automatic priming effects (given that simple short-lived spread of activation could not). Indeed, this was what social cognition researchers set out to do.

SOCIAL COGNITION'S FIRST EFFORTS TO DESCRIBE THE MECHANISMS UNDERLYING PRIMING EFFECTS

Different corpora of data necessitate somewhat different underlying mechanisms, and social-cognitive psychologists proposed different mechanisms for their new data, including those offered by Higgins (1989; 1996; Higgins & King, 1981), Wyer and Srull (Wyer & Srull, 1981, 1986, 1989), Smith (1993; Smith & Branscombe, 1988), Musswemiler and Strack (1999), and more recently Loersch & Payne (2011). For the purposes of the current paper, these can be described very generally as being something along the lines of what is described below.

Given that mental representations that reflect the external environment (accurately enough) exist, they must somehow correspond to it. Hence, these representations should be activated when the things they correspond to (they are about) are presented to the mind (including by symbolic vehicles; see Huttenlocher & Higgins, 1972). These representations have functional dynamics—in the sense that the accessibility and applicability of the information they carry depends on various factors. As stated above, a more recent addition or emphasis in many such studies is that the above happens automatically, by which is meant that the activation occurs without (or even against) the perceiver's intention and/or awareness (Hassin, 2013).

A version of this picture of mind still frequently appears as the theoretical background of studies that employ priming of the social type (e.g., priming of knowledge related to traits, stereotypes, goals). These frequently begin with a statement along the lines of "as other knowledge structures, traits/stereotypes/goals are mentally represented and hence can be activated by relevant external stimuli." More generally, the idea (explicitly or implicitly) that underlies most papers using the priming method to affect social cognition or behavior stems directly from the above picture of mind. As stated, a similar picture of mind was already apparent in the early theorizing of social-cognitive psychologists who used priming (e.g., Higgins & King, 1981). In this sense, the very large number of priming demonstrations in recent years hasn't added a great deal to a new understanding of how the mind works.

It is also notable that social-cognitive psychologists (but not cognitive or neurocognitive psychologists) distinguished among the effect of priming on increasing a stored representation's *accessibility*, the *applicability* of the stimulated representation in relation to some external target (e.g., the degree of semantic relationship between the primed representation and the *to-be-affected* external target), and, finally, the *judged usability* of an activated representation that determined the final stage of actually using the activated representation to do something (e.g., categorization). This last stage had been discussed more generally in the social psychological literature in terms of the perceived appropriateness or relevance of using information that had become activated for some task at hand (for reviews, see Higgins, 1996; Higgins & Bargh, 1987). Finally, it should also be noted that although, as reviewed briefly above, priming's range of effects significantly expanded in the decades that have passed since it became social, not much new mental explanatory machinery was added, with the notable exception of the addition of an evaluative layer to the purely semantic one (Custers & Aarts, 2005).[5]

MENTAL ACTIVATION AS A FUNCTION OF INFORMATIONAL RELEVANCE

Recently, with the aim of explaining the huge body of data that priming studies have generated and clarifying multiple meanings, while proposing the most parsimonious mechanism possible, we proposed the "relevance of a representation" (ROAR) framework for understanding accessibility or, more specifically, the principle of activation of mental representations (Eitam & Higgins, 2010). Surveying the extant literature suggests that not all representations in memory that are stimulated from priming impact downstream thought and action processes; that is, not all will be activated (or their information become accessible). What underlying mechanisms or processes can account for this? We proposed that whether a stimulated representation in memory is activated (or its information becomes accessible) depends on its *motivational relevance*.

Integrating findings from neuroscience and building on a recently proposed taxonomy of motivation (Higgins, 2011), we clustered documented dynamics of inter-

---

5. We qualify this statement as by some this level adheres to exactly the same principles that the semantic one adheres to (e.g., spread of activation; Fazio & Williams, 1986).

nal reward (e.g., striatal activation) and evaluation (e.g., amygdala activation) as reflecting three sources of informational relevance (Eitam & Higgins, 2010; Eitam & Higgins, 2014; Eitam, Miele, & Higgins, 2013): 1) *Value*: the degree that a representation is related to desired or undesired outcomes; 2) *Control*: the degree that a representation is related to how much control one has (can potentially have) on the internal and external environment; and 3) *Truth*: the degree that a representation is perceived as real (in an epistemic sense) or right (in a moral sense). Building on findings from social and cognitive psychological research, we argued that the accessibility of information carried by a representation is a function of the value, control, or truth relevance of that information. We should emphasize that we are proposing that relevance from value, control, or truth moderates the actual accessibility itself and not just whether accessible representations will be used in cognitive or behavioral responses. The latter moderation would derive more from the judged usability mechanism.

Let us begin by providing an example of how each kind of motivational relevance—as an underlying mechanism—can make a classic priming effect appear or disappear. We start with *value relevance* as an underlying mechanism. What happens to the accessibility of a construct that is primed while pursuing a goal after the goal has been attained (i.e., after goal completion)? The classic and general answer is that accessibility decays rapidly after goal completion, which itself is consistent with the relevance-accessibility function (e.g., Förster, Liberman, & Higgins, 2005; Marsh, Hicks, and Bink, 1998; see also Zeigarnik, 1927). Hedberg and Higgins (2011) considered whether this phenomenon would also vary depending on people's chronic manner of approaching desired outcome or avoiding undesired outcomes. Using Förster and colleagues' (2005) paradigm, the participants were shown sets of pictures of common objects, and their goal was to find when a picture of a pair of eyeglasses is followed immediately by a picture of scissors. While pursuing this goal, "eyeglasses" was repeatedly primed. Once a picture of a pair of eyeglasses was followed immediately by a picture of scissors (i.e., goal completion), the accessibility of "eyeglasses" was measured with a response-time lexical decision task for delays ranging from 0 seconds to 180 seconds (between-participants).

What Hedberg and Higgins (2011) found was that the documented phenomenon of "rapid accessibility decay after goal completion" was stronger for participants who had stronger promotion focus concerns with hopes and aspirations (ideals). This effect might be considered as replicating the classic phenomenon with promotion focus strength as a moderator. But this was not all that was found. For participants who had stronger prevention focus concerns with duties and responsibilities (oughts), the classic phenomenon of "rapid accessibility decay after goal completion" *disappeared*. Indeed, for very strong prevention participants, there was some evidence of increased accessibility as the delay increased (see Figure 1).

What is going on here? What Hedberg and Higgins (2011) proposed was that the dynamics of motivational relevance of a goal-related accessible construct is different for those with a promotion focus than for those with a prevention focus. Individuals with a promotion focus are motivated to advance, to make gains. Once one goal is complete, promotion-focused individuals want to move on to make new advancements and new gains, and an accessible construct from the old goal pursuit does not support this and may hamper this new goal attainment. In the mind's eye of a promotor, such information has no value relevance. The stronger

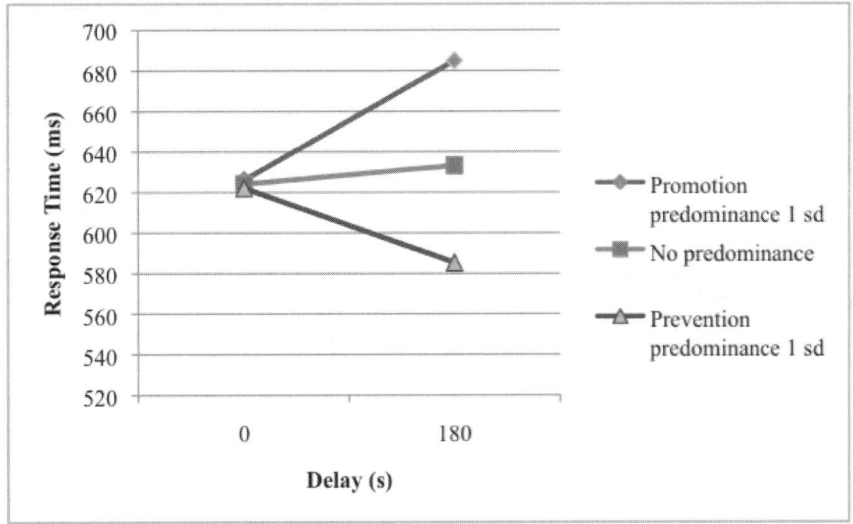

FIGURE 1. Post-Goal Completion Accessibility of "Eyeglasses" as a Function of Delay (Higher Response Times Mean Lower Accessibility)

the promotion focus, the less value relevance the old construct has and the quicker the activation will decay.[6] In contrast, prevention-focused individuals are motivated to maintain a satisfactory state. In the mind's eye of a preventor, its current state (goal completion) *is* satisfactory. Indeed, changing it unnecessarily could be a mistake. Thus, for now, information related to the successful goal pursuit will be maintained because it continues to have value relevance from the recent success, which means there will not be activation decay over this period. Indeed, in this case, valuing maintenance apparently produced higher accessibility for those high in prevention.

Let us now consider *control* as a source of informational relevance. Tools are one of the greatest mental achievements of our species. Using tools, humans have obtained such control over their external (tractors) and internal (medications) environments that it has led to mastering this planet…perhaps. In order to maximize their functionality (their effect over the environment) and their controllability, manufactured tools and artifacts are designed to serve a (today, highly) specific function and hence to be used in a highly specific manner. As an example, imagine an ordinary wine bottle. It shape, size, and weight are all exquisitely balanced to enable a pouring action performed by a human hand connected to a human arm (that is, within arm's length space). If control relevance plays any part in determining activation of mental representations (the accessibility of the concept), then manipulation of control relevance should lead to a change in activation. This is exactly what a study by Costantini, Ambrosini, Scorolli, and Borghi (2011) found.

---

6. Although space limitations will not allow us to develop this point fully, note that the relevance-accessibility perspective opens the possibility for re-evaluating the idea of active maintenance of accessibility. According to ROAR, evaluation of relevance and information accessibility occurs in an ad-hoc manner each time a representation is stimulated (e.g., every time a to-be-judged word appears in a lexical decision task). Hence, maintenance of a representation's activation (i.e., information accessibility) is functionally unnecessary. Accessibility may look *as if* it was temporally extended if the relevance of information has not changed because, in such a case, the activation level will also not change.

Participants were presented with multiple 3D images of tools and artifacts—the same object appearing within arm's reach (i.e., manipulable) and out of reach (nonmanipulable). Immediately after the disappearance of the object, participants saw a verb that was either related to a function ("pour"), to a manipulation ("cork"), or to observation ("look"; that served as the control condition), and was either control relevant or not to the objects they had just seen. Participants had to lift their finger off a key if the verb and the object they had just seen make a reasonable pair (i.e., were control relevant) and to do nothing if they did not (i.e., were control irrelevant). For example, if the object was a wine bottle and the verb "pour" or "cork" appeared, participants were to release the down pressed key, whereas if "dig" or "hammer" appeared, they were to do nothing (observation-related keys were always relevant).

The authors report a main effect for what we termed *control relevance* in that responses to control relevant (functions and manipulation) verbs were faster (i.e., they were more accessible or more "primed" by the object). But interestingly, only the accessibility of control relevant words was modulated by the object's distance. Accessibility of control relevant verbs presented after reachable objects was significantly higher than that of unreachable ones. In fact, control relevant manipulation verbs presented after an unreachable object (i.e., contextually, they were control irrelevant) were not more accessible than looking-related words. What these authors' data show is that (control) relevance must be taken into account when one is measuring the accessibility of concepts (or when one is measuring priming effects for which accessibility is a seemingly necessary but insufficient condition).[7] Does this reflect a failure of experimental rigor or validity? Of course not; if anything, the opposite is true.

Finally, let us now consider *truth* relevance as an underlying mechanism. Priming is not only something that occurs from others exposing us to words (or objects), as in the studies we have reviewed thus far. It is also something that happens from our own verbal responding. An especially interesting version of this is when people tailor or tune their verbal messages to suit the characteristics of their audience (their knowledge, attitudes, goals, etc.). For example, Higgins and Rholes (1978) placed participants in a communication situation in the role of communicator giving a message to an audience. As the communicators, they described the behaviors of a person named Donald to the audience. The communicators are told that the audience belongs to the same club as Donald and that they either *like* or *don't like* Donald very much (the audience attitude manipulation). The communicators are given information about several of Donald's past behaviors, and the behaviors are ambiguous, like the persistent-stubborn behavior we described earlier. They are told that their task is to give a description of Donald to the audience, without mentioning his name, thus allowing the audience to figure out that it is Donald who is the target or referent of the message (a referential communication task). The communicators then describe Donald to the audience. Later, the communicators are asked to recall exactly the behaviors of Donald that they had been originally given.

---

7. Note that although the current example deals with procedural concepts, control relevance applies to any semantic representation; for example, the concept "calm" may have control relevance while reading an annoying review. As parsimony led us to reject adoption of special principles for "trait" as compared to "goal" concepts, it leads us to reject (as far as knowledge activation is concerned) special principles for procedural versus semantic concepts.

The first finding is that participants tailor or tune their message to suit the attitude of the audience, using more positive labels to describe Donald for an audience with a positive attitude toward Donald and more negative labels to describe Donald for an audience with a negative attitude toward Donald. This tuning effect is equivalent to self-induced verbal priming of either positive or negative trait constructs, such as priming "persistent" when the audience has a positive attitude and priming "stubborn" when the audience has a negative attitude. What happens to recall? What Higgins and Rholes (1978) found was that participants with self-induced positive priming had recall reproductions that were positively distorted and participants with self-induced negative priming had recall reproductions that were negatively distorted. This classic priming assimilation effect on memory from audience-tuned messages was given its own phenomenon name—the "saying-is-believing effect."

Many subsequent studies replicated this phenomenon. Then came studies that failed to replicate this phenomenon. Let us discuss one such study. Echterhoff, Higgins, Kopietz, and Groll (2008) had one condition where the communicators' goal was the same as in the Higgins and Rholes' (1978) study (considered the shared reality goal) as well as two other conditions where the goal was different—either an instrumental incentive goal of tuning to the audience's attitude in order to make more money if the audience chose them to be their partner on another task or an entertainment goal of exaggerating the target's traits (positively or negatively) so the audience will have fun. The communicators tuned their message toward the audience's attitude for all three goals. Indeed, the audience tuning effect was significantly stronger for the incentive and entertainment goals than the shared reality goal. This means that the self-induced verbal priming was significantly stronger for the incentive and entertainment goals than for the shared reality goal.

This means that if the saying-is-believing effect phenomenon is a priming assimilation phenomenon, then it should be stronger for the incentive and entertainment goals than the shared reality goal. But that is not what happened. Not only was the phenomenon stronger for the shared reality goal, it actually *disappeared* for the incentive and entertainment goals. Now this can sound like a problem. And it would be a problem if Echterhoff and colleagues were trying to replicate the saying-is-believing effect phenomenon under new conditions—an attempt at generalizing the phenomenon. But that was not the purpose of this study. In fact, the aim was to have a failure to replicate in the incentive and entertainment goal conditions. This is because our concern was to learn more about the mechanism underlying the saying-is-believing effect phenomenon rather than to replicate the phenomenon. Specifically, we believed that the saying-is-believing effect is created by communicators who tune toward their audience in order to create a shared reality with them, and thus tuning for some other goal would eliminate the effect. And creating a shared reality with others is all about trying to be effective in establishing what is real and/or right (see Higgins, 2011)—truth relevance (Eitam & Higgins, 2014; Eitam, Miele, & Higgins, 2013).

Other results of this study provide further support for the importance of truth relevance in understanding how activation occurs from stimulating representations (i.e., recall effects from self-induced verbal priming). The study included questions measuring how much participants considered their message to be the truth about the target person (e.g., How well does your message to your addressee reflect Michael's real characteristics?). As expected, the participants considered

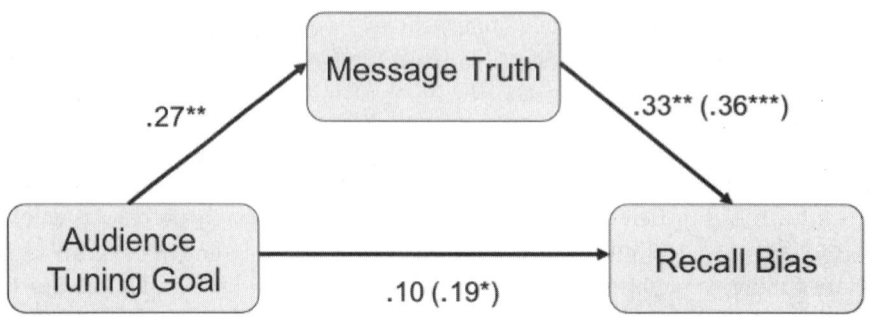

FIGURE 2. Mediation Analysis of Message Truth Mediating the Relation Between Audience Tuning Goal and Recall Bias

their message to be the truth more in the shared reality goal condition than in the incentive goal or entertainment goal condition. And when message truth was included as a potential mediator of the relation between audience tuning goal and recall, message truth was shown to indeed be the mediator (see Figure 2).[8]

This brief review illustrating the role of value, control, and truth relevance to understanding when stimulating representations in memory produces downstream effects on judgment and memory highlights the importance of studying underlying mechanisms and processes rather than being concerned with replicating phenomena per se or even learning *when* a phenomenon will or will not occur (i.e., moderators). It is learning *how* it occurs that is critical. And as you can see from the above discussion, we propose that the mechanism underlying how stimulating representations in memory (i.e., stimulating stored information) produces downstream effects on judgment and memory, that is, activation, is *informational relevance*.

Beyond explanation, the shift from describing phenomena to identifying underlying mechanisms bears other advantages, the central being the ability to link apparently dissimilar phenomena (e.g., priming, implicit memory, and selective attention). In the next and closing section, we attempt to show how this applies to the current case.

RELEVANCE DRIVES SELECTION IN MEMORY AS IT DOES IN PERCEIVING THE WORLD

Ebbinghaus (1885/1964, cited in Roediger, 1990), considered to be the father of the experimental study of memory (Roediger, 1990), differentiated among three forms

---

8. We should note that the motivation to create a shared reality with others can sometimes be more to establish or maintain a relationship with them rather than to establish the truth (an epistemic motive; see Echterhoff, Higgins, & Levine, 2009).

of recollection: 1) *voluntary recollection* in which a person willfully brings to consciousness a "seemingly lost state"; 2) *involuntary recollection* in which a person's previously conscious mental states reappear without their willing it; and 3) when a past experience affects thought or behavior without being consciously recollected itself. Roediger (1990) identified this third type as Ebbinghaus's version of the modern concept of *implicit memory*.

In an important paper, Smith and Branscombe (1987) identified social priming as a case of implicit remembering. In their words: "This category accessibility effect is a form of implicit memory: memory because it constitutes an effect of an earlier experience, and implicit because the task is presented as a judgment rather than a memory task, and in fact the effect can occur without the perceiver's awareness of the prior (priming) episode" (p. 490). One important aspect of Smith and Branscombe's insightful classification is that it places priming in a general class of effects, which allows us to both utilize and contribute to existing knowledge about this class. Specifically, it recasts priming as an unintentional and incidental form of remembering—at least in regard to the conscious perceiver's perspective who (often) has no awareness of the true source of the thought that appears in his mind, and hence *no intention* to access and use the formally primed word or concept in the focal (second) task. From the same perspective, activation is also *incidental* in that it is logically irrelevant to the second task (Förster & Liberman, 2007).

This is exactly the perspective from which the notion of *judged usability* (discussed earlier) is applied: It is the perceiver, unsure about the true source of the activation, who is judging whether to apply the idea active in his mind to the target in question. It is something like asking yourself: "I am thinking 'stubborn,' but should I be using this category to describe this target person's behaviors?" Capitalizing on the "priming as implicit remembering" insight may also enable recasting judged usability in more general terms such as source monitoring (Johnson, Hashtroudi, & Lindsay, 1993) or, even more generally, metacognition of memory (for an interesting example, see Loersch & Payne, 2011). This illustrates how evolving from empirical demonstrations to boundary conditions to *general mechanisms* can serve to link apparently dissimilar phenomena (e.g., automatic stereotyping and eyewitness testimony) and thereby unlock a large body of interrelated knowledge that can now be applied to multiple phenomena.

Before leaving this section, we should emphasize that we are *not* saying that accessibility effects on cognitive processes (e.g., judgment, memory) depend on people being unaware that a priming event has stimulated a particular mental representation. Awareness of the priming event and its causing a representation to come to mind is input to the "judged usability" process, which may or may not lead to a decision that the knowledge is appropriate for the task at hand. Indeed, Higgins and Brendl (1995) found that participants used a primed trait-related representation to categorize a target person's behavior even when they were aware of and remembered the priming event as long as they were also high in chronic accessibility for that representation. As Higgins and Brendl (1995) noted, this is probably because the additional accessibility from the chronic accessibility made the priming event itself no longer perceived as sufficient explanation for the experienced accessibility of the representation, which in turn meant that it was judged usable.

EPILOGUE

Priming has been an important tool in the study of human cognition. As with any experimental task, its ultimate utility will be determined by our ability to utilize it for generating abstract understanding of human cognition. We have built upon uncontested data that priming studies have generated and have argued that a strong focus on general mechanisms will be the most beneficial way to move forward. We have provided one example of such a move using our recently developed ROAR framework.

Given space limitations and the limited power of speculation, we stopped short of demonstrating the degree of generalization that such a mechanism might provide. Relevance, for example, is an important concept in the fields of psycholinguistics (Sperber & Wilson, 1986), information retrieval (Harter, 1992), and cognition. The issue of (selective) activation of representations is also clearly not restricted to memory alone but is at the center of current research on attention as well (Chun, Golomb, & Turk-Browne, 2011; Eitam, Yeshrun & Hassan, 2013), with some current researchers going as far as equating the two (Logan, 2002; see also Neely, 1977; Posner & Snyder, 1975). Relevance of a representation (ROAR) could serve as a bridge not only between topics of study within psychology but also between psychology and other fields. By understanding more about this mechanism, and others as well, we may not only understand particular phenomena more deeply but we can also appreciate how apparently different phenomena actually derive from common underlying processes.

REFERENCES

Aarts, H., & Dijksterhuis, A. (2003). The silence of the library: Environment, situational norm, and social behavior. *Journal of Personality and Social Psychology, 84*(1), 18-28.

Asch, S. E. (1951). Effects of group pressure upon the modification and distortion of judgments. *Groups, Leadership, and Men, S,* 222-236.

Asch, S. E. (1956). Studies of independence and conformity: I. A minority of one against a unanimous majority. Psychological *Monographs: General and Applied, 70*(9), 1-70.

Banaji, M. R., & Hardin, C. D. (1996). Automatic stereotyping. *Psychological Science, 7*(3), 136-141.

Bargh, J. A., Chen, M., & Burrows, L. (1996). Automaticity of social behavior: Direct effects of trait construct and stereotype activation on action. *Journal of Personality and Social Psychology, 71*(2), 230-244.

Bargh, J. A., Lee-Chai, A., Barndollar, K., Gollwitzer, P. M., & Trötschel, R. (2001). The automated will: Nonconscious activation and pursuit of behavioral goals. *Journal of Personality and Social Psychology, 81*(6), 1014-1027.

Bargh, J. A., & Pietromonaco, P. (1982). Automatic information processing and social perception: The influence of trait information presented outside of conscious awareness on impression formation. *Journal of Personality and Social Psychology, 43*(3), 437-449.

Bijleveld, E., Custers, R., & Aarts, H. (2012). Adaptive reward pursuit: How effort requirements affect unconscious reward responses and conscious reward decisions. *Journal of Experimental Psychology: General, 141*(4), 728-742.

Bond, R., & Smith, P. B. (1996). Culture and conformity: A meta-analysis of studies using Asch's (1952b, 1956) line judgment task. *Psychological bulletin, 119*(1), 111-137.

Bruner, J. S. (1957). On perceptual readiness. *Psychological Review, 64*(2), 123-152.

Chun, M. M., Golomb, J. D., & Turk-Browne, N. B. (2011). A taxonomy of external and internal attention. *Annual Review of Psychology, 62*, 73-101.

Collins, A. M., & Loftus, E. F. (1975). A spreading-activation theory of semantic processing. *Psychological Review, 82*(6), 407-428.

Costantini, M., Ambrosini, E., Scorolli, C., & Borghi, A. M. (2011). When objects are close to me: Affordances in the peripersonal space. *Psychonomic Bulletin & Review, 18*(2), 302-308.

Cramer, P. (1964). Successful mediated priming via associative bonds. *Psychological Reports, 15*(1), 235-238.

Custers, R., & Aarts, H. (2005). Positive affect as implicit motivator: On the nonconscious operation of behavioral goals. *Journal of Personality and Social Psychology, 89*(2), 129-142.

DeCoster, J., & Claypool, H. M. (2004). A meta-analysis of priming effects on impression formation supporting a general model of informational biases. *Personality and Social Psychology Review, 8*(1), 2-27.

Echterhoff, G., Higgins, E. T., Kopietz, R., & Groll, S. (2008). How communication goals determine when audience tuning biases memory. *Journal of Experimental Psychology: General, 137*(1), 3-21.

Echterhoff, G., Higgins, E. T., & Levine, J. M. (2009). Shared reality: Experiencing commonality with others' inner states about the world. *Perspectives on Psychological Science, 4*, 496-521.

Eitam, B., Hassin, R. R., & Schul, Y. (2008). Nonconscious goal pursuit in novel environments the case of implicit learning. *Psychological Science, 19*(3), 261-267.

Eitam, B., & Higgins, E. T. (2010). Motivation in mental accessibility: Relevance of a representation (ROAR) as a new framework. *Social and Personality Psychology Compass, 4*, 951-967.

Eitam, B., Miele, D.B., & Higgins, E.T. (2013). Motivated remembering: Remembering as accessibility and accessibility as motivational relevance. In D. Carlston (Ed.), *Handbook of social cognition* (pp. 463-475). New York: Oxford University Press.

Eitam, B., Yeshurun, Y., & Hassan, K. (2013). Blinded by irrelevance: Pure irrelevance induced blindness. *Journal of Experimental Psychology: Human Processing and Performance, 39*, 611-615.

Fazio, R. H., & Williams, C. J. (1986). Attitude accessibility as a moderator of the attitude-perception and attitude-behavior relations: An investigation of the 1984 presidential election. *Journal of Personality and Social Psychology, 51*(3), 505-514.

Fodor, J. A. (1975). *The language of thought*. Cambridge, MA: Harvard University Press.

Förster, J., & Liberman, N. (2007). Knowledge activation. In A. W. Kruglanski, & E. T. Higgins (Eds.), *Social psychology: Handbook of basic principles* (pp. 201-231). New York: Guilford.

Förster, J., Liberman, N., & Higgins, E. T. (2005). Accessibility from active and fulfilled goals. *Journal of Experimental Social Psychology, 41*(3), 220-239.

Förster, J., Liberman, N., & Kuschel, S. (2008). The effect of global versus local processing styles on assimilation versus contrast in social judgment. *Journal of Personality and Social Psychology, 94*(4), 579-599.

Harter, S. P. (1992). Psychological relevance and information science. *Journal of the American Society for Information Science, 43*(9), 602-615.

Hassin, R. R. (2013). Yes it can. On the functional abilities of the human unconscious. *Perspectives on Psychological Science, 8*(2), 195-207.

Hassin, R. R., Ferguson, M. J., Shidlovski, D., & Gross, T. (2007). Subliminal exposure to national flags affects political thought and behavior. *Proceedings of the National Academy of Sciences, 104*(50), 19757-19761.

Hedberg, P. H., & Higgins, E. T. (2011). What remains on your mind after you are done? Flexible regulation of knowledge accessibility. *Journal of Experimental Social Psychology, 47*(5), 882-890.

Herr, P. M., Sherman, S. J., & Fazio, R. H. (1983). On the consequences of priming: Assimilation and contrast effects. *Journal of Experimental Social Psychology, 19*(4), 323-340.

Higgins, E. T. (1989). Knowledge accessibility and activation: Subjectivity and suffering from unconscious sources. In J. S. Uleman & J. A. Bargh (Eds.), *Unintended thought: The limits of awareness, intention and control* (pp. 75-123). New York: Guilford.

Higgins, E. T. (1996). Knowledge activation: Accessibility, applicability, and salience. In E. T. Higgins & A. W. Kruglanski (Eds.), *Social psychology: Handbook of basic principles* (pp. 133-168). New York: Guilford.

Higgins, E. T. (2011). *Beyond pleasure and pain: How motivation works*. New York: Oxford University Press.

Higgins, E. T., & Bargh, J. A. (1987). Social cognition and social perception. *Annual Review of Psychology, 38*(1), 369-425.

Higgins, E. T., & Brendl, C. M. (1995). Accessibility and applicability: Some "activation rules" influencing judgment. *Journal of Experimental Social Psychology, 31*, 218-243.

Higgins, E. T., & Chaires, W. M. (1980). Accessibility of interrelational constructs: Implications for stimulus encoding and creativity. *Journal of Experimental Social Psychology, 16*(4), 348-361.

Higgins, E. T., & Eitam, B. (2014). What's in a goal? The role of motivational relevance in cognition and action. *Behavioral and Brain Sciences, 37*(2), 141-142.

Higgins, E. T., & King, G. (1981). Accessibility of social constructs: Information processing consequences of individual and contextual variability. In N. Cantor & J. Kihlstrom (Eds.), *Personality, cognition, and social interaction* (pp. 69-121). Hillsdale, NJ: Erlbaum.

Higgins, E. T., & Rholes, W. S. (1978). "Saying is believing": Effects of message modification on memory and liking for the person described. *Journal of Experimental Social Psychology, 14*(4), 363-378.

Higgins, E. T., Rholes, W. S., & Jones, C. R. (1977). Category accessibility and impression formation. *Journal of Experimental Social Psychology, 13*(2), 141-154.

Huttenlocher, J., & Higgins, E. T. (1972). On reasoning, congruence, and other matters. *Psychological Review, 79*, 420-427.

Johnson, M. K., Hashtroudi, S., & Lindsay, D. S. (1993). Source monitoring. *Psychological Bulletin, 114*(1), 3-28.

Kleiman, T., & Hassin, R. R. (2011). Non-conscious goal conflicts. *Journal of Experimental Social Psychology, 47*(3), 521-532.

Lalancette, M. F., & Standing, L. (1990). Asch fails again. *Social Behavior and Personality, 18*(1), 7-12.

Loersch, C., & Payne, B. K. (2011). The situated inference model an integrative account of the effects of primes on perception, behavior, and motivation. *Perspectives on Psychological Science, 6*(3), 234-252.

Loftus, E. F. (1973). Activation of semantic memory. *American Journal of Psychology*, 331-337-400.

Logan, G. D. (2002). An instance theory of attention and memory. *Psychological Review, 109*(2), 376-400.

Lombardi, W. J., Higgins, E. T., & Bargh, J. A. (1987). The role of consciousness in priming effects on categorization assimilation versus contrast as a function of awareness of the priming task. *Personality and Social Psychology Bulletin, 13*(3), 411-429.

Mackay, D. G. (1973). Aspects of the theory of comprehension, memory and attention. *Quarterly Journal of Experimental Psychology, 25*(1), 22-40.

Marsh, R. L., Hicks, J. L., & Bink, M. L. (1998). Activation of completed, uncompleted, and partially completed intentions. *Journal of Experimental Psychology: Learning, Memory, and Cognition, 24*(2), 350-361.

Martin, L. L. (1986). Set/reset: Use and disuse of concepts in impression formation. *Journal of Personality and Social Psychology, 51*(3), 493-504.

Mussweiler, T., & Strack, F. (1999). Comparing is believing: A selective accessibility model of judgmental anchoring. In W. Stroebe & M. Hewstone (Eds.), *European Review of Social Psychology* (Vol. 10; pp. 135-167). New York: Wiley.

Neely, J. H. (1977). Semantic priming and retrieval from lexical memory: Roles of inhibitionless spreading activation and limited-capacity attention. *Journal of Experimental Psychology: General, 106*(3), 226-254.

Newman, L. S., & Uleman, J. S. (1990). Assimilation and contrast effects in spontaneous trait inference. *Personality and Social Psychology Bulletin, 16*(2), 224-240.

Perrin, S., & Spencer, C. (1981). Independence or conformity in the Asch experiment as a reflection of cultural and situational factors. *British Journal of Social Psychology, 20*(3), 205-209.

Posner, M. I., & Snyder, C. R. R. (1975). Facilitation and inhibition in the processing of signals. *Attention and Performance V,* 669-682.

Roediger, H. L. (1990). Implicit memory: Retention without remembering. *American Psychologist, 45*(9), 1043-1056.

Rumelhart, D. E., & McClelland, J. L. (1986). *Parallel distributed processing: Explorations in the microstructure of cognition. Volume 1. Foundations.* Cambridge, MA: MIT Press.

Schwarz, N., & Bless, H. (1992). Constructing reality and its alternatives: An inclusion/exclusion model of assimilation and contrast effects in social judgment. In L. L. Martin & A. Tesser (Eds.), *The construction of social judgments* (pp. 217-245). Hillsdale, NJ: Erlbaum.

Smith, E. R. (1989). Procedural efficiency: General and specific components and effects on social judgment. *Journal of Experimental Social Psychology, 25*(6), 500-523.

Smith, E. R. (1993). Procedural knowledge and processing strategies in social cognition. In R. S. Wyer & T. K. Srull (Eds.), *Handbook of social cognition* (2nd Ed., Vol. 1; pp. 99-151). Hillsdale, NJ: Erlbaum.

Smith, E. R., & Branscombe, N. R. (1987). Procedurally mediated social inferences: The case of category accessibility effects. *Journal of Experimental Social Psychology, 23*(5), 361-382.

Smith, E. R., & Branscombe, N. R. (1988). Category accessibility as implicit memory. *Journal of Experimental Social Psychology, 24*(6), 490-504.

Sperber, D., & Wilson, D. (1986). *Relevance: Communication and cognition* (Vol. 142). Cambridge, MA: Harvard University Press.

Srull, T. K., & Wyer, R. S. (1979). The role of category accessibility in the interpretation of information about persons: Some determinants and implications. *Journal of Personality and Social Psychology, 37*(10), 1660-1672.

Srull, T. K., & Wyer, R. S. (1980). Category accessibility and social perception: Some implications for the study of person memory and interpersonal judgments. *Journal of Personality and Social Psychology, 38*(6), 841-856.

Storms, L. H. (1958). Apparent backward association: A situational effect. *Journal of Experimental Psychology, 55*(4), 390-395.

Strack, F., Schwarz, N., Bless, H., Kübler, A., & Wänke, M. (1993). Awareness of the influence as a determinant of assimilation versus contrast. *European Journal of Social Psychology, 23*(1), 53-62.

Tulving, E., & Pearlstone, Z. (1966). Availability versus accessibility of information in memory for words. *Journal of Verbal Learning and Verbal Behavior, 5*(4), 381-391.

Tulving, E., & Schacter, D. L. (1990). Priming and human memory systems. *Science, 247*(4940), 301-306.

Wyer, R. S., & Srull, T. K. (1981). Category accessibility: Some theoretical and empirical issues concerning the processing of social stimulus information. In E. T. Higgins, C. P. Herman, & M. P. Zanna (Eds.), *Social cognition: The Ontario symposium* (Vol. 1; pp. 161-197). Hillsdale, NJ: Erlbaum.

Wyer, R. S., & Srull, T. K. (1986). Human cognition in its social context. *Psychological Review, 93*(3), 322-359.

Wyer, R. S., & Srull, T. K. (1989). *Memory and cognition in its social context.* Hillsdale, NJ: Erlbaum.

Zanna, M. P., & Fazio, R. H. (1982). The attitude-behavior relation: Moving toward a third generation of research. In M. P. Zanna, E. T. Higgins, & C. P. Herman (Eds.), *Consistency in social behavior: The Ontario symposium* (Vol. 2; pp. 283-301). Hillsdale, NJ: Erlbaum.

Zeigarnik, B. (1927). Über das behalten von erledigten und unerledigten handlungen. [The memory of completed and uncompleted actions]. *Psychologische Forschung, 9*(1), 1-85.

UNDERSTANDING PRIMING EFFECTS IN SOCIAL PSYCHOLOGY: AN OVERVIEW AND INTEGRATION

Daniel C. Molden
Northwestern University

> Although much debate has recently focused on the robustness of certain types of priming effects in social psychology, few attempts have been made to examine the full breadth of this literature and consider what is known about priming and what is still left to learn. The goal of this volume was to provide such consideration. This final chapter of this volume provides a brief overview and integration of the insights provided in each of the other chapters included, focusing primarily on revelations about (a) the greater need for clarity and precision in conceptualizing and communicating about priming effects, (b) the issues concerning expectations of replication and when priming effects should occur, and (c) the new insights about the psychological processes by which primes activate stored representations and by which these activated representations are applied to judgment and behavior.

Although much discussion has recently focused on the robustness and replicability of certain types of priming effects in social psychology (e.g., Cesario, 2014; Simons, 2014), this discussion has not truly examined the full breadth of such effects and more carefully considered what is known about priming and what is still left to learn. In bringing together contributions from pioneers in research on priming social impressions and behaviors, as well as recent innovators and critics in this area, this volume aims to provide such consideration.

In this final chapter, I provide a brief overview and integration of the insights presented in each of the other contributions. My comments focus on three primary themes that emerged as challenges priming researchers in social psychology must meet to continue to advance this field: (1) greater precision in conceptualizing and communicating about priming effects, (2) greater attention to when these effects should occur (and when they should not), and (3) better understanding of the

---

Address correspondence to Daniel C. Molden, Northwestern University, 2029 Sheridan Rd., Evanston, IL 60208. E-mail: molden@northwestern.edu.

mechanisms for both the activation of social representations and the subsequent application of these representations during judgment and behavior.

CONCEPTUALIZING AND COMMUNICATING ABOUT PRIMING EFFECTS

Social psychologists have long known that the *automaticity* of a process is not a unitary concept and instead constitutes the presence of several separate qualities, such as lack of awareness that the process is occurring, lack of intention to initiate it, or an inability to control it once initiated (e.g., Bargh, 1989). Despite this knowledge, researchers still often carelessly discuss "automatic" priming effects without specifying which of these qualities such effects are assumed to possess. As Doyen, Klein, Simons, and Cleeremans (2014, this volume) and Newell and Shanks (2014, this volume) both illustrate in their contributions to this volume, such carelessness can breed confusion and even skepticism, particularly among researchers in other areas of psychology.

For example, among researchers who study implicit memory, the question of whether people are completely unaware of perceiving the primes that influence their later responses is of critical importance. Social psychologists also frequently describe priming as occurring "outside of awareness," but here the term almost always refers to the awareness of the *influence* of the prime on subsequent responses rather than of the prime itself (Molden, 2014, this volume). Indeed, many, if not most, priming effects involve conscious processing of the relevant stimuli (see in this volume Bargh, 2014; Ferguson & Mann, 2014; Fujita & Trope, 2014; Higgins & Eitam, 2014; Wentura & Rothermund, 2014). Thus, failing to specify the priming mechanisms under investigation can create misunderstandings that lead researchers more familiar with the implicit memory literature (in which conclusive demonstrations of the complete absence of awareness have proven difficult, see in this volume Doyen et al., 2014; Newell & Shanks, 2014) to doubt any claims that are made. Similarly, when social psychologists describe priming as occurring "without intention," this typically does not further imply the absence of control if one becomes aware of the potential influence of the primes (Molden, 2014, this volume). This too can create miscommunication and skepticism when evidence for control over particular priming effects is observed (see Newell & Shanks, 2014, this volume).

The chapterss in this book by Doyen and colleagues (2014) and Newell and Shanks (2014) also illustrate that beyond better specifying the basic assumptions about the particular priming effects they are studying, researchers need to gather better evidence supporting these assumptions. For example, both chapters describe several limitations in the typical methods used to check for awareness of the prime or its influence and the more stringent tests necessary support claims for the absence of awareness. Newell and Shanks further describe how evidence for a lack of control can be misleading if the methods used to encourage people to exert control are not carefully designed (e.g., broadly manipulating people's motivation to avoid a particular outcome rather than more precisely targeting their motivation to be influenced by the priming process itself).

Finally, as Wentura and Rothermund (2014, this volume) discuss in their contribution, beyond greater care in communicating and evaluating assumptions about the priming effects they are studying, social psychologists should be more precise in how they discuss the mechanisms responsible for such effects. Too frequently, researchers simply explain the priming effects they observe with brief references to some mechanism of "spreading activation" or "increased accessibility" of prime-relevant representations. However, as Wentura and Rothermund detail, such mechanisms on their own can only explain short-term priming effects on the order of seconds rather than the longer-term priming effects social psychologists typically investigate, and more delayed effects must involve some additional encoding processes (see also Molden, 2014, this volume). This is yet another way in which miscommunications that breed skepticism can arise between researchers studying more short-term effects of accessibility and social psychologists studying long-term forms of priming.

THE QUESTION OF REPLICATION AND PREDICTING WHEN PRIMING SHOULD OCCUR

Issues concerning the replicability of priming effects in social psychology are not the primary focus of this book and have been thoroughly addressed elsewhere, but there are a few additional points worth noting here. First, as Ferguson and Mann (2014) discuss in their contribution to the book, given the broad range of effects that can be labeled as "social priming" (see also Molden, 2014, this volume), claims about the lack of evidence for these types of priming effects as a whole are largely nonsensical. Furthermore, although studies that fail to replicate more specific effects of particular primes raise legitimate questions about the robustness of those effects, as Dijksterhuis, van Knippenberg, and Holland (2014) and Wheeler, DeMarree, and Petty (2014) both note in their contributions to this book, it is important not to over-interpret such findings. Even the most robust psychological effects have many variables that qualify their size or occurrence, and research has long shown that priming effects are no exception. If known qualifiers of priming effects are not adequately assessed, direct replication should not be expected (even if these qualifiers were not yet appreciated in the original demonstration of the effect). Indeed, as Wheeler and colleagues further note, because variations in the samples of participants studied or environments in which these studies occur can alter the social representations activated by primes or shift the targets to which the prime is applied, evaluating successful replication also requires verification of the expected activation and application.

However, as Cesario and Jonas (2014) and Higgins & Eitam (2014) emphasize in their contributions to this book, perhaps the most important factor in not only ensuring replication but also predicting and understanding when priming effects should occur is determining the mechanisms responsible for such effects. That is, not fully knowing why a priming effect occurs can create mistaken expectations about when the effect should be observed. Moreover, when the goal is determining the mechanisms of priming effects, failures to replicate the effect can actually provide opportunities to consider what changes in procedures or circumstances might explain this failure. Therefore, priming research will progress more by examining not just variables that might alter when these effects occur but also variables that determine why.

At the same time, the presence of qualifying variables or an incomplete understanding of priming effects should not simply excuse failures to replicate these effects. As both Cesario and Jonas (2014, this volume) and Doyen and colleagues (2014, this volume) discuss, in searching for the boundary conditions and mechanisms of priming effects, social psychologists have favored conceptual replications that extend the original findings over direct replications that simply reproduce them. Despite the value of the former approach for explaining priming effects, it also has costs. The failure of a conceptual replication could reveal new qualifying variables or provide clues to the psychological mechanisms at work, but it also cannot provide unambiguous information about the overall reliability of the phenomenon itself (i.e., does the failure mean the phenomenon is not robust or just does not extend to the new conditions examined?). Therefore, some greater emphasis on direct replication in addition to conceptual replication is likely necessary to maximize what can be learned from further research on priming (but see Stroebe and Strack, 2014, for costs of overemphasizing direct replication as well).

EXPLAINING THE ACTIVATION AND APPLICATION OF PRIMED REPRESENTATIONS

Although new controversy has recently arisen in research on priming effects in social psychology, so too have new developments in theories of how these effects occur. Again, because of the diversity in the priming effects studied, many different accounts for these effects have been offered (Molden, 2014, this volume). However, a consensus is forming that, with the possible exception of phenomena that involve short-term evaluative priming (Ferguson & Mann, 2014, this volume; Wentura & Rothermund, 2014, this volume), priming effects in social psychology must depend on more than the increased accessibility of prime-relevant representations through some form of spreading activation, which, as noted earlier, is often the simple explanation researchers currently invoke.

Indeed, as discussed in this volume by Doyen and colleagues (2014) and Newell and Shanks (2014), one source of the recent controversy over priming effects on behavior is skepticism about the adequacy of spreading activation, or *direct expression*, mechanisms to explain these effects. Moreover, although one can dispute whether Newell and Shanks' critique of direct expression accounts of anchoring effects is truly relevant to the priming effects on behavior typically examined by social psychologists, it is hard to question the broader points their critique raises about gaps between claims of automatic direct expression and the evidence for this mechanism. Nevertheless, this type of skepticism also does not sufficiently credit recent developments in formulating alternative mechanisms, which was the focus of several chapters in this volume.

Higgins and Eitam (2014, this volume) describe an account of priming effects that challenges direct expression perspectives of how primes activate social representations in memory. In their account, the accessibility of primed representations depends on the motivational *relevance* of the primes. That is, although primes may stimulate particular representations whenever they are encountered, these representations only become activated for potential use in impressions and behaviors when they are congruent with one's current motivations. Cesario and Jonas (2014, this volume) present a related account that focuses more narrowly on priming effects on behavior. They discuss how shifts in people's perceived resources for enacting particular behaviors, which can vary with their current states or environments, can determine what representations of behavior primes activate. Thus, Cesario and Jonas outline some specific factors that could contribute to perceived relevance of a prime in Higgins and Eitam's model. The primary implications of both these models, then, is that the primes people encounter in their environments should not be expected to always result in the same direct expression in thought and behavior because they should not always activate the same set of social representations.

Complementing these perspectives on priming effects, Loersch and Payne (2014, this volume) describe an account of priming that challenges direct expression perspectives of how social representations already activated in memory are applied to social impressions and behaviors. That is, they propose that primed representations affect responses only when the heightened accessibility of these representations is further misattributed to a particular source. Different types of sources produce different types of responses (e.g., attributing the accessibility to another person alters social impressions, to one's own desires alters goal pursuit, and to one's choice of actions alters behavior). Similarly, Wheeler, DeMarree, and Petty (2014, this volume) describe an account of priming effects on behavior that involves how accessible social representations temporarily alter what is salient in people's *active self-concept*, which then influences their chosen behavior. Therefore, the primary implication of both these models is that even when primes do activate a shared social representation across different individuals and circumstances, the differential attributions for the source of the prime or differential assimilation of the prime to the self should alter the expression of the activated representation.

In addition to variations in the specific processes of activating and applying primed social representations, Fujita and Trope (2014, this volume) identify other factors that could alter the effects of these primed representations. They first describe mindsets involving what they label *unstructured* regulation, in which the activation and application of primed representations are determined more by the relevance of and attributions from the narrow and concrete goals afforded by people's present environment. They then contrast this with mindsets involving *structured* regulation, in which the activation and application of primed representations are determined more by the relevance of and attributions from the broad and abstract goals people impose on their present environment. That these unstructured versus structured mindsets themselves may be primed adds yet another layer to the challenge of predicting and understanding when primed social representations should influence thought and behavior.

Even though all of these different accounts of priming effects in social psychology complement each other and are not in conflict, Doyen and colleagues (2014, this volume) are correct in noting that integrating these models to anticipate when such effects should arise is complex and daunting. Although only further research will ultimately determine whether this challenge can be met, Schröder and Thagard's (2014) contribution to this book suggests that such a challenge is not insurmountable. Adopting the promising approach of mathematically modeling the simultaneous influence of various factors on the activation and application of primed knowledge (see Sherman, Klauer, & Allen, 2010), they outline a parallel-constraint satisfaction model that describes how variables such as the perceived relevance of a prime, attributions of accessibility to a particular target, and active self-representations can be conceptualized as changes in affective meanings within a connectionist neural network. They then illustrate how the integrated influence of these meanings can be calculated as stable patterns of activation and inhibition into which the network settles and discuss evidence that this model can conceptually reproduce observed priming effects. Thus, while it may be complicated, the possibility of integrating all of the various processes that could influence priming into a single clear prediction does not appear to be entirely out of reach.

Finally, although he too acknowledges that additional processes, such as assimilation to one's self-concept, can influence priming effects, Bargh (2014, this volume) describes a specific set of circumstances in which the direct expression of links between people's perceptions and their primed behaviors is at least more plausible. Rather than focusing on the temporary activation of behavior representations by semantic associates from a previous context (e.g., while reading trait- and stereotype-relevant words), he discusses more naturalistic examples of priming in which these representations are continually activated within one's present environment (e.g., when perceiving an interaction partner's behaviors or the state of one's current environment). These latter cases should still, in theory, be susceptible to influences such as the relevance of the prime or to what the accessibility it creates is attributed, which is inconsistent with the strongest form of direct expression mechanisms for priming effects. However, primes that remain present in one's environment may not require additional encoding and interpretive processes to have their influence in the way that primes encountered in previous, unrelated circumstances do (see Molden, 2014, this volume). Thus, whether such ecological priming effects involve the exact same mechanisms as the more symbolic effects considered in most research and theorizing is an important question for future research. Regardless of the outcome of such research, in reviewing examples of ecological priming effects that arise in real-world contexts, Bargh argues that it is by these effects that the importance and reliability of social priming should be judged.

SUMMARY AND CONCLUSIONS

In conclusion, although questions surrounding various aspects of how robust the priming effects studied by social psychologists are and the mechanisms by which they occur are likely to persist, this book provides the beginning of a blueprint through which such questions can be addressed. First, priming researchers must strive to conceptualize and communicate with greater precision about the specific phenomena they are studying and to provide evidence for the assumptions embedded in their conceptualizations. Second, priming researchers must recognize and assess a variety of factors that are known to qualify the effects they are studying, regardless of whether such qualifiers were present in the original research on a particular effect. Finally, both of these goals can only fully be reached through further research focused solely on how and why different types of priming effects occur (which, as discussed, is well under way).

If this blueprint is followed, then, as illustrated by the contributions to this book by Lakens (2014) and Smith and Mackie (2014) that outline new ways in which priming effects may arise through people's enactment of behavior or their mere simulation of the behavior of others, research on priming in social psychology can continue to expand. That is, by rededicating themselves to determining how, when, and why various priming effects occur, social psychologists will be able to demonstrate that, rather than facing an end-of-life crisis, research on priming is experiencing more of an adolescence in which, after a period of awkwardness following a rapid growth spurt, it is ready to begin developing the maturity necessary for the challenges that await.

REFERENCES

Bargh, J. A. (1989). Conditional automaticity: Varieties of automatic influence in social perception and cognition. In J. S. Uleman & J. A. Bargh (Eds.), *Unintended thought* (pp. 3-51). New York: Guilford.

Bargh, J. A. (2014). The historical origins of priming as the preparation of behavioral responses: Unconscious carry-over and contextual influences of real-world importance. This volume.

Cesario, J. (2014). Priming, replication, and the hardest science. *Perspectives on Psychological Science, 9*, 40-48.

Cesario, J., & Jonas, K. J. (2014). Replicability and models of priming: What a resource computation framework can tell us about expectations of replicability. This volume.

Dijksterhuis, A., van Knippenberg, A., & Holland, R. W. (2014). Evaluating behavior priming research: Three observations and a recommendation. This volume.

Doyen, S., Klein, O., Simons, D., & Cleeremans, A. (2014). On the other side of the mirror: Priming in cognitive and social psychology. This volume.

Ferguson, M. J., & Mann, T. C. (2014). Effects of evaluation: An example of robust "social" priming. This volume.

Fujita, K., & Trope, Y. (2014). Structured versus unstructured regulation: On procedural mindsets and the mechanisms of priming effects. This volume.

Higgins, E. T., & Eitam, B. (2014). Priming... Shmiming: It's about knowing *when* and *why* stimulated memory representations become active. This volume.

Lakens, D. (2014). Grounding social embodiment. This volume.

Loersch, C., & Payne, B. K. (2014). Situated inference and the what, who, and where of priming. This volume.

Molden, D. C. (2014). Understanding priming effects in social psychology: What is "social priming" and how does it occur? This volume.

Newell, B. R., & Shanks, D. R. (2014). Prime numbers: Anchoring and its implications for theories of behavior priming. This volume.

Schröder, T., & Thagard, P. (2014). Priming: Constraint satisfaction and interactive competition. This volume.

Sherman, J. W., Klauer, K. C., & Allen, T. J. (2010). Mathematical modeling of implicit social cognition: The machine in the ghost. In B. Gawronski & B. K. Payne (Eds.), *Handbook of implicit social cognition: Measurement, theory, and applications* (pp. 156-175). New York: Guilford.

Simons, D. J. (2014). The value of direct replication. *Perspectives on Psychological Science, 9,* 76-80.

Smith, E. R., & Mackie, D. M. (2014). Priming from others' observed or simulated responses. This volume.

Stroebe, W. & Strack, F. (2014). The alleged crisis and the illusion of direct replication. *Perspectives on Psychological Science, 9,* 59-71.

Wentura, D., & Rothermund, K. (2014). Priming is not priming is not priming. This volume.

Wheeler, S. C., DeMarree, & Petty, R. E. (2014). Understanding prime-to-behavior effects: Insights from the active-self account. This volume.

INDEX

Page numbers followed by *f* indicate a figure.

Accessibility
 memory activation and, 239, 247
 moderators of priming effects and, 147–148
 overview, 73
 short-term priming and, 56–57
 situated inference model and, 143, 143*f*, 145
ACT model of skill acquisition, 72–73
Activated representation, 191–192
Activation, memory. *See also* Memory
 overview, 234–235, 238–246, 241–246, 243*f*, 246*f*
 from phenomena to boundary conditions to mechanisms, 235–238
 relevance and, 246–247
Activation, spreading
 overview, 18–19, 28–29, 131–132, 139, 255–257
 short-term priming and, 56
 stereotype activation, 23
 structural resources and, 136
Active self-concept. *See also* Active-Self Account; Self-concept
 overview, 9, 120
 priming effects and, 116–119
 replicability and, 120–124
Active-Self Account. *See also* Active self-concept
 overview, 114–116
 priming effects and, 116–119
 replicability and, 120–124
Activity-arousal
 affective meanings, 160
 localist connectionist model and, 161
Adaptation, 240
Affect control theory, 168
Affective meanings
 neural computation of priming and, 168
 parallel constraint satisfaction, 159–160
Affective Misattribution Procedure (AMP)
 overview, 38–39
 response priming paradigms and, 53
 responses from others and, 194
 unintentional prime evaluation and, 39–41

Affective reactions, 191–192
Afforded questions, 143*f*, 144
Aggression, 74
Ambiguity, 73
Amygdala, 165*f*, 167, 167*f*
Anchoring effects
 influence of, 101–105
 long-term semantic priming, 61–62
 overview, 9, 93–95, 109–110
 as priming, 95–97
 processing accounts of, 97–98
 situated-inference model and, 108–109
 subliminal priming and, 99–101
 transfer and, 105–108
Anchoring-and-adjustment account, 98
Anterior cingulate cortex (ACC), 165*f*, 167, 167*f*
Approach, 227
Aspects of the priming event, 145–146
Aspects of the target, 146–147
Assessment
 influence of an anchor and, 102
 measuring awareness and, 16–18, 24–27
 subliminal priming and, 100
Assimilation, 118, 119, 236–238
Associated systems theory (AST), 182–183, 184
Assumptions, 253–254
Attention, 209–210
Attitudes, 38
Attributions. *See* Misattributions
Automatic effects of primes, 21–23
Automaticity
 anchoring as priming and, 97–98
 counterintuitiveness of findings regarding, 208–210
 incidental memory activation and, 239
 influence of an anchor and, 103
 overview, 253–254
 resource computation model of, 132–133
 responses from others and, 196

Automaticity *(cont.)*
  social embodiment and, 184
  subliminal priming and, 99–101
Avoidance, 227
Awareness
  incidental memory activation and, 240
  of the influence of an anchor, 101–102
  measuring, 16–18, 24–27
  overview, 27–28, 253–254
  social psychology and, 24–27
Awareness, lack of, 7, 97

B

Basal ganglia, 167, 167f
Behavior. *See also* Behavioral priming
  evaluation and, 42–44
  long-term semantic priming, 62–63
Behavioral imitation, 197, 222–229
Behavioral plans, 191–192
Behavioral priming
  counterintuitiveness of findings regarding, 208–210
  evaluative priming and, 42–44
  evidence supporting, 206–208
  information leakage and, 212–213
  intentional behavior and, 166–167, 167f
  localist connectionist model and, 160–163
  moderators of, 210–211
  neurocomputational model of, 164–165, 165f
  overview, 36–38, 93–95, 114–115, 205–206, 213, 218–220, 229–230
  perception-behavior link, 222–229
  situated inference model and, 143f
Behavioral responses, 220
Boundary conditions, 235–238

C

Choices, 9–10
Circular reasoning, 209
Cognition
  evaluation and, 42–44
  social embodiment and, 185
Cognitive psychology
  incidental memory activation and, 239–240
  measuring awareness and, 17–18
  overview, 14–16, 30
  priming in, 18–21
  replicability and, 29–30
  response priming paradigms and, 53
  spreading activation and, 27–28
Competence, 160
Competition, 157–158
Computational model, 10
Conceptual metaphor theory (CMT), 178–180, 184, 186

Concrete cues, 184
Confidence judgment, 16
Conscious priming, 143
Consciousness, 209–210
Constraint satisfaction
  affective meanings, 159–160
  intentional behavior and, 166–167, 167f
  localist connectionist model and, 160–163, 161f
  neural computation of priming and, 163–166, 165f
  overview, 157–158, 168–169
  parallel constraint satisfaction, 158–163, 161f
Construal level
  overview, 78–79
  role of in unstructured and structured regulation, 79–82
  situational cues and, 83–84
  traditional priming effects and, 82–83
Construal level theory (CLT), 78–79, 79–82. *See also* Construal level
Construal priming, 74–75, 143f
Constructionist perspective, 74–75
Content, priming process rather than, 72–73
Context-specificity
  situated inference model and, 150–152
  social embodiment and, 181–182
Contingency awareness
  lack of, 73
  replicability and, 131–132
Contrast, 119, 236–238
Control relevance, 244
Core processes, 148

D

Decision-making processes
  neural computation of priming and, 167
  situated inference model and, 145
Direct expression, 9, 255
Dispositional attributions, automaticity and, 23
Dissociation logic, 17

E

Eating behavior, perception-behavior link and, 225–226
Elderly behavior
  long-term semantic priming, 62
  replicability and, 131–132
  research support and, 206–208
Embodiment, social
  associated systems theory (AST) and, 182–183
  empirical data, 177–178
  overview, 175–177, 186
  social inferences and, 182–186
  theoretical frameworks, 178–182
Encoding mechanisms, 9–10, 16–17

Index

EPA space
  affective meanings, 160
  localist connectionist model and, 161
  neural computation of priming and, 164
Evaluation. *See also* Evaluation-valence; Evaluative priming
  behavioral priming and, 42–44
  construal level and, 81
  effects of, 38–42
  overview, 35–36, 44, 253–254
Evaluation-valence. *See also* Evaluation
  affective meanings, 160
  localist connectionist model and, 161
Evaluative priming. *See also* Evaluation
  behavioral priming and, 42–44
  effects of, 38–42
  overview, 44
  social embodiment and, 184
Evaluative priming task (EPT), 38–41. *See also* Evaluative priming
Evolutionary accounts of the mind, 133
Experimental psychology, 221

F

Flexibility, 145
Fluency, 83–84
Forced-choice measures
  measuring awareness and, 16
  subliminal priming and, 100
Functional magnetic resonance imaging (fMRI), 228–229
Funnel debriefing, 24–25, 100
Funnel interview, 16

G

Goal priming, 36–38, 143*f*
Goal-directed adaptation, 240
Goals
  activated representation and, 191–192
  perception-behavior link and, 227
  responses from others and, 192
Goal-undermining temptations, 77

H

High-level construal, 81. *See also* Construal level

I

Identification tasks, 16
Imitation, 197, 222–229
Immediacy criterion, 17–18
Implicit Association Test (IAT)
  overview, 39
  social resources and, 138
  unintentional prime evaluation and, 39–41
Implicit learning, 18
Implicit memory, 16, 247
Implicit-explicit correlations, 150
Impression formation, automaticity and, 23
Incidental memory activation, 238–246, 243*f*, 246*f*. *See also* Memory activation
Individual differences, social embodiment and, 185
Inferences. *See also* Situated-inference model
  metacognitive inferences, 149
  social embodiment and, 181–186
Information leakage, 212–213
Information processing, social embodiment and, 176
Informational relevance, memory activation and, 241–246, 243*f*, 246*f*
Intelligent behavior, long-term semantic priming, 62–63
Intentions
  memory selection and, 247
  neural computation of priming and, 166–167, 167*f*
Interactive competition, 157–158
Interpersonal motivations
  neural computation of priming and, 168
  responses from others and, 197
Intuition, behavioral priming and, 208–209
Involuntary recollection, 247

J

Judgments
  affective meanings, 160
  anchoring as priming and, 98
  automaticity and, 23
  perception-behavior link and, 228
  responses from others and, 196
  situated inference model and, 144, 149
  social priming research and, 5
  transfer and, 105–108

K

Knowledge, construal in priming effects and, 75

L

Learning
  associated systems theory (AST) and, 183
  long-term semantic priming, 60–61
  measuring awareness and, 16, 18

Localist connectionist model, 160–163, 161f, 163
Longevity, short-term priming and, 56–57
Long-term priming, 49–51, 58–63, 63–64
Long-term semantic priming, 59–63
Low-level construal, 81. *See also* Construal level

M

Masked effects, 53
Mechanisms, 235–238, 241–246, 243f, 246f
Medial prefrontal cortex (mPFC), 165f, 167, 167f
Memory. *See also* Memory activation
   long-term semantic priming, 60–61
   measuring awareness and, 16
   prime-to-behavior effects and, 115
   social embodiment and, 184
Memory activation. *See also* Memory
   overview, 234–235, 238–246, 241–246, 243f, 246f
   from phenomena to boundary conditions to mechanisms, 235–238
   relevance and, 246–247
Mental representation systems, 18–19, 197, 255–257
Metacognitive cues, 147–148
Metacognitive inferences, 149
Mimicry, 222–229
Mindset priming, 72–73
Misattributions
   moderators of priming effects and, 145–147
   neural computation of priming and, 169
   responses from others and, 198
   situated inference model and, 143f, 144
Moderators of priming effects
   behavioral priming and, 210–211
   self-other overlap and, 224
   situated inference model and, 145–150
Moment-to-moment transitions, 56–57
Motivated-preparation model, 74–75
Motivations
   memory activation and, 241–242
   neural computation of priming and, 168
   perception-behavior link and, 227

N

Neural computation of priming
   constraint satisfaction and, 163–166, 165f
   intentional behavior and, 166–167, 167f
   overview, 168–169
Neural engineering framework (NEF), 163–164
Neural networks
   long-term semantic priming, 60–61
   perception-behavior link and, 228–229
Neurocomputational model, 164–165, 165f
Nonconscious priming, 143

Numbers
   anchoring and, 95–97, 97–98, 101–105
   overview, 109–110
   situated-inference model and, 108–109
   subliminal priming and, 99–101
   transfer and, 105–108

O

Observed responses from others, 191–192, 193–194, 198–200. *See also* Responses from others, priming from

P

Parallel constraint satisfaction, 158–163, 161f
Parallel distributed processing, incidental memory activation and, 240
Parallel distributed representations, short-term priming and, 56–57
Perception
   active self-concept and, 120
   evaluation and, 42–44
   situated inference model and, 144
Perception-behavior link, 131–132, 222–229
Perceptual symbol systems (PSS) theory
   associated systems theory (AST) and, 182–183
   social embodiment and, 178, 180–182, 184
P-hacking, 212–213
Phenomena, 235–238
Potency-control
   affective meanings, 160
   localist connectionist model and, 161
Predicting when priming should occur, 254–255
Prefrontal cortex (PFC), 167, 167f
Prejudice, 199
Prime exposure, 143f
Prime identification test, 100
Prime numbers
   anchoring and, 97–98
   anchoring as priming and, 95–97
   influence of an anchor and, 101–105
   overview, 109–110
   situated-inference model and, 108–109
   subliminal priming and, 99–101
   transfer and, 105–108
Prime-to-behavior effects
   active self-concept and, 116–119
   mechanisms of, 120
   overview, 114–116, 124
   replicability and, 120–124
Priming effects in general
   anchoring as priming, 95–97
   construal level and, 82–83

Index

history of priming research, 220–222
overview, 3–4, 70–72, 252–254, 257–258
replicability and, 254–255
research and, 220–222
in social psychology, 8–10
Procedural memory, 60–61
Procedural priming, 72–73
Processes, 28–29, 72–73
Publication bias, replicability and, 30

Q

Qualitative visibility judgment, measuring awareness and, 16

R

Reasoning, neural computation of priming and, 167
Regulation. *See also* Structured regulation; Unstructured regulation
construal level and, 79–82
impact of on priming, 75–78
Relevance, 17–18, 241–246, 243f, 246–247, 246f, 255–256
Relevance-of-a-representation (ROAR) account
memory activation and, 241–246, 243f, 246f
neural computation of priming and, 168
overview, 248
Replicability
behavioral priming and, 213
expectations of, 130–132
overview, 29–30, 129–130, 138–139, 254–255
prime-to-behavior effects and, 120–124
self-regulatory account and, 133–134
social resources and, 136–138
structural resources and, 135–136
Representations, 18–19, 197, 255–257
Reproducibility, 150–152
Research practices, 29–30
Resource computation model
overview, 129–130, 132–133, 138–139
self-regulatory account and, 133–134
social resources and, 136–138
structural resources and, 135–136
Response competition, short-term priming and, 55
Response priming designs, 50, 52–53
Responses from others, priming from. *See also* Observed responses from others; Simulated responses from others
compared to other forms of priming, 197–198
evidence supporting, 194–197, 195f
overview, 191–193, 198–200
theoretical frameworks, 193–194
Retrieval account of priming, 57–58

Retrieval mechanisms, 16–17
Rule-governed environment, incidental memory activation and, 240

S

Selective accessibility model, anchoring as priming and, 98
Self-activation theory, neural computation of priming and, 168–169
Self-concept. *See also* Active self-concept
overview, 257
priming effects on, 116–119
responses from others and, 198–199
Self-consciousness, 118
Self-control, 76–77, 80
Self-monitoring, active self-concept and, 118–119
Self–other overlap
perception-behavior link and, 222–229
responses from others and, 194
Self-regulatory account, 133–134, 135–136
Self-report measures, 17
Semantic knowledge, 191–192
Semantic pointers, 163–164, 165–166, 168
Semantic priming
evaluative priming and, 38
long-term semantic priming, 59–63
moderators of, 211
overview, 50, 229–230
short-term priming and, 53–54, 56–57
Semantic processing
measuring awareness and, 25
spreading activation and, 27–28
Semantic representations, 18–19
Sequential priming, situated inference model and, 149
Serial order in behavior, 220–221
Short-term priming
compared to long-term priming, 58–63
core paradigms of, 52–54
mechanisms of, 54–58
overview, 49–50, 51–52, 63–64
Signal detection analysis
measuring awareness and, 26
overview, 219–220
Simulated memory representations, 234–235
Simulated responses from others. *See also* Responses from others, priming from
overview, 191–192, 198–200
priming from, 192–193
theoretical frameworks, 193–194
Situated-inference model
anchoring and, 108–109
context-specificity, 150–152
moderators of priming effects and, 145–150
overview, 74–75, 143–145, 143f, 152
reproducibility and, 150–152

Situational cues
  construal level and, 83–84
  structured versus unstructured regulation and, 75–77
Situational factors, 147
Skill acquisition, 72–73
Social behaviors, 8–10
Social cognition
  affective meanings, 160
  social embodiment and, 186
Social coordination, 199–200
Social embodiment
  associated systems theory (AST) and, 182–183
  empirical data, 177–178
  overview, 175–177, 186
  social inferences and, 182–186
  theoretical frameworks, 178–182
Social impressions, 8–10
Social inferences, 181–186
Social judgments, 228
Social priming in general
  history of priming research, 5–6
  overview, 3–4, 6–8, 36–38, 176
  replicability and, 254–255
  research and, 234–235
Social psychology
  awareness and, 27–28
  history of priming research, 5–6
  measuring awareness and, 17–18, 24–27
  overview, 14–16, 30
  priming effects in, 8–10, 21–23
  replicability and, 29–30
Social resources, 136–138
Spreading activation
  overview, 18–19, 28–29, 131–132, 139, 255–257
  short-term priming and, 56
  structural resources and, 136
Stereotype activation, 23
Stereotypes, 23, 199
Stimulus onset asynchronies (SOA), 51–52
Stimulus-response (S-R) compatibility, 53–54
Stimulus-stimulus (S-S) compatibility, 53–54
Structural resources, 135–136
Structural similarity view, 185
Structured regulation. *See also* Regulation
  construal level and, 79–82
  embodiment and fluency and, 83–84
  impact of on priming, 75–78
  overview, 84
Subjective measures, 17

Subliminal perception, 19–20
Subliminal priming
  anchoring and, 99–101
  automaticity and, 23
  measuring awareness and, 25–26
Supplemental motor area (SMA), 165f, 167f

T

Target of focus, moderators of priming effects and, 147
Temperature, perception-behavior link and, 226–227
Temptations, construal level and, 81–82
Thematic Apperception Test (TAT), 227
Timing, unintentional prime evaluation and, 40
Transfer, breadth of, 105–108
Transitions, short-term priming and, 56–57
Truth relevance, 244

U

Unintentional influence, 37–38, 39–41
Unrelated-studies paradigm, 222
Unstructured regulation. *See also* Regulation
  construal level and, 79–82
  embodiment and fluency and, 83–84
  impact of on priming, 75–78
  overview, 84

V

Valence, response priming paradigms and, 52
Value relevance, 242
Voluntary recollection, 247
Voting behavior, perception-behavior link and, 225

W

Warmth, affective meanings, 160
Weather, perception-behavior link and, 226–227
Willingness-to-pay (WTP) judgment, transfer and, 106
Working memory, long-term semantic priming, 61. *See also* Memory